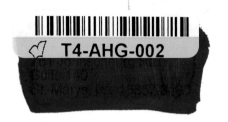

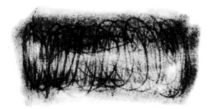

INTERDISCIPLINARY REHABILITATION OF MULTIPLE SCLEROSIS AND NEUROMUSCULAR DISORDERS

Edited by

F. Patrick Maloney, M.D., M.P.H.
Professor and Head, Division of Rehabilitation Medicine
College of Medicine
University of Arkansas for Medical Sciences
Chief of Rehabilitation Medicine Service
John L. McClellan Memorial Veterans Hospital
Little Rock, Arkansas
Formerly, Associate Professor of Physical Medicine and Rehabilitation
University of Colorado School of Medicine
Denver, Colorado

Jack S. Burks, M.D.
Executive Director, Center for Neurological Diseases/The Rocky
   Mountain Multiple Sclerosis Center
Associate Professor of Neurology
Department of Neurology
University of Colorado School of Medicine
Staff Neurologist, Denver Veterans Administration Medical Center
Denver, Colorado

Steven P. Ringel, M.D.
Associate Professor of Neurology
Director, Neuromuscular Section
University of Colorado School of Medicine
Denver, Colorado

27 Contributors

Interdisciplinary Rehabilitation of Multiple Sclerosis and Neuromuscular Disorders

J. B. LIPPINCOTT COMPANY
Philadelphia

London   Mexico City   New York
St. Louis   São Paulo   Sydney

Acquisitions Editor: Lisa A. Biello
Sponsoring Editor: Richard Winters
Manuscript Editor: Leslie E. Hoeltzel
Indexer: Ellen Murray
Designer: Susan A. Caldwell
Production Supervisor: Kathleen P. Dunn
Production Coordinator: Carol A. Florence
Compositor: Progressive Typographers
Printer/Binder: Murray Printing Co.

6   5   4   3   2   1

Library of Congress Cataloging in Publication Data
Main entry under title:

Interdisciplinary rehabilitation of multiple sclerosis and
    neuromuscular disorders.

    Based on the papers presented at a conference, held
June 12–13, 1981, at the University Hospital, in Denver,
Colorado.
    Includes bibliographical references and index.
    1. Multiple sclerosis—Patients—Rehabilitation—
Congresses. 2. Neuromuscular diseases—Patients—
Rehabilitation—Congresses. I. Maloney, F. Patrick.
II. Burks, Jack S. III. Ringel, Steven P. [DNLM:
1. Multiple sclerosis—Rehabilitation—Congresses.
2. Neuromuscular diseases—Rehabilitation—
Congresses. 3. Rehabilitation—Psychology—
Congresses. WL 360 I595 1981]
RC377.I55   1985   616.8′34′06   84-5716
ISBN 0-397-50634-1

To Our Patients, Who Are Our Best Teachers

Contributors

Emmajean Amrhein, R.N., B.S.
Unit Administrator, University of Colorado Health Sciences Center, University Hospital, Denver, Colorado

Richard R. Augspurger, M.D.
Assistant Clinical Professor, Department of Surgery, Division of Urology, University of Colorado School of Medicine, University Hospital, Denver, Colorado

Carole Anne Brammell, O.T.R.
Clinical Instructor, Supervisor, Occupational Therapy, University Hospital, Department of Physical Medicine and Rehabilitation, University of Colorado Health Sciences Center, Denver, Colorado

Gretchen Branowitzer, R.N., B.S.
Assistant Unit Administrator, University Hospital, University of Colorado Health Sciences Center, Denver, Colorado

Surinder Pal Brar, B.S., R.P.T.
Physical Therapist, Department of Physical Medicine and Rehabilitation, Center for Neurological Diseases/The Rocky Mountain Multiple Sclerosis Center, Denver, Colorado

Jack S. Burks, M.D.
Executive Director, Center for Neurological Diseases/The Rocky Mountain Multiple Sclerosis Center; Associate Professor of Neurology, Department of Neurology, University of Colorado School of Medicine; Staff Neurologist, Denver Veterans Administration Medical Center, Denver, Colorado

Nan O'Neal Campbell, B.A.
Formerly Regional Patient Service Coordinator, Muscular Dystrophy Association, Denver, Colorado

Nancy D. Cobble, M.D.
Assistant Clinical Professor, Departments of Neurology/Physical Medicine and Rehabilitation, University of Colorado School of Medicine, Center for Neurological Diseases/The Rocky Mountain Multiple Sclerosis Center, Denver, Colorado

William H. Cooper, M.D.
Instructor, Department of Neurology, Muscular Dystrophy Association; Fellow, University of Colorado Health Sciences Center, Denver, Colorado

Steven L. Dubovsky, M.D.
Associate Professor of Psychiatry, Associate Dean for Academic Affairs, University of Colorado School of Medicine, Denver, Colorado

Gary M. Franklin, M.D., M.P.H.
Clinical Director, Center for Neurological Diseases/The Rocky Mountain Multiple Sclerosis Center; Assistant Professor, Departments of Neurology and Preventive Medicine, University of Colorado School of Medicine, Denver, Colorado

Lyle O. Johnson, Ed.D.
Associate Director of Pupil Services and Special Education, Cherry Creek Schools, Denver, Colorado

Laura L. Knutson, M.S.W.
Psychotherapist in private practice, Denver, Colorado

Joel S. Levine, M.D.
Associate Professor, Department of Medicine, Division of Gastroenterology, University of Colorado School of Medicine, Denver, Colorado

Mark E. Litvin, Ph.D.
Director, Colorado Division of Rehabilitation, State of Colorado, Department of Social Services, Denver, Colorado

F. Patrick Maloney, M.D., M.P.H.
Professor and Head, Division of Rehabilitation Medicine, College of Medicine, University of Arkansas for Medical Sciences; Chief of Rehabilitation Medicine Service, John L. McClellan Memorial Veterans Hospital, Little Rock, Arkansas; Formerly, Associate Professor of Physical

Medicine and Rehabilitation, University of Colorado School of Medicine, Denver, Colorado

Richard J. Martin, M.D.
Assistant Professor of Medicine, University of Colorado School of Medicine; Staff Physician, National Jewish Hospital, Denver, Colorado

Hans E. Neville, M.D.
Associate Professor of Neurology, Codirector, Neuromuscular Section, University of Colorado School of Medicine, Denver, Colorado

Mark G. Pendleton, Ph.D.
Clinical Psychologist, Denver Neuropsychological Associates, Denver, Colorado

Steven P. Ringel, M.D.
Associate Professor of Neurology, Director, Neuromuscular Section, University of Colorado School of Medicine, Denver, Colorado

Neil L. Rosenberg, M.D.
Assistant Professor of Neurology, University of Colorado School of Medicine, Denver, Colorado

Nancy Ruttenberg, M.A., C.C.C.
Clinical Instructor, Department of Physical Medicine and Rehabilitation, University of Colorado School of Medicine; Speech/Language Pathologist, South Valley Rehabilitation Services, Denver, Colorado

Irwin M. Siegel, M.D.
Associate Professor, Departments of Orthopedic Surgery and Neurological Services, Rush–Presbyterian–St. Luke's Medical Center; Chairman, Department of Orthopedic Surgery, Louis A. Weiss Memorial Hospital; Director, MDA Clinics of the above facilities, Chicago, Illinois

Marcia B. Smith, M.S., R.P.T.
Instructor, Department of Physical Medicine and Rehabilitation, University of Colorado School of Medicine; Consultant, Rocky Mountain Neuromuscular Disease Clinic, Denver, Colorado

Marc Mitchell Treihaft, M.D.
Assistant Clinical Professor of Neurology, University of Colorado School of Medicine, Denver, Colorado

Beth G. Wolf, B.S., O.T.R.
Occupational Therapist, University Hospital, Department of Physical

Medicine and Rehabilitation, University of Colorado Health Sciences Center, Denver, Colorado

Carolyn Wangaard, R.N.
Certified Adult Nurse Practitioner (C.A.N.P.), Center for Neurological Diseases/The Rocky Mountain Multiple Sclerosis Center, University of Colorado Health Sciences Center, Denver, Colorado

Foreword

The frequencies of neuromuscular diseases and multiple sclerosis are sufficiently high to create a significant impact on health care facilities in this country. Prevention and specific treatment of these diseases are, of course, immediate and important goals. Despite intensive research, however, these goals have not yet been achieved.

In the absence of specific treatment, current emphasis must be placed on the rehabilitation approach. Such an approach requires the participation of many health professionals working closely together in space and time — an interdisciplinary approach. A description of the complex process is not easy, which probably accounts for the absence of a textbook addressing this problem.

Interdisciplinary Rehabilitation of Multiple Sclerosis and Neuromuscular Disorders is directed toward those professionals who might be involved in managing patients with multiple sclerosis and muscular dystrophy. It successfully achieves its goal because it represents the cooperation needed for managing the complex problems manifest in these patients. The editors are from the fields of neurology and physical medicine and rehabilitation. The contributors have had extensive experience in working as a team providing care for patients, as is apparent from the highly integrated quality of this book, rather than the fragmentation one so often sees in edited books.

Interdisciplinary Rehabilitation of Multiple Sclerosis and Neuromuscular Disorders addresses basic and clinical issues with great clarity and in a practical fashion. It will be the standard of rehabilitation care for patients with muscular dystrophy and multiple sclerosis for many years, and should be within easy access of all professionals who participate in such care.

JEROME W. GERSTEN, M.D.
Professor, Physical Medicine and Rehabilitation
University of Colorado School of Medicine

Preface

The editors anticipate that *Interdisciplinary Rehabilitation of Multiple Sclerosis and Neuromuscular Disorders* will be a valuable addition to the field of rehabilitation medicine and that it will be useful to a wide variety of health care workers who come in contact with similar patients. The book is divided into three sections: The first two review specific rehabilitative aspects of multiple sclerosis and neuromuscular diseases, and the third discusses rehabilitation issues common to many chronic neurologic disorders.

Handicapped rights, laws, and due process are addressed in the chapters on education and vocation. Familiarity with these issues is necessary for effective advocacy of educational and vocational opportunities.

Research in rehabilitation is becoming increasingly important in times of limited research and reimbursement resources. Chapter 29 clarifies the process of obtaining funds in an effort to stimulate interest for the novice and the experienced researcher.

Suggested readings follow each chapter. We have avoided extensive referencing within the text, although some pertinent citations are included by author and year.

Interdisciplinary Rehabilitation of Multiple Sclerosis and Neuromuscular Disorders is an outgrowth of a conference on the rehabilitation of multiple sclerosis and other chronically disabling neuromuscular disorders held at University Hospital in Denver, Colorado, on June 12–13, 1981. The conference was attended by a wide spectrum of health professionals, including physicians, acute- and chronic-care nurses, physical therapists, occupational therapists, speech pathologists, psychologists, and social workers. Many of the chapters in this book are written by the same persons who spoke on those topics at the conference, with additional chapters included for comprehensiveness. Although most participants in the conference were from the Rocky Mountain region, they represented a broad range of perspectives and a depth of experience that, along with their energy and commitment, we hope has been preserved in *Interdisciplinary Rehabilitation of Multiple Sclerosis and Neuromuscular Disorders.*

A great volume and variety of patients are seen at the University of Colorado Health Science Center, and consequently we have had the opportunity to develop a philosophy of patient care that may be useful to other health care professionals. The Neuromuscular Disease Clinic, active since 1950 as one of the first clinics sponsored by the Muscular Dystrophy Association (MDA), is now one of the largest MDA clinics in the United States, treating more than 1500 patients from the Rocky Mountain region. Similarly, the Center for Neurological Diseases/The Rocky Mountain Multiple Sclerosis Center is a regional referral center that treats more than 1000 patients from Colorado and surrounding states.

Each patient is seen by a team of health specialists in order to address the patient's needs with as much breadth and depth as possible. To avoid confusion or misunderstandings that can easily occur when so many people are involved, the health care teams hold weekly meetings to discuss all aspects of each patient's management. The result of this discussion is in-depth communication and analysis of each patient's needs, in-service training and education, and, most important, the development of confidence in being able to treat the patient and family most effectively. From those meetings, a comprehensive, consistent therapeutic approach has evolved that can serve as a useful model for managing other patients with these disorders and those with other chronic progressive disorders.

Our therapy programs encourage independence and self-reliance, thereby fostering the patient's self-esteem. Ultimately, however, the disabled person must also become comfortable with some level of interdependence, since his ability to cope successfully can be enhanced by learning to rely on and utilize the strengths of others. A comprehensive therapy program can never be limited to the patient but must include family, friends, associates at work, and others who relate to the patient but may have had no previous experience working with neurologic disability.

We are grateful for the continued cooperation provided by so many competent and caring people with whom we have the pleasure to interact daily. One message we wish to provide is clear — anyone with almost any chronic illness can and will improve in a hopeful, supportive environment. The sensitive epigraph that follows on page xxi, A Patient's Perspective, emphasizes the importance of how we deliver care. Severely handicapped patients can learn to celebrate the here and now, strengthened by knowing that we will not abandon them.

F. PATRICK MALONEY, M.D.
JACK S. BURKS, M.D.
STEVEN P. RINGEL, M.D.

Acknowledgments

The editors gratefully acknowledge the efforts and assistance of LU-CILLE ENARSON, CANDACE DELAPP, LORENE GRUZDIS, and PENNY McCLAREN.

Contents

PART III
REHABILITATION OF PATIENTS WITH MUSCULAR
DYSTROPHIES

PART IV
ADDITIONAL MANAGEMENT CONCERNS

A Patient's Perspective

Adapting to illness requires a new set of perceptions of a changing personal reality. Thrust into a consuming vortex of new feelings emotionally and a quagmire physically, my battle for survival began against an adversary called multiple sclerosis. Being ill is a lonely, frightening ordeal. Beneath the symptoms beats the being of a vulnerable, traumatized person fighting to survive — each in his own way at his own speed.

At a time of physical and emotional upheaval, the experiences of the medical care system often are pivotal to the patient's perception of his present and future reality. In my own experience traveling through the medical care maze of internists, neurologists, ophthalmologists, vascular specialists, holistic healers, physical therapists, occupational therapists, physiatrists, radiologists, psychiatrists, and a myriad of medical technicians in both private and institutional settings, the scenario became dehumanizing, and at times added to my anxieties. The providers who looked beyond the symptoms stood above the unending crowd.

Because the diagnostic process was "wait and see," I often felt there was a time bomb ticking inside me as I waited for the verdict. The lexicon of medical terminology became haunting in its detached, ambiguous description. The multitude of tests and people taking pieces of me left me as vascillating as the machines that probed my core. Where would help come from? Time would be needed to revise my expectations of a seemingly chaotic system.

I learned that medical personna are also "human" and have difficulty in dealing with chronic disease. Faced with patient expectations and wanting to provide treatment, the physician may withdraw and interact very little in dealing with, as yet, incurable disease. This situation, coupled with an emphasis on research, leads to a feeling of being a medical outcast. Yet, emotional sensitivity is a vital aspect of any physical treatment. The quality of medical care, with technology being equal, comes from the sensitivity of the provider. The finding of the delicate balance between objective care and this sensitivity, although a formidable task, should be a paramount consideration. If you were the patient, wouldn't you want the same?

INTO THE VALLEY

Through the night into darkness
Cajoling the spirit into fear
Fear transforming into terror
A hint of infinity appears
Not the time, not the present,
Somewhere in the entropy of future.
Now to survive the savagery of physical upheaval,
To reach out and touch the hand of rationality
Which calms the gasping, wretching presence,
'Til peace abounds once more
And terror and fear are but memories.
Memories, within the plethora of realities,
Joining the myriad of traumas
Erecting a monument to being
Touching the essence of the unanswerable
'Til once again a valley gives way to majesty
And the sun dawns the light.

MARTIN GOREN

Part I

REHABILITATION PRINCIPLES

F. Patrick Maloney

1

Rehabilitation of Patients With Progressive and Remitting Disorders

Several chronic neurologic disorders that challenge the health professional because of the complexity of their treatment are discussed in this book.

Although multiple sclerosis and the muscular dystrophies involve widely differing parts of the nervous system, rehabilitation of these progressive conditions includes many common, special strategies, techniques, and attitudes for effective management.

Many professionals and the general public think of these disorders interchangeably; for example, witness the frequent errors seen on national telethons when fund raisers mistake multiple sclerosis (MS) for muscular dystrophy (MD). Likewise, medical histories of patients often reveal misstatements of diagnoses within pedigrees. The mislabeling is not only a result of the similarity in letter identification of MS and MD but is often caused by ignorance of the natural history of the disorders and an ingrained feeling of hopelessness of their outcomes.

Although many of these conditions are progessive, their bleak picture has been poorly painted. Partially resulting from professional unfamiliarity with the natural history of these disorders, rehabilitation for people afflicted with MS or MD and their families is usually too little and too late.

Neuromuscular disorders and MS have gained little attention in the rehabilitation literature. A significant reason for such neglect is the pessimism that has permeated the attitudes of professionals. All MS and MD patients tend to be labeled as having the more severe and progressive forms of these disorders. Also, considerable professional frustration and discouragement may be inherent in the treatment process if health professionals are uninformed and unrealistic in their expectations. Such prejudices not only mitigate against providing therapeutic services for these patients but also lead to undue generalizations for the many clinical forms of neuromuscular conditions and varying severity of MS.

Factors that contribute to an underrepresentation of these disorders in rehabilitation practice and literature are

Magnitude underestimations
Ignorance of the prognosis variability
Fragmented delivery of care
Inappropriate goal setting
Unrecognized vocational potentials
Psychological consequences

Disease Magnitudes

MULTIPLE SCLEROSIS

An estimated 250,000 to 500,000 persons in the United States have MS, the most common neurologic disease diagnosed in patients between the ages of 20 and 60 years.

MS is not strictly heritable in a mendelian sense, but is 10 to 20 times more common among family members. The frequency of MS is highest among Caucasians living in temperate climates. In the southern United States, the prevalence is 10 per 100,000 population, whereas in the northern United States, the prevalence is 5 to 10 times higher. Estimates of its prevalence in Colorado run as high as 100 per 100,000 population.

NEUROMUSCULAR DISORDERS

A common fallacious concept is that a physician or therapist who treats neurologic problems in the course of his practice will never see a patient with a neuromuscular disease because of the rarity of these conditions. The frequencies (prevalence) for the more common neuromuscular disorders are listed in Table 1–1. Note the variety of these disorders. Each neuromuscular disorder is often further subdivided into several distinct

Table 1–1 Frequency of Neuromuscular Disorders

Disorder	Frequency*
Werdnig-Hoffman disease	4–7
Duchenne muscular dystrophy	3
Fascioscapulohumeral dystrophy	0.33–1
Myotonic dystrophy	3–5
Amyotrophic lateral sclerosis	2–7

* Per 100,000 population.

entities. McKusick lists 10 spinal muscular atrophies, 39 muscular dystrophies, and 6 types of Charcot-Marie-Tooth disease. Although each condition is rare, when the aggregate is considered, a significant magnitude is attained.

The incidence (the number of new cases per year) of these disorders depends on the population that is being considered. Data collection methods vary, and incidence rates are reported with various denominators, such as births, live births, and male births. The exact occurrence rates for these conditions is unknown, but the most common of these disorders in the general population is estimated to range between 1 per 150,000 live births for infantile spinal muscular atrophy (Werdnig-Hoffman disease) and 5 to 10 per million live births for fascioscapulohumeral (FSH) muscular dystrophy. The incidence for an X-linked disorder, Duchenne muscular dystropy (DMD), is 20 to 30 per 100,000 male births.

Population figures do not give a true picture of the number of cases that can be expected in a particular family. Because many neuromuscular diseases are heritable in a mendelian sense, many patients may be found within a single family pedigree. This factor enhances the need for the rehabilitation health professional to become an expert in at least that disorder affecting the family that he is working with at the present time.

Common characteristics of autosomal dominant, autosomal recessive, and X-linked recessive disorders are listed in Table 1–2. With autosomal dominant illnesses, such as FSH or myotonic dystrophy, on average 50% of family members will be affected in multiple generations. Even a sporadic case (new mutation) can subsequently be transmitted to half the offspring. Autosomal dominant conditions may appear to skip a generation because of a lack of penetrance in clinical findings (careful examination usually reveals some manifestations), although the biochemical abnormality is fully penetrant. Autosomal recessive conditions, such as limb girdle muscular dystrophy, occur in siblings within a

Table 1–2 Common Characteristics of Inheritance Patterns

Pedigree Characteristic	Autosomal Dominant	Autosomal* Recessive	X-linked Recessive
Generations affected	Multiple	Siblings only	Multiple
Offspring affected	50%	0	25%
Female offspring affected	50%	0	0
Male offspring affected	50%	0	50%
Carrier offspring	0†	100%	25% (50% of females)
Male-to-male transmission of disease trait	50% disease†	100% trait	0

* Percentages assume no consanguinity.
† Incomplete penetrance of manifestations may give the appearance of a carrier state.

single generation but not in subsequent generations, because both parents must transmit the genetic abnormality from at least one chromosome in order for offspring to be affected (when recessive disease occurs, the abnormality is present in alleles of a pair of both chromosomes). X-linked disorders may appear to skip a generation because female carriers of the trait are phenotypically normal.

Ignorance of the Prognosis Variability

Much attention will be focused on prognosis in later sections of this book. To understand the rehabilitation process, a knowledge of the natural history of these disorders and practical therapeutic goals are essential. Patients with MS can have widely differing disability and severity of symptoms. Similarly, neuromuscular disorders have various prognosis for life and function.

Fragmented Care

The services of several health professionals are usually required for patients who have any of these neurologic conditions. Nowhere in the practice of medicine can there be found a greater need for communication and coordination of therapeutic effort than with this group of patients. A patient's emotional state can turn a potentially helpful therapeutic regimen into a failure. Medications given for depression or spasticity can alter a patient's response to exercise. Improper equipment may increase the patient's handicap. The list of interrelated factors that can influence function is endless.

Perhaps the most important concept to remember in treating people with these disorders is that the treatment approach is *interdisciplinary*. This term is common in the rehabilitation lexicon but the concept is rarely achieved. *Interdisciplinary* means professionals from various medical fields working *together* for a desired outcome. It must be differentiated from *multidisciplinary* which means varied professionals working *individually* for a desired outcome. For MS and neuromuscular disorders, the approach must be truly interdisciplined, because each professional must know what the other is doing and all must be directed toward developing workable strategies with specific goals.

Inappropriate Goal Setting

A central principle that governs rehabilitation philosophy applies to progressive and relapsing/remitting disorders—namely, the functional restoration of persons to their optimal capabilities. Two factors that cloud the application of this principle are the inability to recognize what is optimal for a particular person and false expectations of therapeutic techniques that were not specifically developed for these disorders.

Therapeutic goals can frequently be inappropriate for the diagnosis or the stage of the disease. Optimal function is not uniform for all persons with MS or from one neuromuscular disease to another; rather, it varies according to the stage of disease progression and with the social and vocational needs of the patient. MS can stabilize with minimal involvement, exacerbate and remit, and be either slowly or rapidly progressive.

Varying distributions of neuromuscular involvement and rates of progression among the neuromuscular disorders warrant caution in transferring the prognosis of a disorder in one patient to another patient.

Positive therapeutic goals are usually possible once the patient's level of involvement is known. Such goals require a flexibility of expectations because the patient's condition may change.

Rehabilitation research concerning the disorders discussed in this book has been sparse. MS itself has not been specifically studied. Only a few studies have examined the value of strengthening exercises and functional improvement potentials for MD, and the results are conflicting. Expectations for rehabilitation outcomes are frequently based on what is known from normal responses to exercise, the results of treatment for other conditions, and reasoned judgments of measures whose validity appears to be self-evident. Although this approach is valuable, goals should be set by the patient's individual response to treatment and not by a preconceived, idealized conception of outcomes that may be inappropriate for the patient being treated.

Function should be judged by a change in or retention of quality of living, not by abnormalities found during a physical examination. Skill at using retained muscle power, improved coordination, the provision of adaptive devices, and educational or vocational capabilities can be determining factors of living style in a static or progressive condition.

Unrecognized Vocational Potentials

In the past, capable students with neuromuscular disorders were denied full educational opportunities. In recent years, this deficiency has changed with the advent of Public Law 94-142. However, the law's mandate to provide an "appropriate education" in the "least restrictive environment" has not been fully met. In higher education, architectural barriers and the lack of program adaptability are still obstacles for handicapped students.

Only 50% of people with MS are estimated to be working 10 years after diagnosis and only 33% after 20 years. Because most of the diseases discussed in this book are not fatal, those people who are affected have an untapped vocational potential.

Psychological Consequences

The psychological impact of these disorders has an overriding influence on all other factors. Psychological problems among families and patients are frequently difficult to confront, not only because of patient reluctance but also because of feelings engendered in the physicians, nurses, psychologists, counselors, and therapists who must work with these handicapped patients.

Rehabilitation measures for MS and the neuromuscular disorders range from simple measures for improving the quality of life to more complex treatment regimens involving interdisciplinary cooperation. People who have these disorders have considerable but commonly unrecognized functional, educational, and vocational potential. Professionals working as a team, by providing hope, counsel, guidance, and treatment, can have an invaluable impact on the lives of these people and their families in their quest for independence and understanding. This book endeavors to provide an increased appreciation of these disorders and practical information to assist the helping professionals in rehabilitation management.

Suggested Readings

BROOKE MH: A Clinician's View of Neuromuscular Disease. Baltimore, Williams & Wilkins, 1977

MCALPINE D, LUMSDEN EE, ACHISON ED: Multiple Sclerosis: A Reappraisal. Edinburgh, E & S Livingston, 1972

MCKUSICK VA: Mendelian Inheritance in Man, 5th ed. Baltimore, Johns Hopkins University Press, 1978

WALTON JN: Disorders of Voluntary Muscle, 4th ed. Edinburgh, Churchill Livingstone, 1981

Part II

REHABILITATION OF PATIENTS WITH
MULTIPLE SCLEROSIS

Nancy D. Cobble
Jack S. Burks

2

The Team Approach to the Management of Multiple Sclerosis

Multiple sclerosis (MS) is often perceived as a progressive disease for which there is little hope of effective treatment but an interdisciplinary rehabilitation approach can offer the patient control over many of the negative effects of the disease. An interdisciplinary team meets the complex challenges of MS management efficiently and comprehensively. The rehabilitation team supports the patient in developing skills and personal strengths to both compensate for loss of function and establish a healthy, positive attitude. With appropriate management and support, MS need not be a burdensome definition of a person's future but only one factor in a strong, productive, and satisfying life.

Why a Team?

In caring for the patient, the rehabilitation team not only documents the physical effects of the disease but also identifies the implications of the symptoms on the patient's life. Team planning unifies team members, patients, and family so that the direction and goals of treatment are consistent, logical, and progressive. Planning adds to both minor and major aspects of the treatment program, from coordinating schedules that minimize patient fatigue to emphasizing treatment of high-priority problems. A patient's newly learned skills, attitudes, and behaviors are supported beyond the treatment setting because the team educates the family and helps to modify the patient's environment at home, at work, and in the community.

Within the team, as team members share evaluations and opinions, professional cross-stimulation and enhanced creative problem-solving occur. Team members also support each other by openly communicating their own feelings, such as anger, frustration, anxiety, guilt, or loss, which interfere with treatment and lower the morale of health-care providers. When understood, these feelings can be channeled to enhance effective, productive treatment and to encourage team members.

What Is a Team?

An interdisciplinary team is a group of health professionals who meet regularly to develop therapeutic goals for their patients. Unlike a multidisciplinary approach in which health-care providers address problems individually, the interdisciplinary team works together to unify individual treatments into a comprehensive plan. Consultants to the primary team provide evaluation and treatment reports that the team members integrate into the treatment plan. The team members and consultants usually include the following:

TEAM MEMBERS

Physician
Nurse
Physical therapist
Occupational therapist
Speech/language pathologist
Counselor
Aides/attendants*
Recreation therapist*

CONSULTANTS

Consulting physicians may include
  Urologist
  Ophthalmologist
  Pulmonary medicine specialist
  Surgeon
Dietitian
Biofeedback technician*
Driving instructor
Vocational counselor*
Legal advisor
Patient
Family

* These may be either team members or consultants.

The primary team may vary in membership. In some settings, the primary physician is not a team member but acts as a consultant; another team member acts as the leader/manager. At the Center for Neurological Diseases/Rocky Mountain Multiple Sclerosis Center (CND/ RMMSC), both a neurologist and a physiatrist are team members and co-leaders.

Each team member's contributions should maximize communication and effectiveness (see Team Member Contributions, below). The

---

TEAM MEMBER CONTRIBUTIONS

Physician
Medical care
Symptomatic treatment
Team leader

Nurse
Self-care skills
Formal education
Skill practice
Encouragement
Off-hours patient observation

Physical therapist
Strength
Tone
Balance
Coordination
Ambulation
Breathing exercises
Bed mobility
Sensory compensation
Adaptive equipment
General conditioning

**Speech/Language
   pathologist**
Dysarthria
Dysphagia
Cognitive dysfunction

Patient/Family members
Goals
Values
Interests

Occupational therapist
Upper extremity strength
Upper extremity tone
Upper extremity coordination
Activities of daily living (ADL)
Adaptive equipment
Homemaking
Prevocational evaluation
Energy conservation
Wheelchair evaluation

Counselor/Social worker
Coping skills
Self-identity
Social roles
Goal attainment
Control over life
Resource identification
Team counseling

Recreation therapy
Skill practice
Motivation
Patient observation

Aides/Attendants
Motivation
Transportation
Skill practice
Patient observation

---

physician defines the overall medical care and symptomatic medical treatment for the patient and alerts the team members to the implication of other health problems, current treatment, and past response to medical intervention. When the physician acts as team leader his functions include the following:

Facilitates communication in formulating goals
Supports the patient's values and goals to the team during planning and treatment
Prevents different plans and treatments from counteracting each other

Assumes responsibility for the team plans with the patient and family

Evaluates the ongoing progress of the team

Mediates intrateam conflicts

Facilitates open discussions with team members concerning their feelings in trying to better understand patients and allowing intrateam support

Supports and protects the team members from themselves (unrealistic expectations) and from any unrealistic pressures and expectations of the patient and his family

The nurse instructs the patient in self-care skills, such as a bowel program and intermittent bladder catheterization. Often the nurse can provide other team members with valuable insights into the patient's problem-solving style, motivation, and family interactions.

At the CND/RMMSC, even the aides who transport inpatients from the ward to the treatment area contribute to the team approach. Although patient contact is brief, aides convey confidence in the rehabilitation process and motivate patients to participate. In other treatment situations in which aides provide some basic care, they encourage patients to practice what they have learned in therapy while being careful not to stress the patient with unrealistic expectations.

Patients and family members are consultants to the team. They provide the crucial information (needs, interests, values, personal goals, and lifestyle) from which the team members identify disabilities and establish priorities.

The Team Approach

GENERAL CONCEPTS

A rehabilitation program combines a structured environment with realistic expectations, firmness, and consistency, with the appropriate encouragement and empathy to help a person achieve his optimal function. The team must be flexible enough to individualize each patient's program because the length of time for evaluation and treatment can vary considerably. Isolated problems may require only a single evaluation by the physician and therapist, whereas multiple problems may require a 2- to 3-day outpatient or inpatient evaluation by several therapists and consultants, with the initiation of a specific treatment regimen and training for a home program.

At the CND/RMMSC, where rehabilitation is carried out in an acute-care hospital, a 2- to 3-week admission allows

A detailed evaluation of complex problems

Observation of response to treatment

Treatment program modifications
Education
Behavior modification
Motivation
Indepth home program development

For more complex physical or emotional problems, a longer hospital stay is justified. Feigenson (1981) reports that patients who have not responded to outpatient rehabilitation benefit functionally from such intensive inpatient attention.

A rehabilitation team should emphasize each person's wellness while resolving specific functional disability problems. When patients identify themselves as being well, they gain a sense of control over their lives and think of themselves as having as full a range of activity as possible. The wellness concept is encouraged indirectly during a rehabilitation admission by having patients wear street clothes and by encouraging them to leave the hospital on passes. Wellness is encouraged directly when patients are challenged to assume responsibility for those areas of their own health that they can control.

Patient responsibility begins before admission, with the agreement to participate in the team's evaluation, identification of problems, cooperative establishment of realistic goals, and the physical/emotional work planned to reach those goals. Responsibility continues after the rehabilitation stay as the patient learns to make safe choices. For example, patients can learn to titrate their own symptomatic medication for spasticity, and they can participte in choices for bladder management.

The experience of working with the rehabilitation team allows patients to better understand themselves, identify problems, and realistically problem-solve. Much of the value of working with a rehabilitation team comes from the patient's experiences.

CONCEPTS LEARNED BY EXPERIENCE

Problem-solving skills
Attitude of focusing on remaining ability (what can be done) rather than on disability (what is no longer possible)
Communication skills
Adaptability
Self-esteem as a valued team participant
Wellness lifestyle
Realistic hope

One outcome of effective patient–rehabilitation team interaction is the patient's improved quality of life. Quality means more than just survival or a mastery of physical skills. Kottke (1982) suggests the following framework for understanding quality of life. First, the patient must re-establish physical and psychological equilibrium. Then he needs to be able to maintain or develop important interpersonal relationships, which means he needs time and energy after basic self-care to spend with family and friends. The patient also needs to be productive, not just interacting with others, but actively contributing to society. The highest quality of life occurs when the patient is involved in creative participation in life. Aspects of Quality of Life, below, lists how goals that are detailed throughout this book enhance quality of life based on this concept.

ASPECTS OF QUALITY OF LIFE

Psychophysiologic equilibrium
Understanding of the disease, the symptoms, and how to manage them
Understanding of limitations and strengths; functioning up to but respecting limits
Maintenance of function with minimum effort and maximum safety (balancing rest and activity appropriately)
Functional improvement in spite of persistent neurologic signs
Return to pre-exacerbation physical status
Altering environment to support independence, diminish disability
Wellness lifestyle
Mastery over potential uncertainty and loss of control

Interrelatedness
Realistic expectations for patient and family
Preservation of family unit
Learning new ways to fulfill family/friendship roles
Knowing and practicing how to be realistically independent — not being a burden — but also being able to communicate when and how help is needed
Avoiding social isolation
Knowing and appropriately using community resources

Productivity
Developing alternative plans to already established vocational goals (job, education, other training)
Establishing a productive life (paid or volunteer)

Creativity
Developing problem-solving skills
Developing avocational interests
Reaching important life goals; focusing on remaining possibilities
Developing an enjoyable, personally meaningful life (MS not being the focus of one's life)

The crucial groundwork for developing personal creativity is established very early in the rehabilitation process so that the patient experiences being a participant whose contributions are valued by team members. As the carefully designed progressive steps are mastered, the patient is motivated to try more. Initial successful participation in basic common activities leads to successful participation in progressively less routine and more self-expressive activities.

The following examples demonstrate good adjustments with resulting successful, satisfying lives.

A 60-year-old patient goes camping and fishing in an electric wheel-chair. He feels it would be a shame to let circumstances interfere with enjoying a normal life.

A nurse with MS was despondent and suicidal over her rapid down-hill course. After working with the team, she understood and better accepted her physical limitation, gained new compensatory skills, found a new job at which she could be successful, and also started dating. Now she is not only ready to go on with life but also looks forward to it.

A 27-year-old mother with relapsing/remitting MS reports that for more than a year after her diagnosis she was afraid to do or plan anything. She saw herself as sick and frail even though all serious medical problems had resolved. The turning point came when she accepted that no one can really predict the course of his or her life, yet everyone goes on living and planning. Since that time, she has become a counselor, community spokesperson for the disabled, and a happy, successful wife and mother.

After a day at a ski clinic for the handicapped, a 50-year-old man with chronic/progressive MS said, "Two years ago I gave up physical activities because I was weak in my legs and tired. Now that I can ski, I will reevaluate the other activities I have given up."

While team members are treating, encouraging, and supporting patients, they must also be listening to and helping patients communicate about what "works." Care-givers can learn from patients who have made good adjustments and subsequently can teach others to use the same adaptive mechanisms.

ELEMENTS OF THE TEAM APPROACH

1. Evaluation
2. Problem identification
3. Goal setting
4. Treatment
   Practical management and problem-solving
   Education and communication
   Motivation
5. Follow-through: discharge planning and home programs

EVALUATION

Each team member should evaluate the patient's problems and physical and psychological adaptive mechanisms. Each patient serves as his own baseline because the course of MS, the location, and intensity of symp-toms are so variable. Although the patient's best performance should be elicited for baseline evaluation, helpful information can be gained by comparing performances of the patient when he is well rested and when he is fatigued.

Disability can be defined as a mismatch between the symptomatic patient and his environment. Symptoms are not always synonymous with the disability. For example, weakness in the left arm is less of a disability in a right-handed person than in a left-handed person. Mild hand incoordination is more likely to be a vocational disability for a concert pianist than for a truck driver.

The following information is needed in the team's evaluation process so that the patient's disabilities can be identified:

Current physical status
  MS
  Residual cardiovascular, respiratory, neuromuscular, skeletal
    function
Psychological status
  Past reactions and coping styles
  Present stresses
  Motivators
Degree of assistance currently required
Family
  Current stresses
  Stability of family unit
Social history
Vocational/avocational history
Resources
  Family
  Community
Physical environment
  Home
  Work
  Community

PROBLEM IDENTIFICATION

A comprehensive list of problems that must be identified by the team is presented in the Team Problem List on page 19.

General Medical Problems

General medical problems include areas of general health apart from MS, such as underlying heart disease, that affect the patient's ability to undergo vigorous rehabilitation. Treatment for these diseases or conditions and for MS may also affect the rehabilitation effort. For instance, osteoporotic bones from chronic steroid administration may be unable

TEAM PROBLEM LIST

General medical problems
Other medical conditions/treatments having a bearing on rehabilitation
Previous reaction (physical, psychological) to medical treatments

Neurologic problems: signs and symptoms
Weakness
Spasticity
Incoordination/tremor/impaired balance
Sensory impairment/pain
Visual impairment
Fatigue
Memory/cognitive impairment

Functional MS problems
Ambulation/transfers
Activities of daily living/community skills
Dysarthria
Dysphagia
Bowel/bladder/sexual impairment
Psychological adjustment/motivation
Medical complications

Nonmedical MS issues
Vocation
Homemaking
Avocation
Finances
Family adjustment

Team business
Education
Equipment
Discharge planning: date
Community resources
Follow-up appointments

to withstand some types of exercise. Knowledge of a patient's past response, both physical and psychological, to previous medical treatments can be a guide to present response.

Neurologic Problems

Neurologic signs and symptoms, which can be caused by specific MS plaques, combine to cause functional MS problems. Treatment of the signs and symptoms should not be an end in itself but should be related to the goal of improvement or amelioration of functional problems.

Functional MS Problems

These disabilities are caused by a combination of neurologic signs and symptoms. Medical complications of MS such as decubitus ulcers, malnutrition, contractures, and respiratory compromise are caused by and often further contribute to functional problems. For example, contractures may be due to immobility associated with other aspects of the disease, such as weakness, spasticity, or depression, or to lack of proper positioning and range-of-motion exercises. When contractures exist, they contribute to functional problems by making independent transfers and dressing difficult or impossible.

Nonmedical MS Issues

These disabilities are related to the person's environment and are the most complex issues to be addressed in order for him to attain a satisfying life. These issues include the ability to be productive (i.e., vocation or homemaking), creative (avocation), and able to fulfill important interpersonal roles.

Team Problems

Certain business details, such as equipment prescription and discharge planning, must be addressed by the team members. Setting the estimated discharge date as soon after evaluation as possible is the key to helping the team set realistic goals that can be accomplished within a reasonable period of time.

GOAL SETTING

Goal setting is crucial in a comprehensive rehabilitation program. Well-defined goals determine the direction of treatment, allow evaluation of progress, refine the identification of patient capabilities, and motivate both the patient and the team members. In the process of setting goals, each team member proposes solutions to the problems that he or she has identified.

Goals should be set according to priority to prevent conflicting treatments and to ensure that high-priority problems are addressed first. The setting of priorities is based on team members' professional opinions about the needs, urgency, safety, efficiency, and steps required to achieve larger goals. The patient provides critical information because his own interests, values, and lifestyle determine which symptoms and problems cause significant disability; symptoms that cause distress in one person may be of no significance to another person. However, when asked directly about his goals, a patient often responds that his goal is "cure" or "looking normal." Therefore, the team must help the patient by providing a structured environment with reasonable alternatives from which to choose. With a set of realistic goals related to his own values, a patient is more likely to be committed to working harder to learn new behaviors and skills.

The example of a 67-year-old woman is instructive. Her only identified goal on admission was to walk normally, which was unrealistic because of longstanding, weakness, imbalance, and spasticity. When questioned directly about bladder function, she replied, "Not bad." She did not identify her bladder function as being a problem, but she really meant, "I do not get wet as long as I am at home near my adapted bathroom." When questioned about her special interests, she revealed that she loved her bridge club but had quit because she was embarrassed to ask for assistance to the bathroom. With that information, the team focused on the goals of a better bladder program, independent transfers, and assertiveness training to enable the patient to ask for appropriate help. When the patient realized the ways in which such rehabilitation would allow her to resume her bridge club activities, she was more excited, interested, committed, and successful in her rehabilitation program.

Goals should be as specific as possible, although initially goals may be somewhat tentative. As the patient responds to treatment, more concrete goals develop. Larger complex goals such as improving gait are broken down into smaller, more manageable and more measurable goals, such as standing balance, parallel bars, walker (first 10 feet, then 20 feet, and so on). The more readily the smaller, measurable steps are achieved, the more motivated the patient and the team members will be. Accurate record-keeping allows both the patient and the team members to document successes or problems so that the patient's program can be refined according to his individual needs.

TREATMENT

Treatment focuses on helping the patient achieve optimal functional capacity and includes physical management and problem-solving, education and communication, and motivation.

Disability can be diminished by

Changing the environment
Learning new physical skills
Compensating with adaptive equipment
Learning new social skills
Modifying symptoms by medication or physical treatment

Areas with a high yield for functional improvement include general conditioning, balance, self-care activities, transfers, bladder and bowel management, bed mobility, wheelchair skills, homemaking, use of adaptive equipment, environmental modifications, and recreational and vocational skills. Functional improvement can occur, although neurologic symptoms (e.g., clonus, weakness) persist.

Practical Management and Problem-Solving

When multiple factors contribute to a problem, the team must assess the relative contribution of each factor in planning specific treatments. Fatigue, for instance, can result from deconditioning, depression, or the neurologic impairment of MS alone. Deconditioning responds to a carefully supervised exercise program with a gradual increase in strength and endurance. A depressed patient may respond to counseling, antidepressants, and successfully learning new skills (see Chap. 8). Fatigue caused by MS is not fully understood; however, patients benefit from learning energy-conservation techniques.

Sexual dysfunction, as another example, can result from impotence, sensory impairments, pelvic floor weakness, lack of lubrication, lack of confidence, and depression. It is complicated by urinary incontinence, spasticity, and tremor. Medical treatment of spasticity, exercise to improve weakness and tremor, appropriate bladder management, artificial lubrication, use of a penile prosthesis, counseling for alternate techniques, and better self-identity can all improve sexual performance.

Table 2–1 summarizes the possibilities of team interaction concerning common MS problems. Specifics are covered in other chapters.

Education and Communication

The educational process is ongoing in a rehabilitation setting. One study noted that more than 60% of rehabilitation chart entries deal with learning, motivation, and behavior change. The patient not only learns directly from each therapist but also learns through formal education dealing with the nature of MS and certain self-care routines, such as through reading and written testing. Factual information concerning specific MS problems can also be conveyed by educational video tapes. Videotapes can be viewed by patients and their families during nontherapy hours, and questions can be answered at the next visit.

When family members and important friends attend some therapy sessions, they gain an understanding of the patient's strengths and weaknesses. At the same time, they can receive training to assist the patient more effectively. The patient should communicate his understanding about his disease to the team. Team members should provide explanations to the patient of the steps in the treatment process that are necessary to reach each goal. Regular team/family conferences are another important aspect of education and communication to address past progress, future steps, and time frame. These conferences also provide a

(text continues on p. 26)

Table 2-1 Examples of Team Interaction on Common MS Problems

Problem	Goals	Team*	Plan
Weakness	Strengthen disuse component Maintain fitness	MD/nurse/OT/PT†	Strengthening exercises, substitution, compensation, protective splints
Spasticity	Normalize tone without causing loss of support	MD/nurse/OT/PT	Medication, stretching, positioning, cold bath or spray, movement techniques, motor point block
Incoordination/tremor/impaired balance	Improve balance and control	MD/nurse/OT/PT	Medication, coordination/balance exercises, joint approximation, adaptive equipment, extremity weights, compensatory techniques, air splints, weighted canes/crutches, gait training
Impaired sensation	Enhance sensory awareness Teach precautions	MD/nurse/OT/PT	Education, visual compensation, developmental sequence exercises, joint approximation, tapping, brushing, weights
Pain	Decrease source of pain Decrease preception of pain	Biofeedback†/counselor/MD/nurse/OT/PT	Medication, improve posture, transcutaneous nerve stimulation, increase activity, stress management, muscle relaxation, diminish pain behavior
Visual impairment	Improve vision Compensate for loss	Blind services/MD/nurse/OT/PT/ophthalmologist	Medication for acute optic neuritis, patch for double vision, compensatory techniques, talking books, home visit
Fatigue	Increase and conserve available energy	Biofeedback/counselor/MD/nurse/OT/PT	Teach energy conservation, treat depression, improve endurance, efficient compensatory techniques and equipment, stress management, have patient keep record of activities and readjustment, rest periods at onset of fatigue
Memory/cognitive impairment	Identify Compensate	Counselor/MD/OT/speech†/neuropsychologist	Evaluation, educate patient and family, teach compensatory techniques, alteration of home environment

(Continued)

Table 2-1 Examples of Team Interaction on Common MS Problems (Continued)

Problem	Goals	Team*	Plan
Ambulation/ transfers	Safe and efficient mobility	Nurse/OT/PT	Decrease spasticity, strengthen and improve balance, improve trunk stability, gait training, gaiting aids, practice on ward, evaluate environment (hospital, home, work) for safety, accessibility, wheelchair evaluation, training
Activities of daily living/ community skills	Efficient and safe self-care Energy conservation Access to community	Driver education/ nurse/OT/PT/ recreation†	Transfers, balance, bed mobility, home equipment, new skills, adaptive equipment, energy conservation, and practice on ward, at home and on supervised recreational outing
Bowel dysfunction	Regularity without constipation, diarrhea, incontinence	Dietitian/MD/ nurse/OT/PT	Diet, decrease constipating medications, manage bladder program, sitting balance, transfers, hand function, increase daily activity
Bladder dysfunction	Freedom from incontinence and infection	MD/urologist/ nurse/OT/PT	Evaluation, medication, teach bladder program, sitting/standing balance, transfers, hand function, treat infections
Sexual dysfunction	Compensation/ education	Counselor/MD/ urologist/OT/PT	Evaluation, education, mobility, balance, decrease spasticity, contractures, hand function, bowel and bladder control, compensatory techniques, prosthesis, support, self-image
Dysarthria	Improve communication Maintain functional communication Compensation Energy conservation	Nurse/OT/PT/ speech	Retraining, teach others to listen, abdominal breathing exercises, oral exercises, decrease spasticity, practice on ward, communication boards, hand function for boards

(Continued)

Table 2-1 Examples of Team Interaction on Common MS Problems (*Continued*)

Problem	Goals	Team*	Plan
Dysphagia	Nutrition Safety Energy conservation	Dietician/MD/ nurse/OT/ speech	Diet, patient and family training and education, evaluation of alternative routes of nutrition if needed
Adjustment/ motivation	Facilitate adjustment Appropriate independence/ dependence Prevent isolation Stress management	Biofeedback/ counselor/MD/ nurse/OT/PT/ recreation/ speech	Supportive counseling, alternative goals, success at valued tasks, improved ability to communicate, antidepressant medication, biofeedback/relaxation, positive social/recreational experiences
Medical complication: decubitus ulcer	Prevent/treat	Dietician/MD/ nurse/OT/PT	Evaluate, educate patient and family, strengthen and position, decrease spasticity, improve nutrition, protective equipment, correct contractures
Medical complication: contractures	Prevent/decrease	MD/nurse/OT/ PT/surgeon	Stretching, positioning, educate patient and family, equipment, strengthen, surgical release
Medical complication: nutrition	Maximize nutrition Avoid fads	Dietician/MD/ nurse/OT/PT	Evaluate, educate, train in swallowing, body position, hand control, treat depression, proper diet
Medical complication: respiratory problems	Improve breath control Avoid respiratory illness	MD/nurse/PT	Breathing exercises, improve posture, increase activity, medical care if needed
Vocation Family adjustment Avocation Home-making	Best and most interesting job and recreation available Strengthen family Mobilize community resources	Counselor/MD/ nurse/OT/PT/ recreation/ speech/vocation counselor	Physical skills, motivation, help to overcome environmental barriers, build bridges to community resources, counseling

* Team members are listed in alphabetical order.
† MD = physician; OT = occupational therapist; PT = physical therapist; speech = speech/language pathologist; biofeedback = biofeedback technician; recreation = recreation therapist.

supportive environment in which to deal realistically with the prognosis of the disease and potential limitations. A written summary of team/family conferences is useful to referring physicians and team consultants and can be sent to the patient after he is discharged to reinforce the team's recommendations.

Motivation

Motivation is crucial for rehabilitation because progress occurs only when the patient is a willing participant. Although education is basic, motivation requires far more than knowledge. Motivation can be suppressed or diminished by the nature of MS. Because of the unpredictable course of MS, a patient may feel "out of control" even when in remission. New physical skills, new self-image, and new social roles as a "disabled person" require adjustments that must be regained with each exacerbation or progression (see Chap. 11). The unending claims of "cures" that patients hear about can eventually contribute to a feeling of hopelessness because promised cures repeatedly fail.

Other motivational issues are raised by the very nature of a rehabilitation admission. Because many patients are initially praised for striving to be independent, they may feel that they are failures when equipment or assistance is needed. The difficulty of facing physical losses during rehabilitation may prompt patients to focus on "when I get better" instead of on "what I can do now," or they may focus on functions they have lost instead of on what is still possible. In spite of rational understanding, most patients at some level hope for "the cure" when they are admitted. As patients realize that they will not be cured and that they may have significant disabilities, motivation and cooperation may diminish.

To understand motivational issues, the team members must understand the patient's feelings, his ideas about his disease, his perceptions of the rehabilitation process, his problem-solving ability, and his interests and values. The team members determine whether the patient responds best to encouragement or to being pushed, limited, challenged, or simply supported empathetically. Finally, the team members must identify and work with those people outside the hospital setting or clinic whose demands, expectations, and assistance may either support or undermine the patient's newly acquired skills and attitudes.

During treatment, the team members help build motivation. Readily attainable short-term goals build confidence. Valued long-term goals build motivation. Positive feedback from significant people and mastery over the environment stimulate further motivation (see Chaps. 7 through 11). The team members listen to the patient and provide consistent and supportive counseling, which helps the patient develop his ability to talk about his feelings. Key words, however, must be used very carefully by the team members. *Better* means "improved, safer, or more efficient" to team members, but it often means "cured" or "normal" to the patient or family. When functional improvement has leveled off in one area, the team members must help the patient and family refocus on other areas without feeling a sense of failure. The team members should remain realistically hopeful, offering better ways of adapting and helping the patient to reduce his disability and to maintain optimal health and function.

FOLLOW-THROUGH: DISCHARGE PLANNING AND HOME PROGRAMS

Because the patient's functional or neurologic status may change, careful follow-through is an integral part of the team approach. If symptoms improve, the patient can tolerate more strenuous exercise and will require less adaptive equipment. If symptoms worsen, an exercise program may have to be curtailed and the patient may need to learn to use more equipment for safety and efficiency. The team members must keep accurate records to compare and evaluate changes and to upgrade patient programs as necessary. Compliance with, understanding of, and motivation for ongoing programs are better with more frequent team/patient contact. Proper follow-through also provides the patient with the sense that the team is "with him" regardless of the disease progression.

Discharge planning, including home programs, begins early in a rehabilitation admission. The patient must understand and agree with his treatment program if he is to follow through after he leaves the structured hospital/clinic environment. Family members play a crucial role in helping a patient comply with his program, and a family setting may be the most cost-effective and positive long-term environment for a patient. Therefore, family unity and family education should be stressed in the program prior to the patient's discharge. Patients, family, or friends must know when to initiate a call to the clinic if questions or problems arise. Also, they must feel welcomed when they do call.

Because the team/patient contact is only the beginning of the treatment program, individualized home programs with regular upgrading ensure that patients will maintain function or improve further after discharge. The team should also identify and mobilize community resources to assist the patient. Follow-through may involve other physicians and therapists (with suggestions and information provided by the rehabilitation team members), MS organizations, visiting nurse services, and other specific community resources. A complete team reevaluation every 3 to 12 months as needed helps the patient maintain control.

How to Develop a Team

One approach to building a team is outlined as follows:

1. Identify the magnitude of the patient problems, the need:
     Number of patients in the serviced area
     Needs assessment for those patients
2. Identify resources required to meet the need:
     Personnel
     Space: hospital/clinic
     Time
     Dollars
3. Discuss the concept with key people.
4. Form a strategy planning committee.
5. Organize team members.
6. Begin with a pilot program and review the results.
7. Open the team concept to all MS patients.

Identification of patients' needs and the resources required to meet those needs is fundamental. Any interested person can begin the process. A needs assessment survey may provide a more accurate idea of the number of patients already seen in a geographical area and the extent of their problems, as well as the number of patients who are unserved or underserved. Local service organizations such as MS societies can also help. Necessary resources include hospital beds, an outpatient clinic area, and the availability of interested team members to provide patient care, education, team meetings, and family conferences. After the needs and resources have been outlined, a strategic planning committee should be formed to develop short-term and long-term organizational plans and the time frame for collecting the needed resources. Organizational plans include identifying team members and their roles, planning their schedules, and identifying potential problems with solutions and alternatives.

A pilot program with a few patients is initially helpful to identify and solve unforeseen problems and to allow the team members to build confidence. Patients with the most potential for success (mild to moderate disability, well motivated) are best for a pilot program. The pilot program outcome is then reviewed, and revisions are made as needed. As the team gains experience, an increasing number of patients with more complex problems can be treated (see Chap. 6). Even if the treatment results are not optimal, some improvement in the patient, the family, and the patient's environment is usual. The only patients who do not undergo at least a trial of rehabilitation at the CND/RMMSC are those who are totally unmotivated or who have never followed through with previous treatment plans.

When no team is currently or potentially available, the care-giver should not feel overwhelmed and hopeless. He can identify many broad patient-care issues using the information presented here and in other literature as guidelines. He can set priorities for problems and, with the patient and family, develop a treatment plan for the most important problems. He can communicate a sense of empathy with the patient and his family. Thus, the care-giver can be a mini-team with the patient and his family. The isolated care-giver can also seek out an interested therapist, nurse, or physician, who can function as an *ad hoc* mini-team for one patient. By discussing different patients repeatedly with the same consultants or therapists, enough interest and confidence may be aroused from experience so that the potential for a full-fledged team may develop.

Ingredients for a Successful Team

Ingredients for a successful team include the following:

Interest
Availability
Leadership
Maintenance of morale
Conflict management
Direction and growth

Experience is not as critical for success as is interest and commitment. Team members need to be available for timely evaluation, team conferences and planning, family conferences, and informal discussions with other team members, families, and patients. As the team members gain experience, a team develops its own style, confidence, expertise, and self-identity. The team leader facilitates team interaction, records team decisions, and coordinates the overall treatment plan (see the list of the team leader's functions, outlined earlier in this chapter). As previously mentioned, a physician often assumes this role, but any other team member may be the leader.

Maintainence of morale when faced with difficulties in treating patients with MS is crucial for effectiveness. Good morale is more critical than pay or benefits in preventing staff burnout. Team members maintain enthusiasm and energy when morale issues are openly discussed and when there is adequate time for team relaxation together. Setting appropriate goals allows team members to feel successful when those goals are achieved and provides guidelines for realistic team expectations.

When disagreement occurs relating to treatment and priorities or when personality conflicts arise among team members, a means for conflict management must be initiated. The team leader can often act as mediator by acknowledging differences and seeking realistic compromises. Finally, the team needs a sense of direction and growth, which is obtained by quality continuing education and judicious expansion of programs.

Cost Effectiveness

The cost of team care and rehabilitation hospitalization (up to 4 weeks once or twice a year) must be weighed against the cost of maintenance medical care without rehabilitation. Maintenance costs may include more frequent outpatient contacts, greater home health-care hours, or the cost of a nursing home. Additional factors include loss of income or loss of family support. Even when a patient must live in a nursing home, decreased intensity of nursing care after rehabilitation can lead to decreased costs. Many patients in nursing homes can, with appropriate therapy, be rehabilitated to live at home.

Feigenson (1981) has shown that MS rehabilitation is cost effective even with severely disabled patients who had not benefited from a multidisciplinary outpatient program. The decrease in care requirements and cost was due to improved functional skills.

Summary

The rehabilitation of MS patients can be successful and rewarding by focusing on the patient's functional abilities. The interdisciplinary team approach allows comprehensive evaluation, planning, and treatment to deal most effectively with the complex problems and issues facing patients with MS. With the team approach concept, the whole is greater than the sum of its parts: the communication between team members allows a truer understanding of the patient and his problems, which results in a coordinated effort at problem-solving. The goal for the patient is to achieve a more functional, productive, creative, and satisfying life.

Suggested Readings

BLEIBERG J, MERBITZ C: Learning goals during initial rehabilitation hospitalization. Arch Phys Med Rehab 64:448–451, 1983

DEJONG G, HUGHES J: Independent living: Methodology for measuring long-term outcomes. Arch Phys Med Rehab 63:68–73, 1982

FEIGENSON JS, SCHEINBERG L, CATALANO M, et al: The cost-effectiveness of multiple sclerosis rehabilitation: A model. Neurology 31:1316–1322, 1981

KOTTKE F: Philosophic considerations of quality of life for the disabled. Arch Phys Med Rehab 63:60–62, 1982

MATSON RR, BROOKS NA: Adjusting to multiple sclerosis: An exploratory study. Soc Sci Med 11:245–250, 1977

MOR V, GRANGER CV, SHERWOOD CC: Discharged rehabilitation patients: Impact of follow-up surveillance by a friendly visitor. Arch Phys Med Rehab 64:346–353, 1983

SCHEINBERG LC, HOLLAND NJ, KIRSCHENBAUM J, et al: Comprehensive long-term care of patients with multiple sclerosis. Neurology 31:1121–1123, 1981

SCHEINBERG LC, GIESSER BS, SLATER RJ: Management of the chronic MS patient. Neurol Neurosurg 4:21, 1983

STOLOV WC: Evaluation of the patient. In Kottke FJ (ed): Krusin's Handbook of Physical Medicine and Rehabilitation, pp 1–18. Philadelphia, WB Saunders, 1982

Gary M. Franklin
Jack S. Burks

3

Diagnosis and Medical Management of Multiple Sclerosis

Multiple sclerosis (MS) is the most common, potentially disabling neurologic disorder of young adults. It is frequently confused with less common disorders such as muscular dystrophy and cerebral palsy. In fact, MS prevalence in some geographic areas in the United States is as high as 100 per 100,000 population, or nearly one patient for every 1,000 people. Including incidental cases diagnosed at postmortem examination, the prevalence may be even higher. It is estimated that there are 250,000 MS patients in the United States.

Although onset of MS usually occurs between the ages of 20 and 40 years, onset in childhood or after the age of 60 years, although rare, is not unknown. Nearly twice as many women as men have the disease, and people living in temperate regions, particularly above the 40th north parallel, are also at greater risk of MS. Although these facts of the disease's occurrence are not currently explained, their elucidation should help unravel the etiology of MS. Other potential environmental risk factors (e.g., diet, pets) have been investigated, but none has a clearly proven association.

The genetic aspects of MS have been investigated in detail, but no specific mode of inheritance has emerged. However, the risk seems to be increased five fold within families, although the increased probability of a child contracting the disease later in life seems to be no greater than 0.5% to 1% (Spielman and Nathanson, 1982). What may be inherited is the susceptibility to develop MS. Exposure to an environmental factor (e.g., viruses) might then allow the disease to express itself in a genetically susceptible individual. Epidemiologic efforts are aimed at more clearly defining additional susceptibility and environmental factors.

Although the pathogenesis of MS is still unclear, the preponderance of evidence indicates that it is a viral-induced immune regulatory disorder, with an etiology similar to that of rheumatoid arthritis or juvenile diabetes. The MS patient's immune system may be stimulated to damage myelin in the central nervous system. The antigenic stimulus for this paradoxical inability of the body's immune system to determine "self" from "not-self" remains unknown. The rationale for most of the current experimental therapies for MS is based on this immunologic hypothesis.

Diagnosis

DIAGNOSTIC CRITERIA

Although formal diagnostic criteria have been suggested, in many cases the diagnosis of MS remains difficult. The principal clinical criterion for the diagnosis of MS is evidence of disordered function in at least two areas of the central nervous system (brain or spinal cord), separated in time and neuroanatomical space. An example of this would be loss of vision in one month and tingling in the legs eight months later. Early in the course of the disease, many patients do not exhibit a pattern of deficits that meet the above criterion. In other patients, symptoms are prominent but neurologic deficits are minimal. For such patients diagnostic testing may be useful.

DIAGNOSTIC TESTING

The diagnostic tests that often serve as critical adjuncts to the clinical picture in diagnosing MS are evoked potential testing and spinal fluid evaluation (Poser, 1983), both of which are available in most communities.

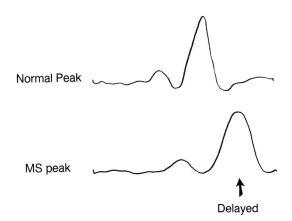

Figure 3-1 Examples of normal and delayed conduction in visual evoked response (VER) caused by demyelination in central visual pathways.

Evoked potentials are computer-averaged electrical impulses that allow measurement of the rate of nerve impulse transmission through the central nervous system (CNS). The myelinated tracts most often investigated are the visual, auditory, and somatosensory pathways. Slowed conduction in any one of these tracts, even in the absence of associated clinical symptoms, is evidence for the presence of demyelination in that tract. Therefore, the test is most useful in identifying "clinically silent" lesions. These tests are expensive and, if abnormal, need not be repeated (Fig. 3 – 1).

The spinal fluid evaluation may be performed in the hospital or in an outpatient setting. Although many parameters may be measured in the spinal fluid, the most productive laboratory analyses are the cell count

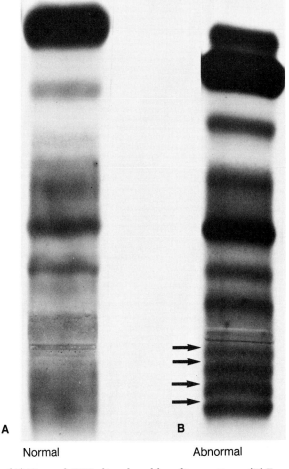

A   **B**

Normal   Abnormal

Figure 3 – 2   (A) Normal CSF oligoclonal banding pattern. (B) Four oligoclonal bands seen in a patient with clinical evidence of disseminated central nervous system lesions.

and oligoclonal banding (Fig. 3 – 2), and tests that measure immunoglob-
ulin (IgG). Although the lymphocyte count may be increased in MS, the
occurrence of an abnormally increased lymphocyte count alone would
not be strong evidence for MS. IgG is increased in the cerebrospinal fluid
(CSF) in 60% to 75% of MS patients. Most of the IgG is synthesized in the
CNS, indicating ongoing immunologic activity. The IgG is usually measured in relationship to the spinal fluid and serum albumin. Oligoclonal
banding is the most sensitive of the CSF tests, although bands may be
seen in other CNS disorders. Lumbar puncture is usually accomplished
with ease, but approximately 10% of patients have significant morbidity
following the procedure. Headache lasting for some days and requiring
bed rest is the most common complication.

Neuroradiologic procedures, such as computed tomography (CT)
scanning, have not proven to be extremely sensitive in the early diagnosis of MS. The CT scan is most useful during acute exacerbations of
MS; specialized CT scans with a double concentration of contrast material and 2-hour delayed views provide the highest yield of MS lesions in
this situation (Fig 3 – 3). The nuclear magnetic resonance (NMR) scan
will greatly improve our diagnostic accuracy for MS. Its yield for demyelinating lesions is three to four times that of the CT scan.

As a result of this new diagnostic technology, the average time from
onset of symptoms to first diagnosis of MS has decreased from 4 years to
less than 2 years in the past decade (Nelson et al, 1983). Most neurolo-

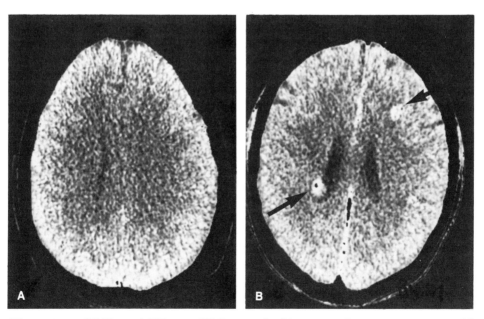

Figure 3 – 3   (A) Normal CT scan. (B) Scattered white matter lesions in a 27-year-old
woman with relapsing/remitting MS.

gists and primary-care physicians are increasingly aware of the condition, and patients are grateful to know the specific cause for their often elusive symptoms. Another direct benefit of the new diagnostic technology is that earlier diagnosis will lead to earlier treatment as more specific therapies become available.

Disease Manifestations and Functional Impairment

THE COURSE OF MULTIPLE SCLEROSIS

The course of MS is most frequently relapsing and remitting. Symptoms come and go, often over a period of many years. Benign forms of MS exist in which attacks are infrequent and complete recovery is the rule. More commonly, however, there is an average of one exacerbation every 2 years (McAlpine et al, 1972). The patient may recover completely, or there may be mild or moderate residual deficit after each exacerbation.

A smaller percentage of patients, perhaps as high as 15%, develop a chronic/progressive course from the very first symptom. Even in this type of MS, symptoms may progress rapidly or slowly. Some patients with a primarily relapsing/remitting course may become chronic/progressive after many years.

When studied in community-based populations, the course of MS is more benign than was once believed. The overall figures suggest that 66% of MS patients are still ambulatory 25 years after disease onset (Percy et al, 1971).

On an individual basis, predictability of outcome is exceedingly difficult. A more benign course in the first five years is more likely to be associated with a better prognosis. Even chronic/progressive patients may stabilize after a certain level of disability is reached. The chronic uncertainty faced by a person with multiple sclerosis may cause a tremendous emotional burden, and this uncertainty often makes planning for the future, in terms of employment or family responsibility, exceedingly difficult.

SYMPTOMS AND SIGNS

MS is the great imitator; its symptoms and signs may mimic those of many other neuropsychiatric disorders. Because demyelination may occur anywhere in the CNS, a great diversity of symptoms and signs may be seen. No two patients present in exactly the same way. Clinical signs may mimic those seen in stroke or with tumors. Lesions may even extend a short distance into the nerve root sleeve, mimicking cranial nerve or spinal root symptoms. The more common and functionally important clinical problems are discussed below. The patient's ability to function is of overriding concern and is stressed in the context of the neurologic examination.

Visual Disturbances

Difficulty with vision is extraordinarily common in MS and takes two primary forms: loss of vision and inability to focus. These two problems are frequently confused, and either may require the patient to stop reading or driving.

Loss of vision most frequently begins with an episode of optic neuritis, one of the most common presenting complaints in MS. The sudden onset of visual loss, usually only in one eye, is accompanied by pain on movement of the eye. Although visual loss may be extreme, return to normal vision and dissipation of pain in 3 to 6 weeks are the rule. A smaller number of patients exhibit a more insidious onset of visual loss that may be more progressive and painless. Demyelination in the visual system occurs in 80% of patients; the visual evoked potential is a highly sensitive test for diagnosis of demyelination in the visual system (see Fig. 3–1). The greatest number of patients in our clinic have either no diminution of visual acuity or only modest loss of vision in the $20/30$ to $20/40$ range.

Inability to focus accounts for the greatest burden of visual disability in our patients. Many patients exhibit a unilateral or bilateral intranuclear ophthalmoplegia with a disturbance of horizontal eye movement resulting from a lesion in the supranuclear connection to the oculomotor nuclei in the brain stem. Patients may see double images, but most frequently they only experience blurred vision, which makes following the printed line when reading exceedingly difficult. Severe nystagmus may also be seen. These rapid to-and-fro movements of the eye cause oscillopsia or the impression that the visual image is not standing still. Reading and other tasks involving visual tracking become difficult.

Motor Disturbances

In MS, the inability to perform motor tasks is due to weakness, spasticity, or incoordination. These findings are frequently present together and thus make functional evaluation of the underlying disturbances difficult.

Weakness and spasticity usually occur together because of myelin damage in the pyramidal tracts. The weakness is usually of an upper motor neuron variety without focal wasting or fasciculations. However, weakness in a specific muscle group accompanied by focal wasting (e.g., intrinsic muscles of the hands) is occasionally seen. Increased tone and hyperactive deep tendon reflexes are the hallmark of spasticity. Paraparesis, which may be asymmetric, is a very common finding. Less commonly, one upper extremity may be involved as well. Weakness and spasticity are important to differentiate and may present in a variety of combinations. The legs may be very weak with a minimum of spasticity, or spasticity may predominate with little weakness noted on direct muscle testing. Therapeutic maneuvers and their efficacy will vary according to the relative distribution of these findings.

Incoordination and tremor are most frequently caused by cerebellar involvement. The tremor is primarily an intention tremor, and it may be so severe as to preclude self-feeding. Strength testing may be entirely normal even in the face of severe tremor. In our experience, cerebellar signs are frequently more marked in the legs than in the arms. A wide-based gait may be seen, often accompanied by truncal instability. The Romberg test, however, is usually normal as long as proprioceptive sense is not markedly decreased in the lower extremities.

Combinations of incoordination with weakness or spasticity often make the neurologic basis of functional impairment difficult to assess. Both paraparesis at the thoracic level as well as truncal incoordination may, for example, lead to poor sitting balance.

Bladder and Bowel Disturbances

Symptoms related to bladder and bowel disturbances most frequently accompany other evidence of spinal cord involvement. The most common bladder complaint is urgency. The ability to get to the bathroom immediately following the initial sensation of having to void may become the preeminent functional problem in many patients' lives. Social life is frequently planned to avoid situations in which urgency may lead to incontinence. Incontinence as a primary complaint, however, is (thankfully) rare except in those few patients with severe paraparesis. Some few patients may complain of hesitancy rather than urgency, and some have experienced both problems (see Chap. 4).

Bowel problems are usually related to constipation. Because of the insidious onset of constipation, patients must be queried directly concerning their bowel habits. Therapy for bowel problems is covered in Chapter 5.

Fatigue

Fatigue, or a sense of total exhaustion, is a prominent complaint in the majority of our patients and may be seen even with a paucity of other neurologic findings. Most patients do well in the morning, but by early afternoon many find it difficult to continue their regular activities. Specific functions may also worsen at this time; examination of the patient in mid-afternoon may reveal significantly more neurologic dysfunction than an examination performed in the early morning hours. Although the basis for fatigue in MS is unknown, disability determination should take full cognizance of its presence.

Sensory Disturbances and Pain

Persistent or fleeting sensory disturbances are common and may be very disturbing. However, functional disability due to sensory disturbances is rare. The most common and well known of these, Lhermitte's sign, is a transient, lightninglike sensation radiating down the spine following neck flexion. Tingling paresthesias or numbness may be noted in the fifth nerve distribution over the face. More unusual localizations, such as bandlike sensations about the trunk, may be encountered as well. The most common finding on examination is mild loss of vibratory sense in the distal lower extremities. More severe loss of proprioception or position sense in the legs is relatively rare but, when present, may significantly jeopardize standing balance.

Pain, on the other hand, is noted in 10% to 20% of our patients and may be extremely disabling. Its origin and presentation are quite variable. Pain of spinal cord and nerve root origin is often extremely searing or burning in quality and may follow a dermatomal pattern. Episodes of trigeminal neuralgia are commonly seen, and laminectomy has at times been mistakenly performed for radicular pain in the lumbar region. Pain related to spasticity is also commonly noted. Patients with moderate spasticity on examination are frequently awakened at night with painful extensor spasms of the legs. Joint pain may be seen as well and is most likely related to mechanical difficulties secondary to weakness and abnormal posturing. Severe quadriceps weakness, for example, may lead to hyperextension and degenerative change in the knee.

Cognitive Dysfunction and Alteration of Mood

Severe cognitive deficits are usually seen only in the chronic/progressive variety of MS. Functionally important loss of cognitive function is relatively rare in the great majority of patients with relapsing/remitting disease. Formal neuropsychometric testing should be performed in all patients in whom such dysfunction is suspected. Although the deficits are not usually striking on clinical mental status examination, their presence should be documented for disability rating, vocational guidance, and family counseling purposes.

Mood disturbances are exceedingly common in MS and usually take the form of depression. Denial, anger, and frustration are appropriate early responses to MS. These feelings may be displaced by severe depression. Usually, however, the depression is moderate and is associated with significant insomnia. This disturbance of sleep may exacerbate daytime fatigue.

Pseudobulbar affect is occasionally seen in MS. "Incontinence of emotion" is noted, with an excessive amount of crying or laughter. This emotional response is involuntary and is a result of bilateral demyelinating lesions in the supranuclear connections to the brain stem. This outburst of emotion is not necessarily associated with cognitive dysfunction. Once again, neuropsychometric testing may be useful in differentiating these two manifestations of MS.

Other Neurologic Problems

As previously mentioned, any symptom or sign of CNS dysfunction may be seen, albeit rare. Seizures, sometimes focal, are seen in fewer than 5% of patients. Autonomic dysfunction, such as severe sweating, is occasionally seen.

Vertigo, usually secondary to brainstem dysfunction, is seen in a modest number of our patients. This symptom may be quite disabling and may make ongoing rehabilitation efforts difficult.

Disorders of sexuality are extremely common in MS and seem to occur with equal frequency in men and women (Lilius et al, 1976). Sensitivity of the sexual organs may diminish, and orgasm may become difficult, although not impossible, for many. Interestingly, some male patients unable to maintain erection may achieve ejaculation. Mood disturbances and waning confidence related to MS may exacerbate these neurologically based sexual disorders.

Medical Problems

Significant medical problems are seen in a large number of moderately to severely disabled patients with MS.

Infections of the urinary tract are commonly seen, particularly in women patients. Urinary tract infections are often difficult to diagnose because the heralding symptoms are not always noted by patients (e.g., dysuria). The only clues may be an increase in urinary frequency, the appearance of hematuria, or a change in the odor or appearance of the urine. Those patients using intermittent catheterization or indwelling catheters are especially at risk for urinary tract infections. Incomplete emptying of the bladder, with associated increased residual urine, is the common denominator in most of these infections. Urinalysis and urine culture should be performed at the slightest hint of infection because serious complications (systemic infection, pyelonephritis) may ensue. Even relatively mild infection and fever in patients already quite disabled or bed-ridden can be catastrophic. Disabled patients may become quite obtunded and barely responsive when infection ensues.

Pneumonia may occur in severely debilitated patients. These patients usually exhibit severe brain stem involvement as well as neurogenic disturbances in respiration.

Skin problems are noted in the more disabled patients and vary from irritation and erythema to decubitus ulcer. The former is a clear warning that steps must be taken to prevent the latter. In some patients with severe brain stem involvement, marked difficulty in swallowing may preclude the maintenance of normal nutritional status. In such cases, enteric feedings or gastrostomy may be indicated (see Chaps. 5 and 10).

EXACERBATING FACTORS IN MULTIPLE SCLEROSIS

The factors that exacerbate MS with some frequency are of considerable importance in that their avoidance may make life a great deal easier for many patients with MS.

Heat

Increased environmental temperature of all origins may exacerbate MS symptoms, even if transiently. Summer heat, hot tubs, and hot baths are all frequently incriminated (in fact, a "hot bath test" was once used as a diagnostic test in MS). Increased internal temperature associated with fever of infectious origin or increased body temperature following rigorous exercise may exacerbate MS symptoms. Exercise, however, is to be encouraged, its only bounds being the patient's own tolerance limits (see Chap. 7).

Stress

Anecdotally, stress is thought to be a precipitant of some MS exacerbations, but it remains for a well-controlled study to relate any association between stress and worsening symptoms in MS. Stress may be positive or negative, including stressful life events (e.g., promotion, marriage, loss of a loved one), physical trauma, or the presence of MS itself. We are all surrounded by stress much of the time; the critical factor is how we respond to stress. The stress response may be mirrored in chronic symptomatology, such as frequent headaches or peptic ulcer pain, but more subtle symptoms may be present as well, including tightening of the paracervical or shoulder girdle muscles or difficulty in falling asleep. Many of our patients complain of worsening symptoms secondary to stress. Although the relationship between stress and the worsening is difficult to document, our approach to these patients is to offer therapeutic modalities aimed at stress reduction.

Trauma

Although many patients can identify traumatic incidents preceding the onset of MS, proof that direct injury to the head or spine plays an etiologic role in multiple sclerosis is lacking. However, injuries are associated with considerable stress, which may contribute to the increased symptoms.

NONEXACERBATING FACTORS IN MULTIPLE SCLEROSIS SYMPTOMS

A great deal of lore exists concerning what MS patients should and should not do. Often, these messages come from ill-informed sources, and the patient's needs for continuing to live life to the fullest are not completely taken into account.

No evidence exists that pregnancy has an adverse effect on MS, and, in fact, the nine months of gestation may have a protective effect. An increased risk of exacerbation is noted in the three to four months following delivery, but long-term outcome in terms of eventual disability is not adversely affected by pregnancy (Thompson et al, 1984).

Too many patients with MS are advised to "rest" most of the time. Prudent rest, tailored to the needs and fatigue levels of each patient, can fit into the ongoing, productive lifestyle of many of our patients. Daily exercise is critical for maintenance of maximal function. We are currently investigating the potential beneficial effects of aerobic exercise on the fatigue in our patients.

MEASUREMENT OF FUNCTIONAL OUTCOME

Functional outcome measures in MS have proven extremely difficult, particularly in clinical trials. A neurologic scale of functional disability (Rose et al, 1968) has been used for many years. (See also Chap. 6 for further discussion of scales.) Recently, an international committee has begun to develop a minimal scale of functional disability encompassing more diverse effects of MS. This new scale includes such factors as sexuality, working ability, and fatigue levels. As this methodology improves, disability-outcome measures for MS will become more accurate.

Medical Management

Pharmacologic manipulation in MS can be divided into symptomatic treatment of specific manifestations and treatment of the overall disease process.

TREATMENT OF SPECIFIC MANIFESTATIONS IN MULTIPLE SCLEROSIS

Spasticity is usually treated successfully with exercise and drugs (see Chap. 7). The most commonly used drugs are baclofen (Lioresal), diazepam (Valium), clonazepam (Clonopin), and dantrolene (Dantrium), which reduce the uninhibited tone that results from demyelinating lesions in the pyramidal tracts. These drugs may unmask underlying weakness in selected patients; that is, spasticity is reduced but strength may decrease as well. Functionally speaking, the use of these drugs depends on the final balance of effects. Their greatest use is in patients with a great deal of spasticity but little underlying weakness. Patients who are extremely weak and are literally "standing on their tone" could be adversely affected. Nocturnal spasms related to spasticity may also be treated very effectively with the use of these drugs. Other major adverse effects of these drugs include excessive drowsiness and liver dysfunction (Table 3–1).

The therapy for incoordination related to cerebellar dysfunction is not usually satisfactory. The drugs in use for incoordination are quite diverse and include isoniazid (INH), an antitubercular drug that may have inhibitory properties in the cerebellum; propranolol (Inderal), a beta-adrenergic blocking agent that is extremely useful in benign essential tremor but only modestly useful in MS; and clonazepam (Clonopin). One can only try each of these in turn, and, over a finite period (4–6 weeks), look for beneficial treatment effects. If none are clearly observed, the drugs should be discontinued.

Bladder problems are very common, and their treatment is often confusing. Specific symptoms may be misleading for an accurate clinical diagnosis. Urodynamic testing is most useful for clarification, especially if the patient does not respond to the first treatment regimen. Baclofen and anticholinergic drugs such as propantheline bromide (Pro-Banthine) and oxybutynin chloride (Ditropan) are helpful for "spastic" bladders, whereas intermittent catheterization is usually required for "flaccid" bladders (see Chap. 4).

Prescription drug treatment for constipation (e.g., stool softeners) is usually unnecessary and may be harmful with long-term use. Over-the-counter preparations that increase bowel motility (laxatives) or bulk (e.g., psyllium hydrophilic mucilloid [Metamucil]) are commonly self-prescribed. Dietary manipulation is also an extremely effective therapy for constipation. Increased fiber (bran, whole-grain products) and water intake as well as regular exercise usually help as much as prescription medication.

A variety of drugs are efficacious in treating sensory disturbances and pain. Carbamazepine (Tegretol) is often effective for dysesthetic, burning pain of central or radicular origin in MS. However, the patient's blood count must be monitored because of potential bone marrow suppression. The use of narcotics is to be discouraged. Nearly all patients with chronic pain have an associated depression and chronic use of narcotics may exacerbate this depression.

Mood disturbances, particularly depression, are best treated by an

Table 3-1 Medications Used in Symptomatic Therapy of Multiple Sclerosis

Symptom	Drug	Usual Dosage Range	Expected Benefit	Potential Adverse Effects
Spasticity	Baclofen* Clonopin Valium Dantrium	10 mg–20 mg tid or qid 0.5 mg tid 5 mg–10 mg tid or qid 25 mg–50 mg tid or qid	Decreased hypertonus; improved movement	Weakness; liver dysfunction; sedation
Cerebellar incoordination	INH Inderal Clonopin	300 mg/day 10 mg–20 mg tid or qid 0.5 mg–1 mg tid	Decreased tremor; improved truncal stability	Liver dysfunction (INH); cardiac effects (Inderal)
Urinary urgency	Ditropan* Pro-Banthine	5 mg bid or tid 15 mg bid or tid	Improved bladder control; decreased urgency	Increased hesitancy of bladder; constipation
Painful sensory disturbance	Tegretol*	200 mg bid or tid	Decreased painful dysesthesia	Bone marrow suppression
Depression	Tricyclic antidepressants* (Aventyl, Elavil)	25 mg bid or tid	Decreased insomnia; improved mood	Dry mouth; constipation; urinary hesitancy; weight gain

* Preferred drugs in our clinic.

44

empathetic health-care professional and, in more difficult cases, by formal counseling and pharmacologic manipulation. Tricyclic antidepressants (amitripyline [Elavil], nortriptyline [Pamelor]) may be especially useful, particularly with associated insomnia. In our experience, tricyclics may also benefit occasional associated symptoms such as pseudobulbar palsy (emotional incontinence). The major side-effects of these drugs include dry mouth and urinary and bowel retention.

TREATMENT OF THE DISEASE PROCESS

At present, no long-term treatment has been proven effective for the disease process in MS. The two mainstays of therapy, ACTH and steroids, should be considered only for short-term use. They may be effective in reducing the severity and duration of a specific exacerbation in certain cases, but they seem to have no effect on long-term outcome. They are most efficaciously used in pulse regimens over a period of two weeks. We see many patients who have been on steroids for months or years and have demonstrated severe long-term adverse effects.

The most promising new mode of therapy, although still experimental, is the use of more powerful immunosuppressive medications. None of these drugs is being used for routine clinical purposes. Azathioprine (Imuran) and cyclophosphamide (Cytoxan) are the two most commonly used of these experimental drugs. Another method of immunosuppression, plasmapheresis, acts by removing immunologically active components from the blood. Most of these treatment regimens have significant side-effects and are currently being evaluated only in progressive MS. In the future, we will need to identify and treat patients earlier in the course of their illness to get the most beneficial effect from any new treatments. A useful therapeutic regimen to stop progression in MS may be available in the near future. However, reversal of existing deficits that have been present for many years may not be possible. Therefore, the early diagnosis of MS becomes vitally important.

A Wellness Approach to a Chronic Illness

As with all other chronic diseases, one must not look at MS, the illness, or its symptoms in isolation. The patient must be considered in the context of his environment and in society as a whole. Chronic illness, for example, is also a family concern, dramatically affecting all who surround the patient. In societal terms, the direct plus indirect costs of a young MS patient having to stop working are enormous in terms of lost income and productivity. Thus, all efforts to maintain productivity become exceedingly important. This view of illness, in contradistinction to the traditional medical model, represents a systems view of disease.

A wellness view of health implies that better health maintenance in an individual may prevent the development of chronic disease. This concept has been strikingly demonstrated in regard to the effect of diet, smoking, and hypertension on the development and effects of coronary artery disease. A wellness view of an illness, such as MS, implies that making one's self healthier may impact positively on the course of the disease. The modalities used in a wellness model might include (1) active patient participation in stress reduction, regular exercise, and energy conservation; (2) the institution of a healthier diet; and (3) decreasing unhealthy behaviors (smoking, excessive alcohol). The goal is for patients to regain a sense of control that permeates many aspects of their lives. This control is of particular importance in MS, where predictability of disease course is nearly impossible and where a sense of loss of control occurs with great frequency. Until a "cure" is discovered for MS, this approach can help a patient tolerate even a severe disease course. Finally, until we "know" the causes of MS, staying healthy overall makes sense.

Conclusion

Caring for patients with a chronic, frequently disabling illness is often extremely difficult and challenging. Health-care professionals must take a hard look at their own mortality in order to effectively deal with the pain and anger of disorders like MS. This often means being able to say, "I can't make this go away, but I can do everything possible, along with the health-care team, to ease your burden."

Many of our patients are survivors and have managed to get beyond severe loss of physical function. The improved personal growth that results from this process often gives us, the health-care team, the motivation to continue.

MS affects those on whose lives it impacts in many ways. The patient with MS is primarily concerned with the burden of the disease: loss of function and self-esteem, impact on family and career, and loss of economic viability. The research scientist is concerned with viruses, the myelin sheaths, and the immune system. The health-care practitioner must attend to the needs of the patient with MS in the context of this current knowledge. Rehabilitation professionals have the closest opportunity to address the primary needs that concern patients on a daily basis and impact positively on their quality of life. Since there is, as yet, no known cure for MS, a clear perspective of the complex ramifications of this disorder is imperative.

Suggested Readings

LILIUS HG, VALTONEN EJ, WIKSTROM J: Sexual problems in patients suffering from multiple sclerosis. J Chronic Dis 29:643–647, 1976

MCALPINE D, LUMSDEN CE, ACHESON ED: Multiple Sclerosis: A Reappraisal. Edinburgh, E & S Livingstone, 1972

NELSON LM, HAMMAN RF, BURKS JS, et al: Higher than expected prevalence of multiple sclerosis (MS) in Northern Colorado. Presented at the Edpidemiological Research Exchange, University of Colorado, Denver, October 13, 1983

PERCY AK, NOBREGA FT, OKAZAKI H, et al: Multiple sclerosis in Rochester, Minn.: A 60-year appraisal. Arch Neurol 25:105–111, 1971

POSER CM, PATY DW, SCHEINBERG L, et al: New diagnostic criteria for multiple sclerosis: Guidelines for research protocols. Ann Neurol 13:227–231, 1983

ROSE AS, KUZMA JW, KURTZKE JF, et al: Cooperative study in the evaluation of therapy in multiple sclerosis; ACTH vs. placebo in acute exacerbations: Preliminary report. Neurology 18, (6):1–10, 1968

SPIELMAN RS, NATHANSON N: The genetics of susceptibility to multiple sclerosis. Epidemiol Rev 4:45–65, 1982

THOMPSON DS, NELSON LM, BURKS JS, et al: The effects of pregnancy in multiple sclerosis (MS): A retrospective study. Neurology 34(suppl 1):244, 1984

4   Richard R. Augspurger

Bladder Dysfunction in Multiple Sclerosis

Multiple sclerosis (MS) often involves the motor and sensory pathways of the bladder. When the innervation to the bladder is affected, a bladder dysfunction called a *neurogenic bladder* occurs. Although the true incidence of neurogenic bladder in MS is unknown, an estimated 50% to 80% of MS patients develop urinary symptoms at some time during the course of their disease. Up to 12% of patients have urinary symptoms at the time of initial presentation, and in 1% to 2% they are the presenting symptoms. The severity of bladder involvement does not appear to be related to the duration of the disease, but rather parallels the severity of the disease.

The symptoms of neurogenic bladder, such as urinary frequency, urgency, urinary incontinence, urinary retention, and recurrent urinary tract infection, are often a major social concern of the patient. Although MS patients may have similar symptoms, they do not necessarily have the same type of neurogenic bladder. Only a 50% correlation exists between bladder symptoms and the type of neurogenic bladder (Blaivas et al, 1979). In the same study by Blaivas and associates, only 27% of the patients were on appropriate and effective therapy with empiric treatment based on voiding symptoms alone.

As with other aspects of the disease, bladder dysfunction can change with relapses and remission. Thus, the MS patient with bladder symptoms needs an initial urologic–urodynamic evaluation so that the appropriate treatment can be selected. Frequent reevaluation is required so that treatment can be adjusted to provide optimal urologic care.

Anatomy and Neurourology

The bladder is the storage organ of the urinary tract. Urine from the kidneys traverses the ureters to the bladder. As urine enters the bladder, the bladder muscle (detrusor) relaxes to accommodate between 450 ml

48

to 500 ml of urine. The urine does not leak out through the urethra because the sphincters are closed. There are two sphincters: the proximal, which is smooth muscle, and the distal, which is skeletal muscle and smooth muscle (Fig. 4–1). At bladder capacity, voiding occurs voluntarily. The detrusor contracts, the proximal sphincter funnels open, and the distal sphincter relaxes, allowing urine to pass from the bladder.

The normal processes of urine storage and voiding are under the control of the central nervous system (CNS). Several theories of neurologic control have been proposed (Wein and Raezer, 1979). The main reflex center for the bladder appears to be located in the mesencephalic–reticular formation — the brain stem micturition center (BSMC) (Fig. 4–2). A less dominant center, the spinal cord micturition center (SCMC), also plays a role.

Sensory, proprioceptive fibers arising in the bladder traverse through the pelvic nerves and then the posterior columns to reach the BSMC. Motor fibers originating in the BSMC travel via the reticulospinal tracts to the detrusor motor nucleus in the intermediolateral gray cell column of the sacral spinal cord (S2–4). From the detrusor motor nucleus, parasympathetic fibers traverse the pelvic nerves, synapse in the pelvic ganglia, and innervate the detrusor muscle. The neurotransmittor is acetylcholine (cholinergic) (Fig. 4–3). Suprasacral interruption of the pathway releases the SCMC from inhibition and can produce a low-capacity bladder with unsustained, uninhibited contraction of the detrusor muscle.

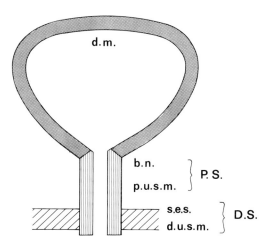

Figure 4–1 Schematic diagram of the bladder, detrusor muscle (d.m.), and urinary sphincters. The proximal sphincter (P.S.) consists of the bladder neck smooth muscle (b.n.) and the proximal urethral smooth muscle (p.u.s.m.) The distal sphincter is made up of the distal urethral smooth muscle (d.u.s.m.) and the skeletal, striate, external sphincter (s.e.s.).

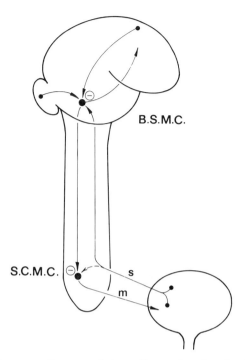

Figure 4–2 Schematic diagram of the reflex arches involved in micturition —motor neuron (m); sensory neuron (s); brain stem micturition center (B.S.M.C.); and sacral cord micturition center (S.C.M.C.).

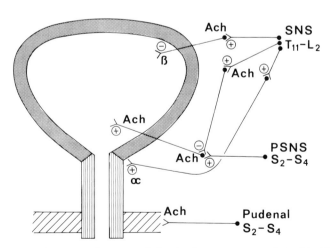

Figure 4–3 Schematic diagram of the dual innervation of the bladder by the sympathetic nervous system (SNS) and the parasympathetic nervous system (PSNS). The neurotransmitters are acetylcholine (Ach) and norepinephrine (alpha, beta). (Inhibitory affect = −, stimulatory effect = +)

Supraspinal areas modulate the detrusor reflex through inputs on the BSMC (Fig. 4–2). The detrusor motor area is located in the prefrontal area. Fibers pass via the internal capsule to synapse at BSMC. Other CNS areas (the thalamus, basal ganglia, cerebellum) have inputs into the BSMC. The overall effect is one of inhibition of the detrusor reflex. Therefore, interruption of these pathways results in loss of voluntary control over the detrusor reflex with resultant sustained uninhibited detrusor contraction.

Sympathetic innervation (see Fig. 4–3) originates in the thoracolumbar spinal cord (T11–L2). The efferent fibers pass via the hypogastric nerve synapse in the inferior mesenteric, hypogastric, and pelvic ganglia. The dome of the bladder is innervated primarily by beta-adrenergic fibers, and the bladder neck is innervated by alpha-adrenergic fibers.

In summary, storage of urine is a sympathetic response with tightening of the bladder neck and relaxation of the dome during adrenergic stimulation. Voiding is under parasympathetic control with contraction of the detrusor and relaxation of the sphincter. An understanding of these neuropharmacologic principles aids in the selection of the appropriate medicines used in the treatment of neurogenic bladder.

The striate (skeletal) external sphincter is under voluntary control. Motor fibers arise in the pudendal motor area in the medial aspect of the central sulcus. Fibers pass through the internal capsule and cortico-

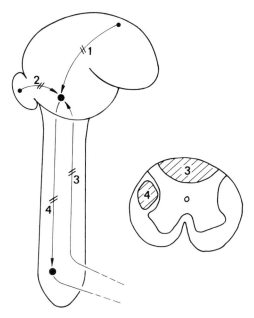

Figure 4–4 The sites of demyelinating plaques frequently seen in MS: CNS (1), cerebellum (2), dorsal columns—sensory (3), lateral columns—motor (4).

spinal tract to synapse on the pudendal motor nucleus in the ventral gray of the sacral cord (S2–4). Motor fibers go by way of the pudendal nerve to the striate external sphincter. Suprasacral interruption of this pathway produces spasticity in the striate external sphincter.

A reciprocal innervation exists between the striate external sphincter and the detrusor muscle. Thus, a detrusor contraction produces reflex relaxation of the striate external sphincter and *vice versa*. To maintain a sustained coordinated detrusor contraction and relaxation of the external sphincter, an intact spinal cord to the level of the BSMC is required. Any lesion below the BSMC can produce a dyscoordination between the bladder and sphincter, or detrusor sphincter dyssynergia. The dyssynergia can be characterized as either intermittent spasm in the striate external sphincter tonic–clonic pattern or a reflex relaxation of the striate external sphincter.

Demyelinating lesions in MS (Fig. 4–4) often involve the bladder pathways (i.e., reticulospinal, corticospinal, and dorsal columns), which accounts for the high incidence of bladder symptoms seen in MS.

Urologic Evaluation

Symptoms that alert the health-care provider and patient that further urologic evaluation is needed fall into several categories (see Urologic Problems and Symptoms in Multiple Sclerosis, below). The poor correlation that exists between bladder symptoms and type of neurogenic bladder mandates a complete urologic and urodynamic assessment.

UROLOGIC PROBLEMS AND SYMPTOMS IN MULTIPLE SCLEROSIS

Irritative Voiding Symptoms
1. Urinary frequency — urinating more often than 6–8 times during the day or awakening at night to urinate (nocturia)
2. Urgency — the sensation of impending need to urinate
3. Urge incontinence — the sensation of the need to urinate associated with the loss of urine

Obstructive Voiding Symptoms
1. Voiding with a weak or intermittent stream
2. Hesitancy — difficulty with initiating voiding
3. Urinary retention — the inability to urinate, requiring a catheter to drain
4. Overflow incontinence — the leakage or urine from a full bladder, often occurring without warning

The urologic–urodynamic evaluation (see below) identifies the specific neurologic dysfunction so that the appropriate treatment program may be instituted.

UROLOGIC–URODYNAMIC EVALUATION

History
Physical examination — neurologic sacral area
Urinalysis
Measurement of residual urine
Cystometrogram (gas or water)
Electromyogram of external sphincter
Other
    Intravenous pyelography
    Cystoscopy
    Voiding cystourethrogram

From September, 1979, to June, 1983, a total of 133 symptomatic MS patients were evaluated urodynamically. Three main patterns emerge (Table 4–1). Normal urodynamic testing was found in 17% of these cases. The majority of the patients had mild irritative symptoms (i.e., frequency/urgency). The significance of the findings is unclear. It may mean that the bladder function was truly normal or that an abnormality could not be detected at that time. The second pattern noted was a flaccid neurogenic or atonic bladder in 14% of the patients.

The third pattern, which accounted for approximately 70% of the cases, was an uninhibited neurogenic bladder. Of patients with this pattern, half had normal coordination between the detrusor and sphincter, while the other half demonstrated detrusor sphincter dyssynergia. Two-thirds of this group had tonic–clonic type of dyssynergia. The other one-third had uninhibited relaxation of the sphincter.

Management

The goals of management of the MS patient with a neurogenic bladder are similar to those of the management of the patient with an injured spinal cord. However, the incidence of renal deterioration and other

Table 4–1. Urodynamic Findings in 133 Patients (Male, 45; Female, 88)

Urodynamic Finding	Percentage of Patients		
Normal	17%		
Flaccid neurogenic bladder	14%		
Uninhibited neurogenic bladder	69%		
Normal sphincter		53%	
Dyssynergia		47%	
Tonic–clonic			2/3
Uninhibited relaxation			1/3

urologic complication in MS appears to be less than in the spinal cord group. The goals of management are

to prevent renal damage
to control urinary infection
to maintain continence
to maintain freedom from catheter use
to maintain social acceptance

A conservative approach is taken because the variable nature of MS precludes the use of irreversible surgical procedures, except in selected cases.

UNINHIBITED NEUROGENIC BLADDER

The uninhibited neurogenic bladder (UNB) is characterized by involuntary detrusor contractions at a lower than normal capacity. However, the involuntary detrusor contractions may occur at normal capacity or above. The symptoms usually encountered are urinary frequency, nocturia, urgency, and urge incontinence. Up to 40% to 50% of this group may also have obstructive symptoms, such as hesitancy, intermittent stream, and elevated residual urines. Obstructive symptoms are often found with detrusor—sphincter dyssynergia.

Urodynamics demonstrate uninhibited detrusor contraction with either a normal coordination between the detrusor and sphincter muscle (Fig. 4 – 5) or dyssynergia (Figs. 4 – 6 and 4 – 7). The upper parts of Figures 4 – 5 to 4 – 7 are electromyographic tracings. For example, in Figure 4 – 5 the first burst of activity is the bulbocavernosus reflex; the smaller bursts on the tracing indicate coughing and voluntary contraction of the urethral sphincter; and the large burst indicates the urge to void. The lower parts of the figures show the pressure in the bladder during bladder filling. Figures 4 – 5, 4 – 6, 4 – 7, and 4 – 9 compare the different types of responses of the bladder with neurogenic involvement.

The patient can apply self-help techniques by establishing a schedule of timed voidings. Usually the bladder should be emptied every 3 to 4 hours, especially in patients who demonstrate uninhibited detrusor contractions at normal or near-normal capacity. The patient must empty the bladder completely, using double or triple voiding, if necessary. The detrusor muscle may be stimulated to contract by applying pressure to the dome of the bladder by pressing over the lower abdomen with a hand or a fist (Credé voiding).

The mainstay of treatment is anticholinergic medicines, such as oxybutynin (Ditropan), propantheline (Pro-Banthine), and atropine (Festalan). These medications exert their action by blocking nerve conduction between the parasympathetic nerve and the detrusor muscle or directly on the bladder smooth muscle. The bladder capacity is increased and

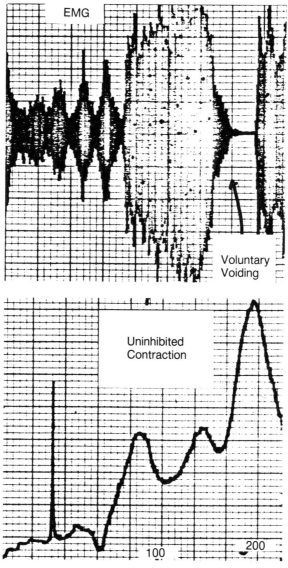

Figure 4-5 Urodynamic testing of a 26-year-old woman who presented with symptoms of urinary frequency, urgency, and rare urge incontinence revealed an uninhibited neurogenic bladder with a normal sphincter. See text for details.

precipitous detrusor contractions are decreased or completely blocked. These drugs treat the symptoms, but they do not alter the basic underlying disease process of demyelination.

Initially a moderate dosage is picked, such oxybutynin (Ditropan), 5 mg 3 times a day, or propantheline (Pro-Banthine), 15 mg 3 times a

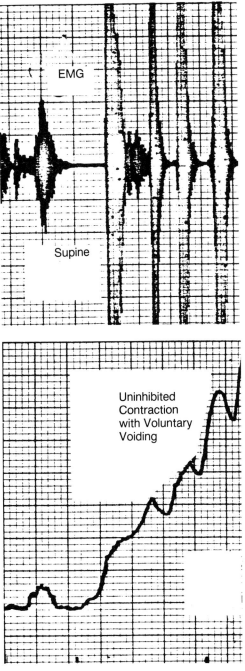

Figure 4–6   Urodynamic testing of a 39-year-old man with symptoms of frequency, urgency, and intermittent stream who has an uninhibited neurogenic bladder with tonic–clonic detrusor–sphincter dyssynergia. See text for details.

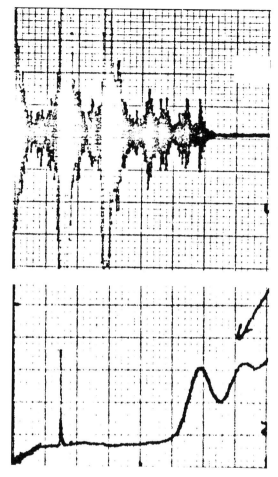

Figure 4-7 Urodynamic testing of a 28-year-old woman with symptoms of urgency and urge incontinence who was found to have an uninhibited neurogenic bladder with uninhibited relaxation of the sphincter muscle. See text for details.

day. The dosage is then titrated up or down until symptoms are improved or intolerable side-effects are encountered. Importantly, the patient may have significant side-effects with one anticholinergic medicine and not another, or may respond better to one than to another. Thus, several types may find use and can be interchanged.

The main side-effects of anticholinergic medicines include dryness of the mouth, constipation, and urinary retention. Blurred vision, blushing, and increased heart rate are encountered occasionally.

The patient with an UNB and normal sphincter (Fig. 4-8) and who has minimal symptoms is untreated (22%). If symptoms are significant,

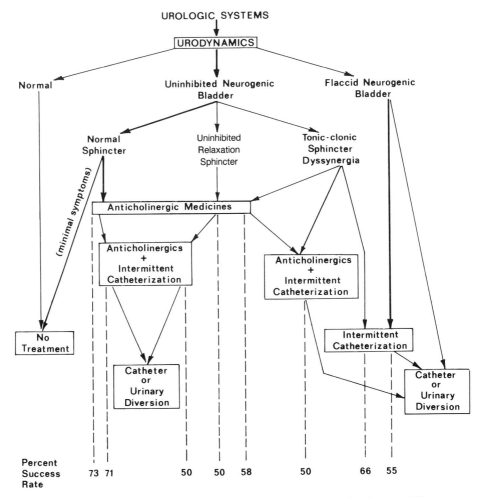

Figure 4–8   Algorithm for the management of MS patients who have voiding symptoms. The success rates are based on patients who have been treated with the above regimens. In all categories, periodic follow-up and reevaluation are mandatory for optimal care.

anticholinergic medicines are employed. A success rate of 70% to 75% can be achieved. Success is defined as complete elimination of symptoms or subjective improvement. However, up to 30% of patients will fail to improve with anticholinergic medicines, most commonly because of elevated residual urines and secondarily because of severe side-effects of the medications.

If the patient develops elevated residual urine, clean intermittent self-catheterization (IC) is initiated, especially if the elevated residual urines are associated with recurrent urinary tract infections. In the group in which anticholinergic medicines fail to provide relief, the combination of anticholinergic medicines and IC is successful in about 70%. Thus, an overall success of 90% can be achieved. Some patients, however, cannot be treated by the above approach and many require an indwelling catheter.

UNB with detrusor–sphincter dyssynergia, characterized by uninhibited relaxation of the sphincter, are treated initially with anticholinergic medicines. The success rate if 50%. IC is added to the failed group, and about 50% of this group can be treated successfully. In 30% of patients all attempts fail, and these patients are treated with an indwelling catheter.

The most difficult problem to manage is UNB with detrusor–sphincter dyssynergia of the tonic–clonic type. Since the condition is commonly associated with elevated residual urines, the initial treatment is either anticholinergic medicines, usually combined with IC, or IC alone. Failures are due to the patients' inability to perform IC or to side-effects of the medicines. Skeletal muscle relaxants (diazepam [Valium], baclofen [Lioresal], dantrolene sodium [Dantrium]) are used to decrease residual urines, but results are discouraging. Sphincterotomy can be used, but only as a last resort, in those cases refractory to medical therapy who have experienced at least 2 years of lower tract dysfunction with unchanging neurologic status.

When elevated residual urines, recurrent urinary infections, or unremitting symptoms persist despite all attempts at treatment, some type of urinary diversion is required.

The Foley catheter has the advantage of being easily maintained by patients who have minimal use of hands. The use of a urethral catheter has no distinct advantage over a suprapubic catheter. However, the presence of recurrent urethritis or epididymitis in the male would favor the use of a suprapubic catheter. With catheter drainage and in the presence of uninhibited detrusor contractions, the patient is maintained with anticholinergic medicines.

Others have recommended supravesicle urinary diversion to preserve renal function and prevent infections. The main disadvantage is the maintenance of an appliance in patients who have little use of their hands.

FLACCID NEUROGENIC BLADDER

The flaccid neurogenic bladder (FNB), or atonic bladder, is characterized by a detrusor muscle that is unable to contract (Fig. 4–9). This pattern can be detected during an acute exacerbation of MS, with significant damage to sensory nerves, or when detrusor–sphincter dyssynergia with elevated residual urine produces bladder muscle decompensation.

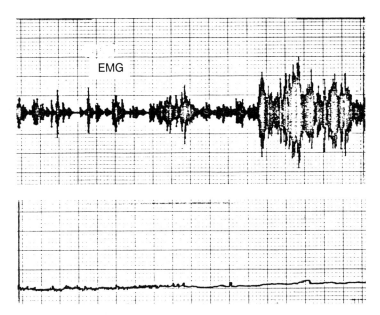

Figure 4-9   Urodynamic testing of a 44-year-old woman with symptoms of frequency, urgency, and urinary incontinence who has a flaccid neurogenic bladder managed successfuly with intermittent catheterization. See text for details.

The symptoms of the FNB are primarily obstructive, that is, infrequent voiding, inability to urinate, and overflow incontinence. However, approximately 50% have irritative symptoms as well. Because the bladder carries a large residual urine, recurrent urinary tract infections are common.

Self-help regimens again include timed voidings every 3 to 4 hours. Since the patient is often unaware of his bladder filling, multiple voidings are needed to ensure emptying. Credé voiding can also be effective.

The mainstay in treating the FNB is clean intermittent self-catheterization (see Fig. 4-8). The catheterizations should be done at 4-hour to 6-hour intervals so that overdistention of the bladder does not occur. During catheterization it is important to empty the bladder completely. Bladder control and prevention of infections can be achieved in 50% to 60% of the cases.

About 50% of patients with IC have bacteriuria. Asymptomatic bacteriuria is not treated, and symptomatic bacteriuria is treated with low-dose antibiotics, such as nitrofurantoin (Macrodantin), 50 mg, or trimethoprim sulfamethoxasole (Bactrim DS) one at bedtime.

Not all patients with MS are capable of performing IC. Many have insufficient manual dexterity to perform self-catheterization. A good rule of thumb to determine if a patient can perform IC is his ability to write his name. If in doubt, a trial of IC is worthwhile.

In those patients who cannot perform IC, an indwelling Foley or suprapubic catheter is employed. Some urologists would prefer supravesicle urinary diversion.

Pharmacologic manipulation of the bladder with cholinergic medicines, such as bethanechol chloride (Urecholine), to stimulate detrusor contraction, or alpha-adrenergic blocking agents, such as phenoxybenzamine hydrochloride (Dibenzyline), to relax the bladder neck, can be tried. However, in my experience and in the experience of others (Blaivas, 1980; Bradley, 1978) these drugs are not helpful.

Summary

The majority of patients with MS and voiding dysfunction can be treated effectively provided a proper urologic evaluation is performed and appropriate treatment is instituted. The variable nature of the disease mandates frequent reevaluation and conservatism in management with avoidance of irreversible surgical procedures.

Suggested Readings

BLAIVAS JG: Management of bladder dysfunction in multiple sclerosis. Neurology 30:12–18, 1980

BLAIVAS JG, BHIMANI G, LABID KB: Vesicouretral dysfunction in multiple sclerosis. J Urol 122:342–347, 1979

BRADLEY WE: Urinary bladder dysfunction in multiple sclerosis. Neurology 28:52–58, 1978

BRADLEY WE, LOGOTHETIS JL, TIM GW: Cystometric and sphincter abnormalities in multiple sclerosis. Neurology 23:1131–1139, 1973

MILLER H, SIMPSON CA, YEATES WK: Bladder dysfunction in multiple sclerosis. Br Med J 1:1265–1269, 1965

PIAZZA DH, DIOKNO AC: Review of neurogenic bladder in multiple sclerosis. Urology 14:33–35, 1979

SCHOENBERG HW, GUTRICH JM: Management of vesical dysfunction in multiple sclerosis. Urology 16:444–447, 1980

SUMMERS JL: Neurogenic bladder in the woman with multiple sclerosis. J Urol 120:535–556, 1978

WEIN AJ, RAEZER DM: Physiology of micturition. In Krane RJ, Siroky MB (eds): Clinical Neuro-Urology, pp 1–33. Boston, Little, Brown & Co, 1979

5

Joel S. Levine

Bowel Dysfunction in Multiple Sclerosis

Bowel dysfunction is a common source of discomfort and disability for the patient with multiple sclerosis (MS). In the late stages of progressive MS, problems with impaction, constipation, and fecal incontinence may be as limiting to the patient's lifestyle as any of the other neurologic sequelae of the disease (Bennett et al, 1977; Bauer, 1978). However, few of the general reviews of MS have directed attention to this problem. In part, this inattention reflects our basic lack of knowledge about how the colon functions in both health and specific disease states. Additionally, many health-care providers are uncomfortable dealing with bowel dysfunction as a clinical problem, and therefore only address the issue when the problem has become intolerable to the patient.

This chapter provides information that allows the physician who is not a gastroenterologist to (1) understand the normal process of defecation and controls of anal continence; (2) understand how MS disrupts the normal bowel habit; (3) systematically approach the differential diagnosis of bowel dysfunction in the MS patient; and (4) implement bowel care programs for the MS patient with few bowel problems and those who have significant neurologic disability.

Physiology of the Large Bowel

In humans, the colon acts as an efficient storage organ, where the semi-liquid effluent from the ileum accumulates and substantial absorption of water and electrolytes occurs. The following brief overview of colonic physiology will focus on the neuromuscular controls of the storage, containment, movement, and defecation of feces, since these are commonly disrupted in the MS patient.

STORAGE

Although all segments of the colon are able to store contents, radiologic studies suggest that feces remain in the right side of the colon for long periods of time. There appears to be a dominant electrical pacemaker in the transverse colon that initiates myoelectrical activity that tends to move feces back toward the cecum. In addition, a number of observations have suggested that passage of stool into the left colon depends on the right colon being distended by a critical volume of stool (Phillips and Devroede, 1979). Nonpropulsive segmenting contractions, occurring throughout the colon, tend to mix the colonic contents and increase absorption of water and electrolytes. Another high-pressure zone and increase in basal electrical rhythm occur at the rectosigmoid area, offering a further barrier to the anal movement of feces. The mechanisms that maintain rectal continence also contribute to storage.

CONTINENCE

Fecal continence is maintained by a variety of mechanisms. Constant tone in the levator muscles and the rectopubalis sling are important factors in forming an angle between the rectum and the anus. This angle prevents the weight of the fecal mass from being transmitted directly to the anal canal. Two sphincters encircle the anal canal. The internal anal sphincter is composed of involuntary smooth muscle, which resists stretching forces and provides a strong barrier. Voluntary control of continence is provided by the muscles of the pelvic floor, the puborectalis muscle, and the external anal sphincter. Rectal distention causes a transient involuntary contraction of these muscles that helps maintain continence during sudden brief increases in rectal pressure. Voluntary contraction of these muscles is the final barrier against involuntary defecation, but can only be maintained for a minute at most.

MOVEMENT

In contrast to the well-characterized storage capabilities of the colon, less is known about the mechanisms by which stool moves into the rectum. The observation that a bowel movement commonly follows the ingestion of a meal has been called the *gastrocolic reflex* (GCR). However, GCR is a misnomer because these events can be initiated by a meal entering the proximal small intestine. Humoral as well as neural mediators are involved. Nevertheless, the timing of a meal and the subsequent bowel movement have therapeutic importance, requiring further discussion of the response. The GCR is initiated by large meals that have a high fat content. Within a short period of time the ileocecal valve, which is tonically contracted, relaxes, and ileal contents move into the right colon. This distention initiates passage of stool out of the right colon into the transverse colon. Coincident with these events, a mass peristaltic movement of colonic contents begins in the transverse colon. In contrast to the segmenting contractions that mix colonic contents, three or more segments contract simultaneously, and the fecal mass is then moved toward the rectum. This highly coordinated sequence of events is easily disrupted by diet, emotions, and drugs (Christianson, 1981).

DEFECATION

The conscious appreciation of the need to move one's bowels is elicited when a threshold volume of stool reaches the rectum. The fine sensory discrimination of the nerve endings in the anal canal is attested to by the internal sphincter's ability to distinguish between solid, liquid, and gaseous material. During voluntary defecation intra-abdominal pressure increases, leading to a decrease in the anorectal angle that is so important in maintaining continence. Hip flexion, as that which occurs when the individual is in a squatting position, further straightens the anorectal angle. When this angle has been straightened, the bolus of stool moves further into the rectum, initiating a reflex inhibition of the resting tone of the internal anal sphincter. At this point the individual gives voluntary consent to the act, eliminating those voluntary muscular impediments to defecation. This process of normal defecation requires an intact lumbosacral cord.

Pathophysiology of the Colon in Multiple Sclerosis

Only recently has any attempt been made to directly measure parameters of colonic function in patients with MS. In 1982, Glick and co-workers measured somatosensory evoked responses, volume–pressure curves of the colon (the colonometrogram), and colonic motor and myoelectric activity in a small group of patients with far-advanced MS. All of the patients had symptoms of bladder and bowel dysfunction. These authors demonstrated that the inability to sense the presence of stool in the rectal ampulla is most likely secondary to a lesion central to the lumbosacral portion of the spinal cord.

The colon in these patients was "hyperreflexic" or showed an inappropriately rapid and pronounced rise in intraluminal pressure with the instillation of water into the large bowel. This type of volume–pressure curve has been ascribed to lesions of the motor tract in the brain or descending spinal tracts. These findings are much the same as those demonstrated by cystometrograms in bladders of MS patients. Finally, the normal increase in colonic motor and myoelectric activity that occurs after eating was not present. This abnormal gastrocolic reflex may be a contributing factor to the constipation experienced by these patients. The study by Glick and co-workers provides insights into the causal relationship between CNS lesions in advanced MS and the observed bowel complaints. These observations should be extended to a group of MS patients who are more representative with respect to disability, immobility, diet, and emotional status.

Other abnormalities can contribute to bowel dysfunction in MS patients, such as

Diminished anorectal sensation
Loss of the gastrocolic reflex
Weakness of the abdominal wall muscles
Spasticity of the pelvic muscles
Immobility
Exogenous depression
Medications

For example, any associated weakness of the abdominal musculature will dimish the ability to increase intra-abdominal pressure and to defecate. If the muscles of the pelvic floor are spastic and unable to relax, defecation is further impeded. As the associated neurologic abnormalities worsen, the patient with MS is more likely to become bedfast and immobile. As a result, two factors lead to constipation. First, because physical activity *per se* is an important factor in establishing a normal bowel habit, the transit time of stool through the colon is delayed. Second, the patient may not get to a bathroom quickly enough when the urge to defecate is appreciated, and as a result, defecation is voluntarily suppressed and the fecal mass dries out, leading to further constipation. Rectal incontinence may occur if voluntary muscular function is diminished.

Increasing neurologic disability is commonly accompanied by an exogenous depression that can initiate or worsen a state of constipation. Finally, most of the drugs that are being used to diminish muscle spasticity (propantheline bromide, oxybutynin chloride, flavoxate hydrochloride) have the potential to worsen constipation.

Diagnosis of Bowel Dysfunction

Bowel dysfunction may be quite easy to diagnose when the patient with MS spontaneously complains of incontinence, impactions, or obstipation. The diagnosis is more difficult in the earlier stages of the disease. A number of population studies have attempted to define the "normal" bowel habit as ± 3 standard deviations from the mean of the population interviewed. In most Western countries, "normal" bowel habit is less than 3 bowel movements per day and more than one every three days (Connell et al, 1965). These broad ranges are used to reduce overcompulsive attitudes about bowel habits, which create problems where none really exist. However, a growing body of epidemiologic data suggests that bowel habits in industrialized areas of the world, where refined, low-fiber diets and laxatives are commonly used in conjunction, do not represent an optimal state of health (Gooding, 1980). For the purpose of discussion, a healthy bowel habit is defined as a once-a-day defecation of a soft stool associated with complete rectal evacuation.

Ideally, the health-care provider's concern about the MS patient's bowel function will antedate the onset of severe symptoms, so that therapeutic interventions are more likely to be efficacious. The patient's affirmative answer to the question "Are your bowels working normally?" provides little assurance that "normal" means "healthful." A structured interview about the patient's bowel function, diet, physical activity, and associated neurologic symptoms is necessary. A series of directed questions that will help in the diagnosis, differential diagnosis, etiology, and therapy of bowel dysfunction in the MS patient is given below

Is Bowel Dysfunction Present?
1. How often do you move your bowels?
2. Is your bowel movement hard or pebbly?
3. Do you ever feel that you don't completely empty your rectum?
4. Have you ever soiled yourself?
5. Do you take laxatives, enemas, or other preparations for your bowel?

What is the Etiology of the Bowel Dysfunction?
1. Does your bowel problem antedate the onset of your multiple sclerosis?
2. What medicines do you take? Any recent changes in medication?
3. Does your daily schedule or a physical impairment make it difficult getting to a bathroom when you have the urge to defecate?
4. Can you tell when you need to move your bowels?
5. Describe a typical day's diet.
6. Any blood in your bowel movement?

Similarly, the physical examination can be made more helpful by specifically evaluating for (1) signs of hypothyroidism (bradycardia, hoarseness, delayed deep tendon reflexes), (2) palpable feces in the colon on abdominal examination, (3) hemorrhoids or fissures by carefully spreading apart the anal canal (4) anal sphincter tone by asking the patient to act as if he is preventing a bowel movement while the examiner performs the rectal examination, and (5) occult blood in the stool using guaiac-impregnated paper (Hemoccult).

Differential Diagnosis of Bowel Dysfunction in the Multiple Sclerosis Patient

DIARRHEA

Diarrhea is an uncommon problem in the patient with MS unless a second disease process (e.g., gastroenteritis, giardiasis, inflammatory bowel disease) is superimposed. However, diarrhea may occur secondary to a fecal impaction. If the patient's constipation has not been treated properly, the onset of loose stools should initiate a careful search for an impaction by rectal digital examination and sigmoidoscopy, followed by appropriate therapy (see below). If an impaction is not found, stools for culture or ova and parasites are indicated.

CONSTIPATION

The presence of constipation with abdominal cramps that antedates the onset of MS suggests irritable bowel syndrome, which is very common in the general population. Evaluation and therapy, however, are identical to those used for MS bowel dysfunction.

The onset of constipation is the most frequently encountered new bowel dysfunction in the MS patient. Even though the most common cause of bowel dysfunction is likely to be the MS itself, certain diagnostic tests are worthwhile to look for treatable disorders. These disorders are listed below:

1. Diarrhea
   a. Fecal impaction
   b. Otherwise same evaluation as in non-MS patient
2. Constipation
   a. Drugs
      (1) Narcotics
      (2) Anticholinergics
      (3) Antidepressants
   b. Metabolic
      (1) Hypothyroidism
      (2) Hyperparathyroidism
      (3) Hypokalemia
   c. Perirectal disease
      (1) Hemorrhoids
      (2) Anal fissures
   d. Structural obstruction of the colon
      (1) Cancer
      (2) Stricture (ischemic)

A careful history and physical examination may indicate a specific diagnosis. Tests for serum potassium, serum calcium, and thyroid function should be done. If perirectal examination reveals hemorrhoids or fissures, these can be treated (see below). These simple steps should be considered each time the MS patient with constipation comes to medical attention.

A difficult question arises as to when to test for a structural lesion of the colon. The recommended tests, a sigmoidoscopy and air-contrast barium enema, can be uncomfortable and expensive. My approach has been to do a sigmoidoscopy in all patients when constipation is diagnosed for the first time, and to reserve further evaluation of the colon to (1) patients above the age of 40 years, (2) patients with positive tests for occult blood in the stool or with iron-deficiency anemia, and (3) patients who do not respond to an initial therapeutic trial.

Patients with MS are living longer with progressively worsening disease and persistent bowel problems. After the age of 40 years, the incidence of colon cancer begins to increase rapidly with each succeeding decade of life. Because the signs of cancer, such as change in bowel habits, may be blunted by MS, some reasonable screening program will aid in making decisions regarding retesting of these patients. Following the American Cancer Society guidelines for the general population, yearly screening of evacuated stools for occult blood beginning at age 40 and sigmoidoscopy at age 50 and every 5 years thereafter should suffice. Obviously, acute worsening or new symptoms should initiate a more aggressive diagnostic evaluation that may include colonoscopy (e.g., if bright red blood per rectum ensues).

Therapy of Bowel Dysfunction in the Multiple Sclerosis Patient

The management of constipation during the lifetime of a MS patient is not easily packaged into simple solutions that will apply equally when the patient first presents and when he is severely disabled. MS patients can be separated into three groups (asymptomatic, mild constipation, and severe constipation), which generally represent the spectrum of bowel dysfunction. For every patient, clearly defined goals are established at the onset of treatment.

THE MULTIPLE SCLEROSIS PATIENT WITH NORMAL BOWEL FUNCTION

The potential for the greatest long-term benefit from therapy exists in the patient with MS who still has relatively normal bowel habits. A short educational intervention can be made that may prevent or delay the onset of bowel dysfunction. The goals are to have the patient understand the long-term importance of a "healthy" bowel habit of 1 to 2 soft, easily evacuated stools per day, and to understand the relationship between diet and bowel function. Specifically, the patient must comprehend the importance of an adequate intake of fiber in preventing constipation. Specific recommendations about daily fiber intake should be to

1. Eat 1 bowl of a bran cereal plus 4 slices of a bran-containing bread (not simply whole wheat), or
2. Use the equivalent of 3 tablespoons of miller's bran in ordinary cereal or home-baked bread

Fibrous foods such as fruits and vegetables, which should be used in addition to the whole bran, are not adequate replacements alone. In addition, patients should be encouraged to maintain an adequate intake of fluids (8 glasses of water per day) to ensure that the fecal mass does not dry out. The patient should understand that a natural consequence of a diet high in fiber is an increase in abdominal bloating and flatulence. The patient can be reassured, however, that these symptoms should resolve within the course of several weeks.

THE MULTIPLE SCLEROSIS PATIENT WITH MILD CONSTIPATION

This category includes patients who have evidence of bowel dysfunction, but who have not resorted to laxatives or enemas over a protracted period, have not had a fecal impaction, and have not developed fecal incontinence. The goal of therapy for this group is to restore and maintain a normal bowel habit. Alternative causes of constipation should be excluded or treated. When possible, constipating drugs should be discontinued or their dosage reduced. Hemorrhoids or fissures can be treated with topical hydrocortisone cream, Sitz baths, and increased dietary fiber to soften the stools. Dietary instruction is provided that is identical to that given the asymptomatic patient. In addition, at this time it is appropriate to educate the patient concerning the following:

1. Laxatives and enemas. In a society where innumerable approaches to a daily bowel movement are advertised on television, and over $200,000,000 is spent annually on laxatives sold over the counter, reeducation is necessary. Patients should understand that the role, if any, of laxatives in the management of their bowel dysfunction will be for a short course prescribed by their health-care provider. Avoiding the chronic use of laxatives and enemas should be stressed because they impair the ability of the patient to have normal bowel movements. The bulk-forming agents that can be prescribed to supplement or replace bran in the diet should be differentiated from the osmotic, secretory, and stimulant laxatives (e.g., bisacodyl, cascara,

magnesium salts). The judicious use of laxatives as well as enemas may be necessary in the severely constipated patient.

2. Emotional state. Patients should be aware that their state of mind can affect their bowel habit. I have seen patients who have become depressed because of their disease develop constipation secondary to the depression, take the constipation as a sign of worsening MS, become more depressed, and so forth. The health-care provider, by being aware that constipation may be a sign of endogenous depression, will attend to the primary problem, the depression, rather than just treating the symptom.

3. The importance of taking enough time for the daily bowel movement. Both patients and health professionals often ignore this simple admonition. Commonly, patients will try to maintain a normal lifestyle despite progressively worsening disability and will suppress the urge to defecate to attend to other matters. These patients should be encouraged to set aside 20 to 30 minutes each morning, usually after their morning coffee or breakfast (to use the gastrocolic reflex to greatest advantage), when they can have their bowel movement without interruption. The patient may need to arise earlier in the morning to accomplish this activity.

If dietary manipulations to increase the amount of ingested fiber do not alleviate the constipation, the patient is not ingesting enough fiber. For many patients, this intolerance to fiber is secondary to the associated bloating and flatulence that can occur. Others cannot ingest the required amount of bran products. A careful history should be able to separate the former from the latter. If a high-fiber diet cannot be tolerated, an attempt should be made to prescribe bulk in the form of psyllium hydrophilic muciloid, calcium polycarbophil, psyllium, and senna, or any of the other available fiber compounds. In general, the quantity of these compounds needed to provide a daily, soft stool will be greater than noted on the package insert. For instance, patients commonly require 4 to 6 tablespoons of psyllium per day to normalize bowel movements. Patients should be told that (1) they cannot be hurt by taking additional fiber; (2) each person's fiber needs are different; and (3) the quantity and quality of their bowel movements are directly related to the amount of fiber ingested. Patients are then instructed to begin at a low dose and increase the amount of bulk ingested each week until normal bowel movements ensue. Diarrhea or too frequent stooling is an indication to reduce fiber intake. Close telephone contact with the patient will be needed during this time.

THE MULTIPLE SCLEROSIS PATIENT WITH SEVERE BOWEL DYSFUNCTION

A patient may be considered to have severe bowel dysfunction if he has (1) severe constipation that requires laxatives or enemas to initiate a movement; (2) presents with a fecal impaction; or (3) develops fecal incontinence. Although these events may overlap, they will be discussed separately.

Severe Constipation

Frequently, patients with severe constipation present to the health-care provider dependent on laxatives or enemas for a daily bowel movement. They usually have not had medical supervision for the problem nor have they had the dietary and other instructional material presented above. When the constipation has proceeded to this point, the goal remains to restore a normal bowel habit without drugs. However, the combination of the MS and chronic laxative use may compromise this expectation.

The initial evaluation should exclude an impaction or other reversible cause of constipation. This evaluation should be thorough to avoid repeated evaluations each time the same complaint arises. Consultation with a gastroenterologist may be advisable at this stage. Once other processes are excluded, full attention can be directed at "retraining" the patient to have normal bowel movements without the aid of pharmaceutic agents.

Our approach to this difficult therapeutic problem is presented in outline form below (see Retraining Bowel Habits in the Severely Disabled MS Patient).

RETRAINING BOWEL HABITS IN THE SEVERELY DISABLED MS PATIENT

1. Optimize the mechanics of defecation.
   a. Decrease the anal—rectal angle.
      (1) Avoid the use of bedpans.
      (2) Try to maximize hip flexion during defecation.
          With standard toilet or bedside commode, have the patient raise his feet on a step stool
   b. Attempt a trial of digital stimulation of the anal canal to initiate bowel movement in patients with pelvic and perineal spasm.
   c. Have the patient gently massage his abdomen to increase intra-abdominal pressure during defecation.
   d. Ensure that help is available to get the patient to the bathroom when needed.
2. Discontinue all laxatives and enemas.
3. Institute a high-fiber diet with or without a bulk agent.
4. Have the patient sit on the toilet for 30 minutes each morning after breakfast, in spite of a lack of urge to defecate.
5. Administer tap water enema to avoid impaction if there is no bowel movement by the second day.
6. Repeat steps 4 and 5 until bowel habits normalize.

The majority of patients who have this degree of bowel dysfunction also have considerable disability from their MS in other systems such as motor or bladder. As a result, our initial concern is to ensure that the patient can get to the bathroom and that the mechanical factors known to improve defecation are optimized. For example, a decreased angle between the rectum and the anus when the hips are maximally flexed, as when squatting, helps initiate defecation. Thus, bedpans promote improper defecation, and yet for convenience or the lack of skilled help the bed-ridden patient may be forced to use a bedpan. If movement to a bathroom is impossible, a bedside commode is much preferable to the bedpan. Even then, the commode or the toilet in most homes is too high off the ground for optimal defecation. Ideally, a seat should be no more than 12 to 15 inches from the floor. If a low-rise fixture is not feasible because of the motor limitations of the MS patient, the patient should be instructed to place his feet on a footstool 12 to 15 inches high when trying to defecate.

When patients have obvious spasm of the pelvic and rectal muscles, a trial of digital stimulation of the anus during defecation may initiate a bowel movement. All patients should be instructed to gently massage the abdomen while trying to defecate to increase intra-abdominal pressure. Additionally, adequate help from within or outside of the family group should be provided, so that the patient can be brought to the toilet before the urge to defecate is suppressed or incontinence ensues. Careful planning with an occupational therapist may be required to modify the home environment.

Once the mechanics for adequate defecation have been addressed, laxatives and enemas are stopped. High-fiber diet with or without bulk agents is initiated, and the patient is instructed to set aside 30 minutes each morning after breakfast to sit on the toilet. Since a common cause of constipation in MS is the inability to sense the presence of stool in the rectal ampulla, time should be spent on the toilet in spite of a lack of the urge to defecate. If a bowel movement has not occurred by the second day, a gentle tap water enema should be administered to reduce the risk of an impaction. This daily regimen is repeated until spontaneous defecation has ensued or until it has become obvious that the regimen has failed. If, even with high-fiber and water intake, the stools appear dry and hard, the use of milk of magnesia (30 ml at bedtime) to osmotically draw water into the stool should be tried.

Stimulants or secretory laxatives are unlikely to be needed. Increasing doses and numbers of laxatives in an attempt to initiate a bowel movement is discouraged. In the majority of patients treated as outlined, some normalization of bowel habits is likely. In some patients a dependence on laxatives or enemas will persist, but the use of these agents should be limited and controlled by a health professional and not by the patient. Drug therapy of constipation is not innocuous. Laxatives can lead to fecal incontinence, hypokalemia, idiosyncratic drug reactions, and acidosis. In contrast, carefully and judiciously administered enemas rarely cause injury (Godding, 1980).

Fecal Impaction

Fecal impaction is a troublesome, recurrent complication that can occur in any patient with chronic constipation. In the MS patient, the inability to sense the presence of stool in the rectum may increase the likelihood of impaction. Essentially all fecal impactions occur in the rectal vault. Thus, the condition should be readily apparent during digital examination of the rectum. Since the symptoms of impaction can be quite subtle prior to the onset of obstipation (abdominal distention, rectal fullness), the importance of the rectal examination as a routine part of the office visit becomes apparent. Uncommonly, impaction will present as diarrhea, an intestinal obstruction, or a pressure ulcer of the bowel wall.

An impaction requires immediate therapy. Unless true obstruction is present, attempts should be made to lubricate the fecal mass by giving mineral oil orally (30 ml per hour while awake) (Klein, 1982), or as a retention enema (150 ml twice daily) for two days. Oral mineral oil should never be used in patients with swallowing abnormalities or fluctuating levels of consciousness because aspirated mineral oil causes a severe lipoid pneumonia. If the impaction has not broken up and passed, then bisacodyl (Dulcolax) can be given to stimulate propulsive movements in the colon. Manual disimpaction can be quite painful, requires pretreatment with a narcotic analgesic, and should only be employed as a last resort. Once the acute impaction is resolved, the patient is begun on the regimen for severe constipation noted above.

Fecal Incontinence

The most common cause for fecal soiling in patients with MS is the presence of an impaction in the rectal vault. The large fecal mass presses down on the internal sphincter, intiating a relaxation response, and continence cannot be maintained by the voluntary anal and pelvic musculature, which is so commonly weakened in MS. Thus, careful examination for a fecal impaction is the initial approach to the complaint of diarrhea or incontinence. Avoidance of an impaction by careful bowel retraining or the use of enemas should be attempted.

In a few patients who lose all continence mechanisms, incontinence without an impaction or an organic diarrheal illness may occur. In the past, little has been available for these patients other than trying to constipate the stool by using a low-fiber diet and providing scrupulous nursing care to avoid perianal tissue breakdown. Recently, biofeedback has been used to improve continence by sensitizing patients to the presence of stool in their rectum and strengthening anal sphincter tone (Cerulli et al, 1979). The value of biofeedback in the patient with MS has not been ascertained at present.

Summary

As a consequence of the damage to the CNS, many patients with progressively disabling MS develop bowel dysfunction. Usually this is characterized by constipation, caused by decreased peristaltic movements in the colon after a meal as well as by the inability to sense stool in the rectum. This chapter emphasizes the importance of carefully questioning the patient about bowel function so that therapy can be initiated early in the course of the disease. The foundation of our therapeutic regimen is a high-fiber diet and the manipulation of the patient's environment to optimize the chances of having a spontaneous bowel movement without the use of laxatives. More direct investigations of bowel dysfunction in a large heterogeneous group of patients with MS should ultimately lead to improvement in our management decisions in the future.

Suggested Readings

AMERICAN CANCER SOCIETY: Recommendations for screening for colo-rectal cancer. Cancer 30:208–215, 1980

BAUER HJ: Problems of symptomatic therapy in multiple sclerosis. Neurology 28:8–20, 1978

BENNETT L, HAMILTON H, NEUTEL CI, et al: Survey of persons with multiple sclerosis in Ottawa, 1974–1975. Can J Pub Health 68:141–147, 1977

CERULLI MA, NIKOOMANESH P, SCHUSTER MM: Progress in biofeedback conditioning for fecal incontinence. Gastroenterology 76:742–746, 1979

CHRISTIANSON J: Motility of the colon. In Johnson LR (ed): Physiology of the Gastrointestinal Tract, pp 445–470. New York, Raven Press, 1981

CONNELL AM, HILTON C, IRVING G, et al: Variation of bowel habits in two population samples. Br Med J 2:1095–1098, 1965

GLICK ME, MESHKINPOOR H, HALDEMAN S, et al: Colonic dysfunction in multiple sclerosis. Gastroenterology 83:1002–1007, 1982

GODDING EW: Physiological yardsticks for bowel function and the rehabilitation of the constipated bowel. Pharmacology 20(Supp 1):88–103, 1980

KLEIN H: Constipation and fecal impaction. Med Clin North Am 66:1135–1141, 1982

PHILLIPS SF, DEVROEDE GJ: Functions of the large intestine. In Crane Rk (ed): International Review of Physiology: Gastrointestinal Physiology III, Vol 19, pp. 264–290. Baltimore, University Park Press, 1979

Rehabilitation of the Patient With Multiple Sclerosis

Rehabilitation can be highly successful for people with multiple sclerosis (MS) if there is a team effort, a motivated patient, and attainable goals. A team approach provides added emotional support, with results often surpassing any expected from treatment provided by therapists working independently.

Although the clinical impressions of physicians and other therapists who frequently treat MS support such an optimistic view, careful and rigorous documentation of effective strategies is lacking because of the multiple variables that influence outcomes. A reliance on clinical impressions in the design of programs has many pitfalls. Alternatively, randomized clinical trials using carefully chosen outcome measures are infrequent because they require meticulous planning. Most existing therapeutic strategies are difficult to evaluate because they have included MS patients with a variety of symptoms, varying clinical courses, and a mixture of treatment methods. Additionally, placebo effects of treatment, predetermined expectations, and poor patient selection have blurred conclusions.

These factors are mentioned not as a deterrent to the design of individualized therapeutic programs but to emphasize the care that should be taken in interpreting conclusions of published data. A rationale for individualized treatment requires that attention be given to three general factors that establish a therapeutic framework: (1) an understanding of the varying clinical spectra and courses in MS; (2) an assessment of functional levels; and (3) a reasoned selection of short-term goals.

Clinical Course in Multiple Sclerosis

TYPES OF MULTIPLE SCLEROSIS

The course of MS can be divided somewhat arbitrarily into four clinical types: (1) benign; (2) relapsing/remitting/nonprogressive (RRN); (3) relapsing/remitting/progressive (RRP); and (4) progressive (Fig. 6–1).

A person with benign MS frequently experiences one or two acute episodes of neurologic dysfunction with little or no residual impairment. Occasionally, a patient classified as benign may experience worsening of his condition several years later, so that "typing" of patients is always tentative when established prospectively. However, with each year that the patient remains symptom-free, the chance of his disease remaining as a "benign form" of MS increases. Relapsing/remitting MS can be further separated into two clinical courses: following an exacerbation a person may return to his prior level of neurologic function (RRN), or he may retain increased neurologic deficits (RRP). Following a remission, patients with RRP may be stable between episodes or progress (see different slopes between exacerbations in Fig. 6–1). Progressive MS rapidly or slowly progresses without remitting after an insidious onset. The slowly progressive form usually begins after the age of 35 years and may remain relatively unchanged for years. The rapid form has a grave prognosis, although, fortunately, this form is rare.

RATE AND FREQUENCY OF CHANGE IN NEUROLOGIC DEFICIT

The rate of progression varies within each clinical type of MS. The frequently imagined image of a rapidly progressive course is incorrect for the majority of MS patients because many MS patients stabilize indefinitely or only progress slowly. Some improvement is to be expected following most exacerbations or interventions, or even with chronic progressive MS. The slopes of the MS courses shown for RRP and progressive forms of MS in Figure 6–1 depict *potential* courses. Stable periods with no deterioration are commonly seen, so that 100% disability is never reached.

The frequency of relapses varies from none or few (benign form) to several within a year. Patients with an increasing frequency of relapses have a higher risk of converting to progressive MS and deteriorating neurologically. Conversely, a decreasing frequency of relapses may herald more stable neurologic impairment, (i.e., "burning out" of an active disease process).

The neurologic examination may be normal in benign or RRN MS during remission. Improvement in signs occurs with remissions of RRP MS and occasionally in progressive MS. Gains from therapy cannot be distinguished readily from spontaneous neurologic improvement. How-

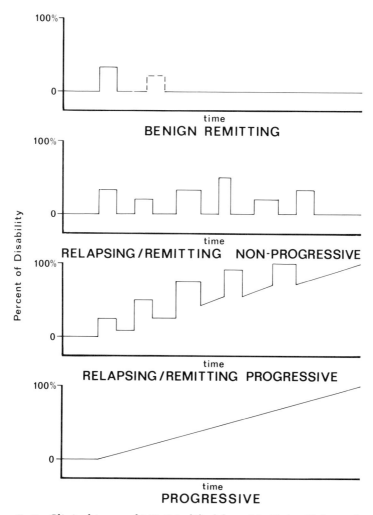

Figure 6-1 Clinical types of MS. (Modified from McAlpine D, Lumsden CE, and Acheson ED: Multiple Sclerosis—A Reappraisal, 2nd ed. Edinburgh, Longman Group Ltd, 1973)

ever, some improvement in function is more clearly attributable to therapy. Improved gait, coordination, speech, and activities of daily living are expected with intervention regardless of neurologic deficits noted on examination (Fig. 6-2).

PROGNOSTIC INDICATORS

Several factors, although clearly unreliable when applied to an individual patient, have been reported as prognostic indicators for MS:

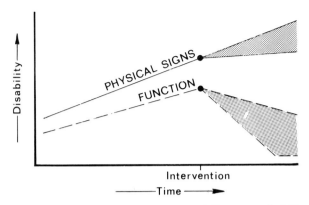

Figure 6-2 Idealized depiction of outcomes following rehabilitation intervention. Although disability may stabilize or worsen with respect to physical signs, improved function is expected.

Onset with a single symptom or absence of motor symptoms has a better prognosis.

The patient's disability status at 5 years can be a useful predictor. Functional status before 5 years is a poor predictor.

Minimal or absent cerebellar and pyramidal signs at 5 years carries a more favorable prognosis.

Cerebellar, pyramidal, and multiple neurologic functions/signs usually have a poorer prognosis.

Functional Assessment

A myriad of disability, mobility, and functional scales have been developed that primarily describe locomotor abilities. Progression in all of these scales is similar, beginning with independent ambulation and followed by ambulatory aids, then a wheelchair, and finally complete helplessness. The functional level established with these scales in combination with the rate of progression has valuable prognostic implications. Since the best indicator for the future in individual patients with MS is past performance, predictions are difficult early in a patient's course. Patient status 4 or 5 years after onset of symptoms is a more useful predictor. For example, a person whose rate of progression requires that he use a wheelchair 4 years after the onset of neurologic symptoms has a worse prognosis than the diagnosed MS patient who is still ambulating with crutches 10 years later.

Following is a list of functional locomotor events (functional mobility levels) that permits evaluation of the need for intervention:

1. No restrictions; minimal signs
2. Definite impairment, but fully ambulatory without aids

3. Limited ability (distance) without aids; able to climb stairs
4. Needs cane or brace; stair-climbing equivocal
5. Requires crutches or walker
6. Uses wheelchair but may use crutches or walker in the home
7. Wheelchair independence
8. Wheelchair independence but cannot transfer
9. Requires motorized chair (or could manage motorized chair)
10. Wheelchair dependent — specialized chairs; cannot manage motorized chair
11. Bed-ridden but still has arm and hand functions
12. Bed-ridden, helpless

This scale can be used not only to show the progression of MS but also to identify milestones where treatment may be beneficial.

Scales are points of interruption along a disability continuum. However, scales provide no reasons for the level of ability, the quality of performance, or how nearly a patient approaches the loss or gain of a level of function. Therefore, as each level is approached, a patient should be assessed to establish whether or not the clinical reasons for the imminent change warrant intervention to maintain a higher level (see Chaps. 7 and 8 for specific evaluations).

Framework and Guidelines for Intervention

A framework for program design can be established by first considering an optimal situation for a patient whose MS is diagnosed early and who remains in contact with the MS team throughout his illness. Although ideal programming for each patient is rarely achieved, the program should include an evaluation early in the patient's disease process and reevaluation at specified intervals. If subsequent evaluations show further impairment, the patient should be treated aggressively to return him to as near his prior neurologic level as possible. A person with stable impairment should still be placed on a maintenance exercise program to prevent deterioration caused by inactivity. Intervention is indicated following any exacerbation as well as at points along the functional scale when a change to a lower level is imminent. If progression significantly reduces the patient's function, new adaptive skills must be taught using appropriate adaptive equipment, including mobility aids and vocational training.

Intervention goals should be designed according to the following desired outcomes:

1. Improvement in the presenting neurologic signs of MS. This category includes lessening of paresis, ataxia, or other neurologic signs. For example, improvement in spasticity during remissions or baclofen treatment may permit therapy to become effective in further inhibi-

tion of spasticity or can enhance measures to improve strength and balance.

2. Improvement in neurologic *function*. The physical disability may persist but new skill or function is gained through training. For example, dysmetria of upper extremities may be lessened with wrist weights but further improvement in hand function can be obtained with training.

3. Compensatory training
   a. Learning new and unaccustomed skills has special importance in vocational retraining when functional progression warrants job reclassification. The attainment of independent wheelchair transfers or the learning of one-handed activities for hemiplegia are other examples.
   b. Equipment. Mobility aids (cane, brace, wheelchair) and devices that facilitate activities of daily living can significantly improve function. For example, a person with footdrop and impaired balance may be prevented from frequent falls by an ankle–foot orthosis and cane (Chap. 7). Adaptive equipment (Chap. 8) may allow independence in household activities such as cleaning and cooking.

4. Retardation of progression. Modification of a program to maximize neurologic function can be especially helpful for patients whose disease is worsening. This category includes short-term work for persons progressing to a lower functional level (see list of functional mobility levels, above). For example, a person who is wheelchair independent may have this independence threatened by increased fatiguability and may require transfer assistance, which may improve with short-term therapy (Chaps. 7 and 8). Self-catheterization and bowel programs can maintain independence in spite of worsening neurologic function (Chaps. 4, 5, and 10).

Several goals can be addressed simultaneously with emphasis changed to reflect a patient's current clinical picture. Following an exacerbation, the initial emphasis is given toward improving neurologic features. After a fair trial of treatment, other guidelines take precedence if impairment persists.

Intervention Strategies

1. Every person with MS should receive a baseline functional assessment by a physical and occupational therapist and by a speech/language pathologist. The range of possible benefit will vary from simple suggestions to aggressive programming dependent on the patient's level of disability.

2. Patients with stable neurologic impairment benefit from a home maintenance exercise program with periodic reviews to prevent deterioration and a continued sense of well-being. Group exercise programs, including adaptive swimming programs, are helpful both physically and psychologically.

3. During relapse, all patients are treated with the aim of restoring prerelapse neurologic function. Treatment should continue until that level is reached or until 2 to 3 weeks of stable but lesser function is attained.

4. Patients should be reevaluated if a change to a lower functional level appears imminent. Each patient must be initially assessed for the constellation of findings responsible for his particular alteration of function.

5. Patients with progression to a lower functional level need a sensitive therapist to help them adjust to increasing disability.

6. Often, an initial evaluation is best performed in the hospital so that extended observation can be performed and response to therapy adequately assessed. In patients who have progressive MS, but who have never received rehabilitative treatment, initial consideration should include realistic short-term goals based on an assumption that disuse atrophy, low motivation, and a skill level lower than their potential function all exist. A decision whether or not to initiate ongoing therapy can usually be determined within one week after inpatient or intensive outpatient observation.

Psychological Factors in Planning Rehabilitation

A reasonable estimate can be made of the maximal functional outcome for a patient if physical potential is considered separately. A separate psychological evaluation may identify additional factors that prevent effective physical rehabilitation. By modifying common psychological obstacles, the attainment of more optimal physical performance is possible. For example, antidepressant medications or the successful achievement of a first step in a staged rehabilitation program may sufficiently improve a depressed MS patient so that he can participate in remaining steps designed toward an optimal outcome (Chaps. 11 and 20).

Summary

The variation in clinical course, functional status, prior treatment, and patient motivation make the design of rehabilitation programs for patients with multiple sclerosis complex. In spite of permanent neurologic deficits, function can be improved in patients with MS. Although rehabilitation programs must be highly individualized, there are useful general principles that facilitate the design of effective treatment strategies.

Suggested Readings

KRAFT GH, FREAL JE, CORYELL JK, et al: Multiple sclerosis: Early prognostic guidelines. Arch Phys Med Rehabil 62:54–58, 1981

KURTZKE JF: Clinical manifestations of multiple sclerosis. In Vinken PJ, Gruyn GW (eds): Handbook of Clinical Neurology, Vol 9, pp 161–216. New York, American Elsevier, 1970

McALPINE C: Clinical studies. In McAlpine D, Lumsden CE, Acheson ED (eds): Multiple Sclerosis: A Reappraisal, pp 59–238. Edinburgh E & S Livingstone, 1965, 1972

SCHNEITZER L: Rehabilitation of patients with multiple sclerosis. Arch Phys Med Rehabil 59:430–437, 1978

Surinder Pal Brar
Carolyn Wangaard

7

Physical Therapy for Patients With Multiple Sclerosis

Multiple sclerosis (MS) patients provide physical therapists with one of their most challenging professional experiences. Almost all MS patients, regardless of their physical status, can benefit from a physical therapy evaluation and treatment program. For the treatment program to be successful, the physical therapist must thoroughly understand the patient's abilities and limitations and exhibit a positive yet realistic attitude toward the patient and the disease. For the program to be successful, a motivated patient is essential.

MS patients often are not referred to physical therapy until their disease becomes so severe as to significantly affect activities of daily living. However, most patients can benefit from a physical therapy evaluation and a formal treatment plan at the time of diagnosis. An exercise program recommended early in the course of the disease will help patients attain some control of their physical well-being. Physical therapists should emphasize the delicate balance between exercise and fatigue and suggest the most appropriate recreational activities.

Because of the variety of MS symptoms, no one specific treatment plan for rehabilitation exists. Therefore, an individualized plan using an interdisciplinary approach aimed at achieving the highest functional level is recommended. All members of the team must work closely together to meet the goals of the treatment program. As the disease remits or progresses, this potential must be reevaluated on an ongoing basis.

Evaluation of the therapeutic effects of treatment techniques is difficult because of the unpredictability of MS. Consequently, the physical therapist must recognize that improvement may result from fluctuations of the disease and not necessarily from physical therapy. Despite these obstacles, physical therapy can play an important role in maintaining the patient's highest level of independence and in improving the patient's overall quality of life.

Evaluation

A baseline evaluation usually requires one hour to complete. In those patients in whom fatigue is a major problem, the evaluation is more accurate when performed in multiple sessions. For best results, the therapist should schedule the evaluation at the time of day the patient usually has the most energy. The evaluation should be repeated every 3 to 6 months depending on the patient's functional status. When recording the data, objectivity is important. A functional muscle test using a standard scale helps differentiate actual muscle weakness from fatigue or underlying depression.

Many evaluation forms are available. A sample initial evaluation form and explanation of items intended to provide guidelines for baseline data is included at the end of this chapter. The following outlines the information on the form:

EVALUATION

1. Historical data
2. Physical examination
   a. Historical data
      (1) Hand dominance
      (2) Natural history of the disease
      (3) Previous rehabilitation programs
      (4) Sensory symptoms
      (5) Motor symptoms
   b. Physical examination data
      (1) Functional muscle strength
      (2) Range of motion
      (3) Proprioception
      (4) Muscle tone
      (5) Gait
      (6) Balance
      (7) Activities of daily living (transfers)
      (8) Functional mobility grade

Once the data base has been completed, the patient and therapist review the information and establish common goals. During the goal setting, the patient should be encouraged to discuss activities that are important to him. The therapist is responsible for recommending realistic goals based on the patient's functional status. Active participation by the patient and joint planning result in better overall compliance.

Specific Clinical Problems

FATIGUE

Fatigue is one of the most common and least understood of all MS symptoms. Even patients with minimal disability can be plagued with this problem. Fatigue is a subjective phenomenon that is often misinterpreted by the patient's relatives and friends. Other MS symptoms such as incoordination, spasms, and muscle weakness are clearly visible and therefore may be considered more "legitimate."

Herndon and co-workers (1981) describe four types of fatigue in MS. The first type is "normal" fatigue occurring after excessive physical activity. Patients with MS experience this type of fatigue more frequently and more rapidly than normal people. The second type of fatigue can be attributed to underlying depression, which affects the energy level of the patient. Depression may go unrecognized because of the patient's labile affect or pseudobulbar euphoria. The third type of fatigue results from muscle weakness and strain. When one limb is weakened the second must work harder to compensate, resulting in more fatigue. Using walking aids (e.g., crutches, canes, walker) expends more energy than an unimpaired gait. Walking aids probably conserve energy when severe lower extremity muscle weakness exists. "Nerve fiber fatigue" is the fourth type of fatigue. In certain situations, such as with increased body temperature, demyelinated nerve fibers fail to conduct impulses effectively. The early afternoon fatigue that many MS patients experience may be related to an elevation in the core body temperature. Other undefined biochemical changes may occur that contribute to fatigue. "Neuronal fatigue" is a concept based on the theory that more energy is required to transmit impulses in a demyelinated area.

Fatigue should not hinder the accomplishment of realistic goals provided that short rest periods are interspersed with exercise and excess body temperatures are avoided. Therapists should be specific about the frequency and duration of each exercise and the maintenance of an exact balance between moderate exercise and rest. Energy conservation in activities of daily living is essential. A few minutes of rest during a task helps avoid undue fatigue and allows the patient to complete the work. The physical therapist should work closely with the other team members to reinforce energy conservation in all aspects of the patient's life (see Chap. 8). Family members as well as the patient must be educated on specific energy-conservation measures.

A regular exercise program improves endurance and may lessen fatigue. Exercising muscles to the point of fatigue seems to increase endurance; however, exceeding that point consistently may result in increased weakness. Each patient quickly develops awareness of his own exercise tolerance.

CONTRACTURES

Contractures occur secondary to prolonged immobilization of an extremity and limit the normal range of motion. Patients confined to bed may develop flexion contractures at the hip or knee if these joints are not regularly moved. Muscle shortening, which results in limited range of motion, may be due to spasticity and decreased mobility.

Prevention remains the best treatment for contractures. Spasticity can be reduced with physical therapy and medication. The physical therapy program includes daily passive range-of-motion exercises and stretching. These exercise programs can be taught to the family members or to the nursing home personnel. Each major body joint should be moved through its full range of motion. Another method to prevent contractures is to employ splints or braces to maintain joint alignment. Proper positioning techniques in beds or chairs are also helpful. Once contractures occur, passive exercises are less helpful and surgical intervention may become necessary.

WEAKNESS

Weakness can be one of the most disabling symptoms in MS. Although most often occurring in the lower extremities, the upper extremities may also be involved. The manifestations vary from a vague sense of inability to total paralysis. Weakness is usually secondary to an upper motor neuron lesion. However, when the patient is put to bed voluntarily or at the doctor's request, the inactivity leads to further weakness secondary to disuse. Fatigue also may play a role in the patient's inability to perform muscular activity.

In physical therapy, muscle exercise is the most important modality for improving impaired muscle function. To enhance function, the physical therapist attempts to substitute the use of uninvolved muscles for the use of involved ones. Depending on the degree of impairment, the most frequently used techniques at the Rocky Mountain Multiple Sclerosis Center (RMMSC) are as follows:

1. Active assistive exercise, active exercises
2. Proprioceptive neuromuscular facilitation (PNF) technique
3. Therapeutic exercises
4. Resistive exercises

The patterns of facilitation of PNF are used for active motion, guided active motion, or resisted motion depending on the degree of weakness present. When weakness is minimal, resistive exercises are included. Because of the fatigue factor, regular rest periods must be incorporated into the program. The exercise program may be performed whenever convenient, but the morning is generally recommended because decreased energy in early afternoon is a frequent problem. The therapist must remember that an overly vigorous program can elevate core body temperature and enhance weakness and fatigue. Each program must be individualized for the specific patient.

The goals for a daily home exercise program to strengthen muscles are to

Maintain physical fitness even in asymptomatic patients
Enhance activities in patients with fluctuating status
Maintain function as long as possible

Because of the exacerbating/remitting nature of MS, the exercise program may need to be reevaluated and updated monthly. Regular visits with the therapist offer reinforcement and encouragement in a program that might be lifelong. The therapist should offer enough variation to prevent boredom or discouragement.

SPASTICITY

Altered muscle tone is a common finding in MS, especially in those patients with spinal cord lesions. Although hypotonicity may be present, hypertonicity is more common. The stretch reflex may be pathologically altered in MS. According to Burke (1980), this reflex is velocity dependent in spasticity. Damaged muscles that are slowly stretched have little reflex response and minimal increase in tone. With faster stretching, the reflex response increases linearly with the stretching activity and the exercised muscle undergoes increased shortening (spasticity).

The MS patient has difficulty inhibiting primitive reflex patterns and initiating normal movement. Peterkin (1969) explains that some reflex mechanisms partially lose their cortical control and are not integrated into functional movement. Particularly at risk are the static postural reflexes, whose overactivity prevent movement rather than provide background stability. The stretch reflexes are activated, and changing limb or trunk position becomes more difficult.

The effects of spasticity are readily apparent. The inability to relax alternating agonist and antagonist muscle groups results in difficulty initiating movement and maintaining normal posture. In those patients too weak to stand with muscle strength alone, spasticity may provide stability to joints surrounded by weakened muscles, allowing some patients to stand who otherwise would be unable to do so. They literally "stand on their spasticity." In these cases, liberal use of antispasticity drugs may worsen the patient's functional status.

In managing spasticity the physical therapist must consider the following interrelated points:

Reflex dominance
Hypertonicity
Abnormal movement

Positioning techniques are used to inhibit primitive reflex patterns that
do not allow normal movement. For example, head and neck positions
can elicit strong postural reflex mechanisms (e.g., asymmetrical tonic
neck reflex [ATNR] and tonic labyrinthine reflex [TLR]; Figs. 7 – 1 and
7 – 2). Additionally, higher-level reflexes (e.g., ATNR, symmetrical tonic
neck reflex, TLR) may influence the pattern of spasticity in MS patients.
Therefore, side-lying positions are suggested (Fig. 7 – 3).

The application of cold with ice packs or ice massage has been used to
reduce hypertonicity. Miglietta (1973) studied the effect of cold on spasticity and concluded that cooling delays or blocks conduction along
muscle and nerve membranes. The end result is depressed muscle-
spindle activity, probably from afferent cutaneous stimulation and resultant alteration in alpha or gamma motor neuron activity. Watson
(1959) used immersion in cold water (70° F – 80° F) to reduce spasticity
and reported improvement in other MS symptoms. A core temperature
decrease of at least 1° F was needed for beneficial results.

Spasticity can also be modulated through movement techniques. Patients must experience the sensation of normal movement and normal
position. The earlier that treatment is initiated, the more likely the
patient will retain normal movement. Some of the techniques found
useful are

Rhythmic passive and assisted active trunk rotations
Reduction of volitional activity until it can occur without associated
abnormal movements
Encouragement of movement when the effect of the reflex mechanism is minimal

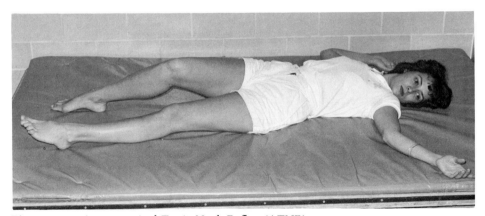

Figure 7 – 1   Asymmetrical Tonic Neck Reflex (ATNR).

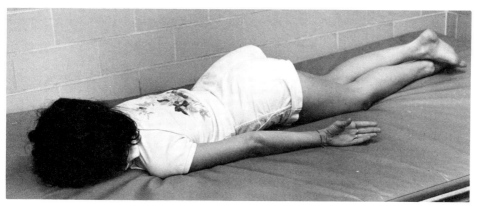

Figure 7–2 Tonic Labyrinthine Reflex (TLR). These abnormal reflexes may dominate MS patients' posture.

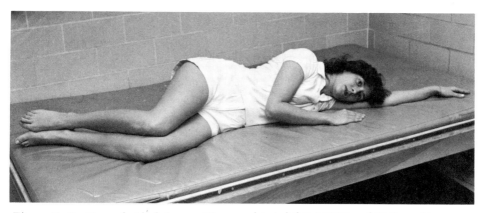

Figure 7–3 Normal side-lying position used to inhibit ATNR and TLR positions.

Spiral rolling patterns with head and shoulder girdle

Performance of basic functional movements through the developmental sequence (see Fig. 7–4A–H)

Normalization of tone and facilitation of movement with traction, approximation, gentle body rocking, and repeated controlled precision movements

Encouragement of weight-bearing in a normal position to enhance postural awareness

All of these techniques reinforce the sense of normal movement and ultimately help reduce hypertonicity.

When spasticity is severe, the entire treatment team must cooperate to prevent deformity and decubitus ulcers. Daily passive range-of-mo-

(text continues on p. 92)

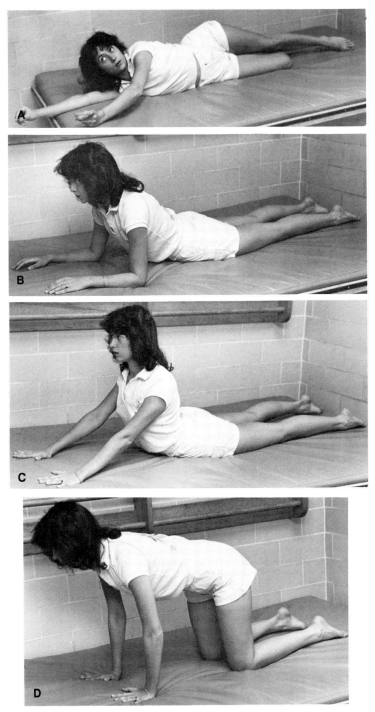

Figure 7-4 Use of basic functional positions and movements of the developmental sequence: (A) prone to supine, supine to prone, rolling; (B) prone on elbows; (C) prone on hands; (D) creeping (hands and knees);

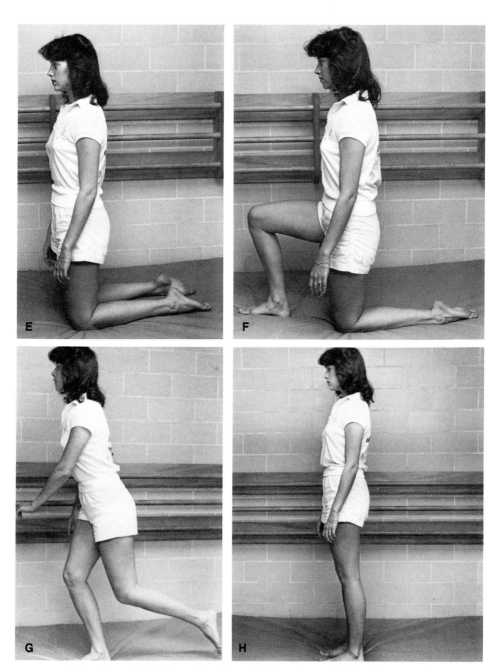

(E) kneeling; (F) half-kneeling; (G and H) standing. The developmental sequence allows the patient to progress from positions of wide base and low center of gravity to more mature positions.

tion exercises can minimize contractures and maintain joint mobility. The physician can simultaneously adjust the antispasticity medications to attain the maximum effect. The speech pathologist can develop a program for the dysarthria associated with spasticity (Chap. 9). At times, however, all conservative modalities may fail to control spasticity. Under these conditions, tendon-release surgery and motor-point blocks have been implemented.

ATAXIA

In MS, demyelination can occur in the cerebellum and cerebellar tracts, resulting in ataxia or incoordination of varying severity. Poorly coordinated muscle activity underlies slurred speech, intention tremor, and staggering gait. Ataxia can be mildly troublesome or severely disabling, depending on the degree of involvement. Symptoms resembling cerebellar ataxia may result from proprioceptive sensory loss. Ataxia is often associated with weakness and spasticity.

The physical therapist attempts to improve coordination and balance in all activities of daily living (ADL). Teaching compensatory techniques is of paramount importance. Adaptive equipment such as wrist weights or ball-bearing feeders may be suggested to make feeding easier and safer (see Chap. 8). Personal safety is always a consideration. For that reason, weighted canes or crutches are often employed to stabilize balance. Some potentially beneficial treatment techniques include the following:

Use of basic functional positions and movements of the developmental sequence (e.g., prone to supine, supine to prone, rolling [Fig. 7–4A]; prone on elbows [Fig. 7–4B]; prone on hands [Fig. 7–4C]; creeping [hands and knees] [Fig. 7–4D]; kneeling [Fig. 7–4E]; half-kneeling [Fig. 7–4F]; standing [Fig. 7–4G and H]). The developmental sequence allows the patient to progress from positions of wide base and low center of gravity to more mature positions.

Joint approximation techniques applied in the direction of weight bearing. This technique gives rise to co-contraction of muscles around the weight-bearing joints, increasing their stability.

Use of alternative sensory feedback. In cases of vibratory and position sense loss, the eyes particularly can be used to facilitate walking.

Use of weighted utensils or cuff weights. These adaptive devices reduce tremor and make feeding and other activities of daily living more efficient (see Chap. 8).

Gait training with weighted walking aids. The patient is taught to widen the base of support and walk with weighted canes or walkers to increase stability and enhance safety.

Regular coordination and balance exercises

All of these techniques are useful to help the patient remain functional and independent.

GAIT ABNORMALITIES

Gait abnormalities are common problems in MS. Keeping patients ambulatory and upgrading their current functional level are important responsibilities for the therapist. Abnormalities of gait occur for the following reasons:

Altered muscle tone
Decreased muscle strength
Impaired sensation
Balance disturbance
Rapid onset of fatigue

Because the therapist strives to keep the patient upright and independent, proper use of ambulation aids becomes an important consideration. The treatment program to improve gait can be divided into two major training categories: (1) independent gait training without aids, and (2) gait training with ambulatory aids and equipment.

The physical therapist uses stretching exercises, muscle-strengthening exercises, and balance exercises. Stretching exercises are particularly important when spasticity interferes with normal walking. The muscle groups most frequently affected by spasticity are the gastrocnemius–soleus, the hip adductors, and the hamstrings. Muscle weakness most often occurs in the lower extremities, but the upper extremities, including the hands, may be weakened as well. An increase of repetitions in the exercise program may be more beneficial than adding resistance. Both sitting and standing balance exercises are helpful. The goal is to increase trunk stability in preparation for a more stable gait.

Ambulatory aids and equipment are varied. Those most commonly used are

Ankle–foot orthosis (AFO) (Fig. 7–5)
Canes, crutches, walkers
Rocker shoes (Fig. 7–6)

Ankle–foot orthosis are used to improve footdrop or to stabilize the ankle. Most MS patients do well with the AFO, although other braces may also be used. Plastic AFO braces are helpful for the following:

Weakened or absent dorsiflexor or plantar flexor muscles
Moderate spasticity
Adequate knee extensors and hip muscle strength (i.e., greater than grade 3). Plastic AFOs are not generally used in patients with significant foot or ankle edema.

The physical therapist helps the patient decide when a walking aid is needed. Patients frequently resist initially and will not accept the walk-

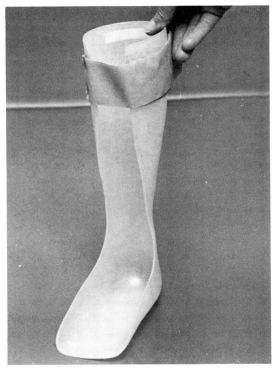

Figure 7–5   Ankle foot orthosis (AFO).

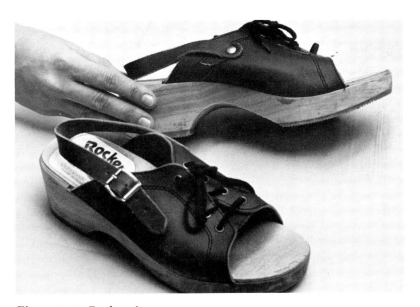

Figure 7–6   Rocker shoes.

ing aid until they realize resultant improvement in their mobility. The therapist should select the type and size of the appropriate aid. After selection, training the patient with the walking aid is essential, and regular reevaluations of the gait pattern with the walking aid are equally important. A patient using a cane who begins to fall probably needs additional support to improve balance and augment weakened muscles. Crutches or a walker might be recommended.

Rocker shoes (see Fig. 7 – 6) are clog-type shoes that have been found to be helpful in a select group of MS patients. According to Perry and associates (1981) the elevated heel neutralizes the plantar flexed position while the curved forefoot sole passively initiates knee flexion in a normal manner. The patient then uses a mass flexion pattern for swing and mass extension pattern for stability during stance. Perry described energy conservation and fatigue reduction as the most beneficial effects. Before rocker shoes are suggested the patient must first be able to walk independently, with adequate hip and calf strength.

IMPAIRED RESPIRATION

Breathing problems in severe MS contribute to difficulties with speech and swallowing and increase the incidence of respiratory infections and anxiety. Causes of impaired respiration can be linked to poor posture, inactivity, and weakness of the respiratory muscles including the diaphragm, intercostals, and abdominal muscles. The physical therapist and speech pathologist cooperate to improve breath support through a breathing exercise program by concentrating on diaphragmatic breathing and prolonging inspiratory and expiratory time. Sitting posture is evaluated and strengthening exercises for abdominals and accessory muscles are provided as needed.

ACTIVITIES OF DAILY LIVING

If a patient is no longer ambulatory, the physical therapist attempts to increase independence and maintain the highest functional level in activities of daily living (ADL), working closely with the occupational therapist (Chap. 8). The two disciplines cooperate in the evaluation of what equipment might be most useful. The physical therapist provides training in effective and safe transfer techniques from bed to wheelchair, wheelchair to toilet, wheelchair to car, and *vice versa*. Training the patient to progress from supine to sitting and sitting to standing positions is important. Exercises to improve sitting and standing balance make ADL safer. Bed mobility training is also helpful. The recommendation of appropriate equipment to increase independence and safety is best accomplished with home visits so that specific suggestions will match each patient's particular needs. An overhead trapeze for a bed to help with rolling and bathroom grab bars may be helpful. When a wheelchair is needed, each patient is evaluated individually. Important considerations are what is ideal, what is essential, and what is financially reasonable for each patient (Chap. 25).

DECUBITUS ULCERS

Bed-ridden patients with severe spasticity are prone to develop decubitus ulcers. Severely disabled MS patients are particularly vulnerable because of sensory deprivation, generalized wasting, contractures secondary to spasticity, and involuntary movements causing excessive friction over boney prominences. Prolonged pressure and resultant tissue ischemia are the etiologic factors. Particularly prone to decubiti are the areas over the ischial tuberosities, the sacrum, the greater trochanters, and the heels (see Fig. 10-1). The goal of treatment is prevention and requires the cooperation of the nursing staff, the family, and the physical therapists. Position changes should be accomplished at least every 2 hours, with attention paid to proper positioning techniques to prevent pressure and to enhance the comfort of the patient. Protective devices such as alternating air pressure mattresses, flotation pads, and sheepskin in bed or chair are helpful. The physical therapist takes a primary role in educating both nursing staff and family members in decubitus ulcer prevention.

SENSORY DISTURBANCE

The success of any rehabilitation program may be directly related to the patient's sensory awareness. Although severe and prolonged pain is not commonly seen in MS, sensory loss secondary to demyelination is common. Treatment programs should focus on improving sensory awareness and teaching precautions to avoid trauma to the skin from cold, heat, pressure, and other noxious stimuli. Vision should be used as a substitute for proprioceptive loss even in simple automatic activities. Developmental sequence postures can be used to provide additional sensory input (Fig. 7-4A-H). Repeated stimulation of nerve endings in muscles and joints by approximating joint surfaces and using hands for tapping and brushing can also be helpful. Coordination exercises in combination with sensory stimulation enhance sensory awareness and are frequently used as a treatment tool. Weighted belts are also helpful in providing more sensory input.

Other General Considerations

ROLE OF PHYSICAL THERAPIST

All patients with MS can benefit from regular physical therapy. The role of the physical therapist will vary according to the patient's degree of impairment. Functional levels are divided into three groups: mildly impaired, moderately impaired, and severely impaired. Those with mild impairment have few if any physical symptoms other than fatigue. They are independent in ambulation and ADL. Patients with moderate impairment require one or more walking aids intermittently or continuously and require some assistance with ADL. Severely impaired patients require wheelchairs for mobility and may be completely dependent in ADL.

The physical therapist's role with the mildly impaired is that of an educator. Explanations about disease manifestations and the usefulness of physical activity are helpful in patients' adjustment process. Teaching patients to deal with fatigue and teaching activity planning are extremely useful. General health promotion, physical fitness program guidelines, and advice regarding recreational activities should be emphasized (see Chap. 27 and Table 27–1).

The benefits of physical therapy are most readily apparent in the moderately impaired MS patient. Appropriate intervention can make a difference in the patient's functional level (e.g., from crutches to cane; see Chap. 6). Exercise programs can delay progression of functional disability in some cases. Adaptive techniques are used when a lower level of function is unavoidable. Education continues to be important but the emphasis shifts to the maintenance or improvement of independent function.

The severely impaired patient requires increased nursing care at home or in extended-care facilities. Nursing home personnel require and usually welcome instruction about the disease process, positioning techniques, range-of-motion exercises, and other maintenance programs. Special equipment needs should also be considered.

GROUP ACTIVITIES

Physical therapy group sessions can be an important adjunct to the rehabilitation program and can be directed by any member of the rehabilitation team. Some treatment goals are more readily achieved in a group setting. Psychological support and encouragement from other patients with MS help the group members achieve their own specific goals. Coping mechanisms in ADL are shared within the group. Groups can be oriented toward very specific goals such as improving sitting balance or dressing skills. Group settings are ideal for patient education regarding the disease process. Patients with the same disability level can work together to achieve similar goals.

RECREATIONAL ACTIVITIES

Supervised recreational activities such as pool therapy, yoga, and handicapped skiing have proven extremely beneficial for our MS patients.

The physical therapist provides consultation and supervision for these activities. Those patients with minimal or moderate disabilities benefit the most, but some facilities also provide services for the severely impaired. Ideally, these special programs should be offered at least weekly.

Pool therapy uses the buoyancy of water to help patients exercise more easily, walk with less difficulty, practice balance activities, and relax spastic muscles. Swimming also improves strength and endurance. Yoga programs increase flexibility, strength, and coordination as well as teach valuable relaxation techniques. Handicapped skiing offers an outdoor experience with opportunity to enjoy a sport usually perceived as only for the physically fit. Specialized equipment and trained instructors work on a one-to-one basis with the handicapped. If needed, two instructors per patient can be provided. The development of better balance and increased endurance and the increase in confidence to try other activities are the major advantages of this program.

With all recreational activities, fatigue can be an important factor and should be anticipated. Gaining independence and enjoying new experiences increases a patient's confidence and self-worth, which extends into all areas of the patient's life (see Chap. 27). Specifics concerning these programs are available through the RMMSC.

Conclusion

Physical therapy can be very valuable to the MS patient. It should be initiated at an early stage of the disease and directed toward maintaining the highest functional level. The success of a rehabilitation program depends on the motivation of the patient and on the attitude of the therapist as much as on the disease course. A multidisciplinary team approach provides for the most comprehensive care. The physical therapist helps manage spasticity, weakness, ataxia, fatigue, ADL, and gait problems. Education regarding the disease process and health promotion is incorporated into the treatment sessions.

Rehabilitation of MS patients provides a continuing challenge. Achievement of small goals should be regarded as a major accomplishment. The entire therapeutic milieu provides psychological support for the patient. An open mind, a positive attitude, and a sense of humor are of unlimited benefit to the patient and the therapist. How patients deal with their disease and their resultant disabilities will affect their entire lives. Most MS patients are people with courage and fortitude who usually earn the respect and admiration of the treatment team. These patients make the battle for health worth fighting.

RMMSC PHYSICAL THERAPY EVALUATION FORM (AND EXPLANATIONS)

Hospital-Number _____ – ___   Date: Year 19____ Mo____ Day____

Name_____   Sex___ (M = Male, F = Female)
        (Last, First)

Date of birth: Year 19____ Mo____ Day____   Hand dominance___ (R = Right, L = Left)

Age at first symptom___   Year of diagnosis 19____

Physical status___ (R = remission, E = exacerbation, P = progression, S = stable, U = other)
    (Definitions below.)
Most involved extremity . . . UE___ . . . LE___(R = Right, L = Left, E = Equal)
Have you ever received physical therapy before? [___] (Y = Yes, N = No)

Current sensory symptoms (check all that apply):
    Paresthesia/numbness . . . . Right UE___   Left UE___   Right LE___   Left LE___
                                            Trunk___
    Dysesthesia/pain . . . . Right UE___   Left UE___   Right LE___   Left LE___
                                            Trunk___

Definitions of Items Regarding Physical Status
Remission: Patient has recovered from an exacerbation and has resumed normal function.
Exacerbation: Patient is in an acute attack.
Progression: Patient is experiencing slowly or rapidly progressing MS.
Stable: Patient is in a stable condition with some residual symptoms of MS remaining.

Functional Movement Evaluation
    (Use standard scale of 0 to 5. For + or −, use second box.) (If strength in an extremity is normal, record only for extremity as a whole. If not normal, record individual muscle groups.)

Right UE___ – ___   Left UE___ – ___   Right LE___ – ___   Left LE___ – ___

Right	Muscle Groups	Left	Right	Muscle Groups	Left
___ – ___	Shoulder flexors	___ – ___	___ – ___	Hip flexors	___ – ___
___ – ___	Shoulder extensors	___ – ___	___ – ___	Hip abductors	___ – ___
___ – ___	Shoulder abductors	___ – ___	___ – ___	Hip extensors	___ – ___
___ – ___	Elbow flexors	___ – ___	___ – ___	Knee extensors	___ – ___
___ – ___	Elbow extensors	___ – ___	___ – ___	Knee flexors	___ – ___
___ – ___	Wrist flexors	___ – ___	___ – ___	Ankle dorsiflexors	___ – ___
___ – ___	Wrist extensors	___ – ___	___ – ___	Ankle plantarflexors	___ – ___
___ – ___	Back extensors	___ – ___	___ – ___	Abdominals	___ – ___

Range of Motion
(Check functional range in each extremity below. 0 = Absent, 5 = Normal. If ROM is abnormal, check the appropriate range for the categories given.)

Right UE___   Left UE___   Right LE___   Left LE___

Shoulder abduction . . . . Right UE___   Left UE___
    (A = 0–90, B = 90–180)

Ankle dorsiflexion/plantarflexion . . . . Right LE___   Left LE___
    (A = 10–15 of dorsiflexion, B = neutral to +5 or −5, C = 10–20 plantarflexion, D = 25–35 plantarflexion)

List specific contractures (*e.g.,* 20-degree hip flexion in contracture):_____

Sensation
Proprioceptive loss (1 = none, 2 = mild, 3 = severe. Explanation below.)
Right UE___   Left UE___   Right LE___   Left LE___

Definitions of Sensation Classifications
None: No loss of proprioception
Mild: Any loss at PIP joints in upper extremities and MP joint in toes.
Severe: Any loss at ankles or wrists.

Muscle Tone

Tone Grade	Spasticity Grade
(1 = normal, 2 = hypotonic, 3 = spastic)	(1 = mild, 2 = moderate, 3 = severe)
Right UE. . . . ___ Left UE . . . . ___	Right UE. . . . ___ Left UE . . . . ___
Right LE . . . . ___ Left LE. . . . . ___	Right LE . . . . ___ Left LE. . . . . ___

(If spasticity exists, check appropriate categories to indicate amount of spasticity.)

Gait

Does vision affect your gait? ___ (Y = Yes, N = No)
   If Yes, check all that apply: Blurred vision ___ Double vision ___
                   Loss of vision ___

Patient ambulatory? ___ (Y = Yes, N = No)

Appliances used for ambulation (Check all that apply.)
   Shoes/braces ___   Crutches ___   Walker ___   Cane ___
         (Check all listed items that definitely are present.)

	With Appliances and shoes		Without Appliances or shoes	
	Right	Left	Right	Left
Independent reciprocal gait.	___	___	___	___
Recurvatum at mid stance	___	___	___	___
Toes in/out at mid stance	___	___	___	___
Circumduction on swing	___	___	___	___
Lack of reciprocal arm swing.	___	___	___	___
Footdrop.	___	___	___	___
Wide base.	___	___	___	___
Ataxic	___	___	___	___

   Additional comments: _____

Explanation of Gait Evaluation

   Most items of gait are evaluated by checking whether a type of gait, gait component, or structural change is present or absent. Gait is observed front, back, and side for all determinants. Patients are assessed with and without shoes, with and without aids, wearing clothing that permits easy view of the trunk, hips, and legs. Rather than setting up a several-point scale, the items that are used are assessed as definitely present, which means that mild tendencies on items that may cause disagreement among evaluators as to their presence would usually be termed absent. Also, for the item to be listed as present, it must be observed for at least 5 to 10 consecutive complete strides (heel strikes of the same foot).
   Specifics of gait are as follows: Write "Y" if patient is ambulatory and "N" if nonambulatory. If nonambulatory, go on to "Balance." Check the appropriate numbers for appliances used. Please evaluate gait with shoes and appliances and without either.

1. Independent reciprocal gait is defined as the absence of all the factors evaluated.
2. Recurvatum is present when the knee is obviously thrown back on weight bearing or is curved more than 180 degrees visually at mid to late stance.
3. Toes in and out are judged from the front by watching the plane of the foot during stance as the foot strikes a line on the floor. A neutral or greater adduction position is considered toe in, and an angle greater than 15 degrees of toe out is marked as toe out.
4. Circumduction is determined by obvious pattern of swing phase. Very mild and equivocal circumduction is termed as absent.
5. Person walks without reciprocal swing.
6. Foot drag assessment is either absent or present.
7. Wide base is present if the patient walks with greater than 9 inches between feet. The 9" is measured using the standard 9" floor tile width. This may be due to mild limb ataxia or proprioceptive loss.

8. Ataxic—present if for any reason other than weakness the person cannot keep balance during gait especially during sharp turns, or base is wide because of balance impairments; equivocal assessments are listed as absent. This would indicate a more severe form of incoordination.

Balance

Sitting balance___ (G = good, F = fair, P = poor, N = none)
Standing balance___ (G = good, F = fair, P = poor, N = none)
   Standing on right foot___ (A = 1 min, B = 10 sec, C = 1–9 sec, D = N/A or 0 sec)
   Standing on left foot___ (A = 1 min, B = 10 sec, C = 1–9 sec, D = N/A or 0 sec)
Romberg Test (see definition below): Positive___   Negative___

Balance
   Independent sitting and standing balance are evaluated:
Good—maintains balance in all directions even with moderate pushing from evaluator
Fair—cannot maintain balance with moderate push in any direction
Poor—cannot maintain balance with mild push in any direction
None—no balance

For evaluating one-leg standing balance choose one of the listed categories.

Romberg Test: Patient stands with comfortable stance with eyes open.
   Positive Romberg is moderate to marked worsening of standing balance with eyes closed. Negative Romberg is no change in patient's standing balance. The Romberg tests proprioceptive loss rather than cerebellar ataxia.

ADL Status

ADL status determined by: ___ (D = demonstration, H = history) (use ADL scale below)

Roll side to side. . . . . ___   5 = independent and in optimal manner
Sit up in bed . . . . ___   4 = independent, but less than optimal manner
Transfers:
          Bed–W/C . . . . . . ___   3 = independent, but impractically
          W/C–Toilet. . . . . . ___   2 = with standby attendant only
          W/C–Car . . . . . . ___   1 = with human assistance
Operate W/C . . . . ___   0 = unable to perform

Functional mobility grade___ (range 0–12, use scale below)

Functional Mobility Grade:

(Choose one or more items to signify present functional level. Use "Comments" space for further explanation of functional mobility level.)

1. No restrictions; minimal status
2. Definite impairment, but fully ambulatory without aids
3. Limited ability (distance) without aids; able to climb stairs
4. Needs cane and/or brace; stair-climbing equivocal
5. Requires crutches or walker
6. Uses wheelchair, but may use crutches or walker in the home
7. Wheelchair independent
8. Wheelchair independent, but cannot transfer
9. Requires motorized wheelchair (or could manage motorized chair)
10. Wheelchair dependent (specialized chairs)—cannot manage motorized
11. Bed-ridden, but still has arm and hand functions
12. Bed-ridden, helpless

Comments on functional mobility grade: _____

_____

Additional comments: _____

_____

Recommendations: _____

_____

_____

Suggested Readings

ABRAMS MW: A comprehensive physical therapy program for the treatment of multiple sclerosis patient. Phys Ther 48:337–341, 1968

ABRAMSON A: Physical management of the patient with multiple sclerosis. Geigy Symposium, Part IV, pp 16–20, 1980

BAUER MJ: Problems of symptomatic therapy in multiple sclerosis. Neurology 28:8–20, 1978

BLOCK J, KESTER N: Role of rehabilitation in the management of multiple sclerosis patients. Modern Treatment 7:930–940, 1970

BURKE D: A reassessment of the muscle spindle contribution to muscle tone in normal and spastic man. In Feldman RG, Young RR, Koella WP (eds): Spasticity: Disordered Motor Control, pp 261–279. Chicago, Year Book Medical Publishers, 1980

BURKS JS, THOMPSON DS: Multiple sclerosis. In Earnest M (ed): Neurologic Emergencies, pp 361–385. New York, Churchill Livingstone, 1983

GORDON EE (ed): Multiple Sclerosis: Application of Rehabilitation Techniques, pp 8–21. New York, National Multiple Sclerosis Society, 1951

HERNDON R, RUDICK R: Fatigue. MS Quarterly, pp 4, 5, 14, 1981

KELLY-HAYES M: Guidelines for rehabilitation of multiple sclerosis patients. Nurs Clin North Am 15:245–256, 1980

KNOTT M, VOSS DE (eds): Proprioceptive Neuromuscular Facililitation: Patterns and Techniques, 2nd ed, pp 13, 14. New York, Harper & Row, 1968

MIGLIETTA O: Action of cold on spasticity. Am J Phys Med 52:198–205, 1973

MOOR FB, PETERSON SC, MANWELL EM, et al (eds): Manual of Hydrotherapy and Massage, pp 22–23. Mountain View, California, Pacific Press Publishing Association, 1964

NOSWORTHY SJ: Symposium on multiple sclerosis: Physiotherapy. Nursing Mirror 143:53–55, 1976

PERRY J, GRONLEY J, LUNSFORD T: Rocker shoe as walking aid in multiple sclerosis. Arch Phys Med Rehabil 62:59–65, 1981

PETERKIN HW: The neuromuscular system and the re-education of movement. Physiotherapy 55:145–153, 1969

SARNO J, LEHNEIS N: Prescription considerations for plastic below the knee orthosis. Arch Phys Med Rehabil 52:503–510, 1976

SCHEINBERG L, HOLLAND N, KIRSLENBARUM M: Comprehensive long-term care of patients with multiple sclerosis. Neurology 31:1121–1123, 1981

SCHNEITZER LM: Rehabilitation of patients with multiple sclerosis. Arch Phys Med Rehabil 5:430–437, 1978

SMITH WD: Combining wall pulleys and mat activities to total pattern movement. Phys Ther 54:746–747, 1974

WATSON C: Effects of lowering body temperature on the symptoms and signs of multiple sclerosis. N Engl J Med 261:1253–1259, 1959

WOLF BA: Effects of temperature reduction on multiple sclerosis. Phys Ther 50:808–810, 1970

8

Beth G. Wolf

Occupational Therapy for Patients With Multiple Sclerosis

Occupational therapy (OT) is concerned with the functional disabilities of multiple sclerosis (MS). This therapy's focus is to improve the quality of a patient's life by developing or maintaining those abilities essential to productive living. The occupational therapist determines objective levels of dysfunction and defines problem areas that are not usually addressed by the physician or other health-care personnel. Examples include how the patient brushes his teeth, combs his hair, or dresses himself. OT seeks to rehabilitate the areas of the patient's dysfunction that affect the performance of daily life tasks.

OT focuses on five areas of treatment for MS. These are (1) energy-conservation and work-simplification techniques; (2) upper extremity coordination and strength; (3) activities of daily living (ADL) and adaptive equipment; (4) homemaking and vocational evaluation and training; and (5) wheelchair evaluation and training. Each area is equally important, but the focus may be on one particular area as individual patient needs dictate.

Patients should be referred to OT for deficits in any of these five areas. Common patient concerns include, "How do I button, cut meat, turn pages, or get out of bed? How do I manage housework better? How do I modify my job?" Frequently only the MS patient who suffers obvious dysfunction is referred to the occupational therapist for treatment. However, many patients with mild impairment suffer from extreme fatigue. These patients can benefit from occupational therapy instruction in work simplification, energy conservation, and stress management. An OT referral is appropriate when there is a question about patient functioning in daily tasks.

103

Evaluation

A comprehensive OT evaluation serves as a baseline of objective information. This evaluation provides an understanding of the functional difficulties the patient is having and what is responsible for these difficulties. The recommended evaluation (Fig. 8–1A–C) takes approximately one hour. It should be done initially and repeated every 6 to 12 months or when an exacerbation occurs. The assessment includes date of onset of symptoms, type of MS, current living situation and responsibilities, vocational status, hand dominance (and whether this has changed since the onset of the disease process), which hand the patient feels is more functional, as well as any previous therapy, adaptive equipment used, and ambulation status. Additionally, there are formal tests of grip and pinch, coordination, and ADL.

Upper extremity muscle tests done by a physical therapist need not be duplicated. If a test has not been done, the occupational therapist should do a muscle test as described in Figure 8–2. Grip and pinch measurements are done with a hand dynamometer and pinch gauge. A test of two-point discrimination is done by the physician or by the occupational therapist. The results should be evaluated in terms of decrease in functional ability.

A test of hand coordination is used as a tool to indicate the level of functional ability and disability, and as an indication of progression of disability (for retests). The Jebsen Test of Hand Coordination was selected for use with MS patients because it evaluates each hand separately, distinguishes between the dominant and nondominant hand, allows for age and sex variance in scoring, and can be administered easily and rapidly. This test measures the patient's ability in writing, simulated page turning, manipulation of small objects, simulated feeding, stacking checkers, and manipulation of both light and heavy cans. The results give an overall picture of both gross and fine motor coordination and are scored by computing the number of standard deviations below the norm. For MS patients a score of 0 to 2 standard deviations below normal is considered to be within normal limits; a score of 2.1 to 4 standard deviations below the norm is considered a mild coordination disturbance, 4.1 to 6 standard deviations below norm a moderate disturbance, and 6.1 or more standard deviations below norm, a severe disturbance. Severe ataxia may result in scores considerably below these values.

The ADL evaluation was designed to be a comprehensive test of ability without repetition of information. The six subcategories assessed are communication, eating, mobility, hygiene, dressing, and miscellaneous. Patients are scored on a scale of 0 to 5, with 5 being independent and 0 being unable to perform. The ADL evaluation includes questions related to homemaking and job skills. If an alternate ADL evaluation is used that does not include this information, separate tests should be done. Patients should perform tests of functional abilities because many may deny or exaggerate disabilities.

Once the evaluation is complete, the occupational therapist determines areas of dysfunction, establishes goals, and develops a treatment plan.

Fatigue

Although the pathophysiology of fatigue in MS is unknown, more energy is required for nerve impulse conduction between two points in a demyelinated nervous system. Therefore, daily activities performed by MS patients will use more energy than is normal. Treatment of fatigue is very important in order to allow a patient maximum ability to perform daily life tasks. The following are some basic work-simplification and energy-conservation techniques that patients can use:

1. Organize your activities before you start them. If you begin to get frustrated or confused, stop what you are doing and gather your thoughts.
2. Allow enough time to complete an activity so that you do not get rushed. Rushing wastes energy and promotes anxiety, and can quickly cause fatigue.
3. Analyze what you are going to do. Is it necessary? When should it be done and by whom? Eliminate all unnecessary work. Simplify the necessary operations.
4. Space activities to decrease fatigue. If you become tired or fatigued, stop the activity and rest for 15 minutes and then continue.
5. Use both hands and arms whenever practical.
6. Slide rather than lift or carry.
7. Use proper work heights according to the job and the individual. Jobs requiring hand activity will need a higher work surface than those requiring arm motion.
8. Sit to work whenever possible. Standing uses oxygen, which uses energy and can cause fatigue.
9. Use the assistance of gravity and momentum whenever possible. Toss instead of placing unbreakable items.

These basic concepts are then demonstrated and discussed with each patient.

Work-simplification and energy-conservation instruction should include a stress management program. Occupational therapists are particularly suited to teaching stress management because of their dual training in physiologic and psychological functioning.

OCCUPATIONAL THERAPY EVALUATION
MULTIPLE SCLEROSIS   Date ____/____/____

Patient's name _____ Hospital # _____

Address _____

Phone (H) _____ (W) _____

Birthdate ____/____/____   Date of onset of symptoms ____/____/____

Date of diagnosis ____/____/____   Type of multiple sclerosis _____

Hand dominance R( ) L( )   More functional UE R( ) L( )

Living arrangement
   House ( )   Apartment ( )
   1 Story ( )   1st Floor ( )
   2 Story ( )   Elevator ( )
   Basement ( )

Lives alone ( )   Lives with other adult ( )

Lives with young children ( )

Previous therapies
   O.T. ( )   P.T. ( )   Speech/Language ( )

Adaptive devices _____

Ambulations
   Walks independently ( )   Walks holding walls ( )
      Cane ( )   Walker ( )   Crutches ( )   Wheelchair ( )

Employed Yes ( )   No ( ) _____

Previous employment Yes ( )   No ( ) _____

A

Figure 8–1 Occupational therapy evaluation form. *(A)* History. *(B)* Functional hand strength and hand coordination form. *(C)* Activities of daily living form. (Used by permission. University of Colorado Health Sciences Center. All rights reserved)

Figure 8–1. Continued.

Name _____

Hospital # _____

FUNCTIONAL HAND STRENGTH

Date	Date	Date	Date		Date	Date	Date	Date
		Left					Right	
				Grip				
				Lateral pinch				
				3-Point pinch				
				Thumb–index pinch				

Coordination: (Jebsen Test of Hand Coordination)
(Circle dominant hand for each subtest.)
SUBTEST   Date:

SUBTEST		RS	SD	RS	SD	RS	SD	RS	SD
Writing	RT.								
	LT.								
Cards	RT.								
	LT.								
Small Object	RT.								
	LT.								
Eating	RT.								
	LT.								
Checkers	RT.								
	LT.								
Empty Cans	RT.								
	LT.								
Full Cans	RT.								
	LT.								
Total	RT.								
	LT.								

RS = Raw Score
SD = Standard Deviation

B

(Fig. continues on next page)

Figure 8–1. Continued.

UNIVERSITY OF COLORADO MEDICAL CENTER
Department of Physical Medicine and Rehabilitation
Evaluation of
ACTIVITIES OF DAILY LIVING

Date
Ward
Name
Hosp. No.
Address

		Date	Date	Date	Comments	METHOD OF SCORING
C	Summon aid					Performs activity:
O	Speak intelligibly					5 — independently and
M	Read and interpret					in optimal manner
M	Turn pages					4 — Independently but in
U	Write adequately					less than optimal
N	Complete phone call					manner in relation to
E	Eat with spoon/fork					time and adaptations
A	Drink from cup/glass					3 — independently but
T	Cut with knife					impractically
	Carry own dishes/tray					2 — with standby
	Roll side to side					attendant only
	Sit up in bed					1 — with human assistance
M	To W/C and back					0 — unable to perform
O	Operate W/C					
B	Site-stand-sit					*SUMMARY:*
I	Ambulation					
L	Stairs					
I	Toilet on/off					
T	Shower in/out					
Y	Tub in/out					
	Braces/prosthesis on/off					
	Car in/out					
	Bus on/off					
H	Wash hands and face					
Y	Brush teeth					
G	Comb hair					
I	Shave/make up					
E	Bathe					
N	Care for nails					
E						
D	Dress/blouse/shirt on/off					
R	Slacks on/off					
E	Manage fastenings					
S	Socks/stockings/shoes on/off					
S	Clothes in/out of storage					
M	Operate radio and TV					
I	Manage eyeglasses					
S	Pick up object from floor					
C	Operate light switch					
E	Operate doors					
L	Wind watch					
L	Use matches safely					
A	Use money					
N	Object from pocket/purse					
E	and replace					
O	Prepare snack					
U						
S						

C

Left				Right		
Date	Date	Date		Date	Date	Date
			Scapula Protraction			
			Extension			
			Abduction			
			Adduction			
			External rotation			
			Internal rotation			
			Elbow Flexion			
			Extension			
			Wrist Flexion			
			Extension			
			Radial deviation			
			Ulnar deviation			

Figure 8-2   Suggested upper extremity muscle test for MS patients.

A group stress management program is recommended. A psychologist should serve as a consultant and the program should include lectures, discussion, and group activities. Patients are taught that stress can be negative "distress" or positive "eustress." Stress can be caused by a person, an event, or the environment, and can be experienced mentally, physically, emotionally, spiritually, socially, or intellectually. These patients should then be educated about the stages of stress, stress-provoking situations, and ways to reduce stress.

Weakness

Two components of weakness are observed in MS: weakness caused by reduced nerve transmission due to an upper motor neuron lesion and muscle atrophy caused by disuse. OT treatment cannot alter the former, but should focus on improving the disuse aspect.

Treatment of upper extremity weakness in the MS patient is done by exercise and activities that may involve the use of theraplast. Fatigue should be avoided, and exercises should be designed in conjunction with physical therapy to avoid an overstrenuous cumulative effect.

Static splints such as resting-pan or wrist-extension splints may be helpful. A resting splint (Fig. 8–3) is indicated where there is weakness of the finger extensor muscles. This splint allows the finger flexor tendons to remain at full length and prevents overstretching of the finger extensors as strengthening is attempted. A wrist-extension splint (Fig. 8–4) is used in the presence of weak wrist extensors and provides optimal positioning for the function of the finger flexors. A mobile arm support or ball-bearing feeder (Chap. 17) can be used successfully to compensate for upper extremity weakness. This device facilitates motion in the presence of shoulder or elbow weakness. The mobile arm support can be used when muscle strength is limited or where rapid fatigue is a factor. If wrist extension is weak, a wrist-extension splint is used along with the ball-bearing feeder and may require a utensil insert or universal cuff.

Ataxia

Upper extremity ataxia differs greatly from patient to patient and requires individualized treatment. It is important to evaluate whether the ataxic tremor is distal or proximal, or both, and in which area it is more pronounced.

When mild ataxia is present, the patient should be started on a daily program of theraplast exercises and coordination activities. These activ-

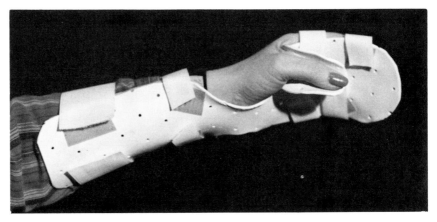

Figure 8–3 Resting splint used to prevent flexion contractures in the presence of weak finger extensors.

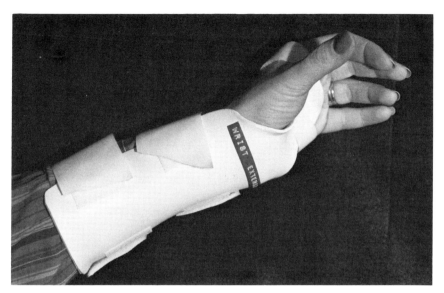

Figure 8–4   Wrist extension splint, which holds wrist in optimal functioning position in the presence of weak wrist extensors.

ities include pegboard manipulation, picking up coins and buttons, rolling objects between the fingers, and manipulating jar lids.

Recently the use of an air splint (as described by Margaret Johnstone in her book on motor restoration for the stroke patient) has been used to stimulate coordination and increase functional ability. The full or half arm cuff is applied once or twice a day for 15 to 20 minutes. However, there is no conclusive evidence of any beneficial effects of this procedure on MS symptoms.

Various methods have been tried to compensate for arm and hand tremors as seen in MS. All methods are successful for some patients but ineffective in others. Two 2-pound cuff weights applied, one proximal to the other, above the wrist have been found to be effective in decreasing forearm tremor. This technique, however, has little effect on wrist or finger tremors. A specially designed hand cuff weight (Fig. 8–5A and B) is used for hand tremors and is particularly useful for feeding activities. A wrist-extension splint with a metal brace and a 1- or 2-pound cuff weight (Fig. 8–6) has also been used. As ball-bearing feeders are used to compensate for weakness, when ataxia is present friction feeders have proven successful in enabling some patients to attain control of the upper extremities. A trial of several days with these feeders is indicated when there is upper arm, forearm, wrist, and finger tremors.

Head and neck ataxia interferes with the ability to eat, drink, and swallow. An adapted soft cervical collar can promote independent feeding and swallowing skills. This collar is custom adapted for each individ-

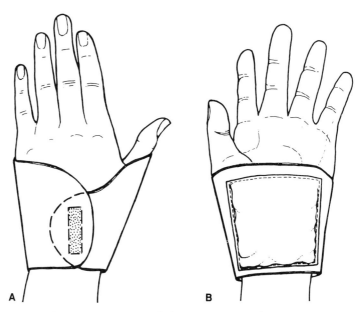

Figure 8–5 (A) Dorsal view and (B) volar view of hand cuff weight. The stitched area on the volar surface represents two 1-lb steel plates that have been inserted between the cuff and leather patch.

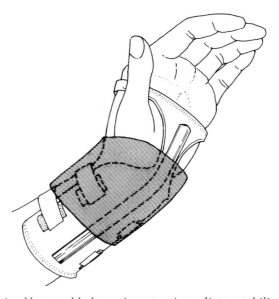

Figure 8–6 Metal brace added to wrist extension splint to stabilize wrist when ataxia is present. Wrist weight may also be added.

ual and allows support without interfering with neck flexion and swallowing. A ½-inch area over the laryngeal musculature at the top front of a standard cervical collar and the bottom front of the collar over the laryngeal musculature is cut out, angling the cut to the middle of the clavicle. Approximately 1½ inches of material is left between the two cut portions (Fig. 8–7).

Activities of Daily Living

The treatment of ADL problems and the use of adaptive equipment requires cooperative problem-solving between the occupational therapist and the patient. Because variety and severity of symptoms may differ greatly from patient to patient, the procedures may involve trial and error. When functional limitation exists, the goal is to compensate for the lack of functional ability by adapting methods and providing adaptive equipment. Table 8–1 and Figures 8–8 to 8–17 represent common problems and possible solutions encountered when treating the MS patient.

Because of the individual variation and severity of symptoms, it is important to try different methods and equipment, selecting and discarding as individually appropriate.

(text continues on p. 120)

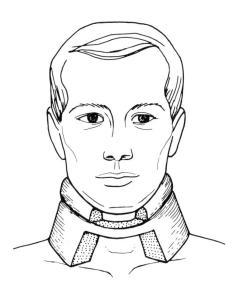

Figure 8–7   Adapted soft cervical collar supports head while allowing for neck flexion and swallowing.

Table 8-1 ADL Problems and Possible Solutions

Function	Neurologic Problem		Disability	Adaptive Method	Adaptive Equipment	Comments
	Weakness	Ataxia				
Feeding	*	*	Bringing cup or glass to mouth	Use both hands to hold cup or glass	Long straw	
		*	Spilling from cup		Tupperware tumbler; (Fig. 8–8); tommy tippee cup; long straw	Finger foods may be easier to eat.
		*	Stabilizing arm to bring food to mouth	Tuck upper arm against side of body and use elbow motion to feed	Weighted utensils	
				Using spoon to eat vegetable and/or rice, etc.		
	*		Holding eating utensil		Built-up utensil handle with cylindrical foam or metal tube (Fig. 8–9)	
	*	*	Getting food from plate to utensil		Spork (Fig. 8–8); plate guard (Fig. 8–8)	
	*	*	Cutting meat	Human assistance	Rocker knife; pizza cutter	Have patients try both.

		Activity	Technique	Equipment	Remarks
*	*	Feeding independently		Ball-bearing feeder, Friction feeder	OT supervises training and starts with one meal per day.
*	*	Completing a full meal		Ball-bearing feeder, Friction feeder	Patients frequently tire during the meal.
*	*	Holding head for feeding		Adapted cervical collar (Fig. 8–7)	
Dressing					
*	*	Putting on a shirt or blouse	Patient places arms into the shirt sleeves, pulls sleeves up over the elbows, and then slips shirt over his head		When learning dressing techniques, patients should wear loose-fitting clothing.
*	*	Putting on pants	Put pants on in bed, rolling from side to side	Pants spreader (Fig. 8–10)	
*	*	Buttoning	Replace buttons with Velcro	Button hook (Fig. 8–11)	
*	*	Putting on socks		Sock aid (Fig. 8–12)	
*	*	Putting on shoes		Long-handled shoe horn, elastic laces, Velcro closure	
*	*	Getting clothes from closet bar		Lowered bar or shelf attachment	

(Continued)

Table 8–1 ADL Problems and Possible Solutions (Continued)

Function	Neurologic Problem		Disability	Adaptive Method	Adaptive Equipment	Comments
	Weakness	Ataxia				
Hygiene	*	*	Getting off commode		Grab bars	
	*	*	Getting out of bathtub or shower; tiring when bathing		Grab bars; bath bench with seat, hand-held shower hose (Fig. 8–13)	
	*	*	Dropping soap		Bath mitt (Fig. 8–14); soap on a rope	
	*	*	Bathing feet		Long-handled sponge (Fig. 8–14)	
	*		Holding toothbrush		Built-up handle	
	*	*	Not fully brushing teeth		Electric toothbrush	
	*	*	Washing hand or arm		Suction brush (Fig. 8–14)	
	*		Clipping finger or toe nails		Adapted nail clipper (Fig. 8–15)	
	*	*	Dropping razor or cutting self		Electric rather than straight edge razor	

Miscellaneous

		Equipment
*	Writing	Typewriter, built-up writing tool, pencil grip (Fig. 8–16), ball-bearing feeder
*		Pencil grip, friction feeder, built-up writing tool
*	Picking up objects from floor	Reacher (Fig. 8–17)
*	Holding playing cards	Playing card holder (Fig. 8–16)
*	Turning pages	Electric page turner
		Pencil eraser to turn pages
*	Holding a book for reading	Book holder
*	Cutting with scissors	Loop scissors (Fig. 8–16)
*	Dialing a phone	Phone adapters (Fig. 8–16)

* Indicates principal causes of functional disability. Suggested adaptive methods or equipment is found by reading across the table.

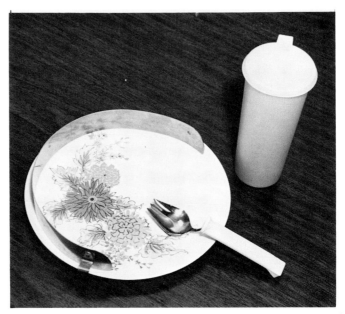

Figure 8-8 Adapted eating equipment. *(From left to right)* Plate guard, which assists in getting food onto the utensil; spork, which enables use of only one utensil; tupperware tumbler with spout lid to prevent spills.

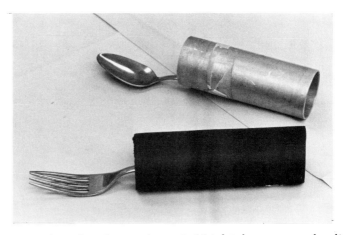

Figure 8-9 Adapted eating equipment. Metal tube spoon and cylindrical foam around utensil are both used to compensate for poor grasp.

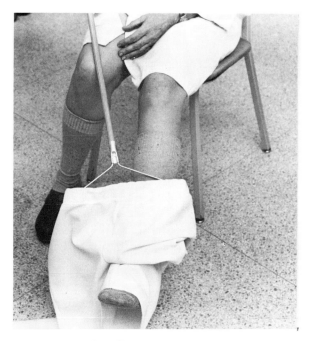

Figure 8-10   Pants spreader allows patient to put on pants without trunk flexion.

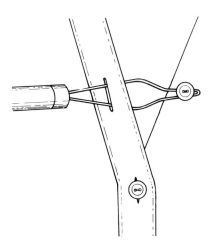

Figure 8-11   A button hook alleviates the most common difficulty in dressing encountered by MS patients.

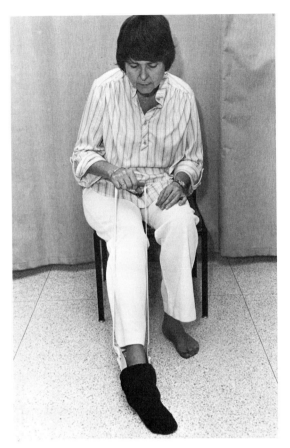

Figure 8–12 Sock aide allows increased functional ability in putting on socks.

Homemaking

OT treatment for the MS patient includes a comprehensive homemaking instruction program. All aspects of homemaking are considered. To supplement the instruction, patients are given a manual called *A Guide for the Homemaker with Multiple Sclerosis*. Homemaking tasks are divided into ten areas:

1. General rules — work simplification and energy conservation
2. Grocery shopping
3. General shopping
4. Laundry
5. Kitchen organization
6. Cooking

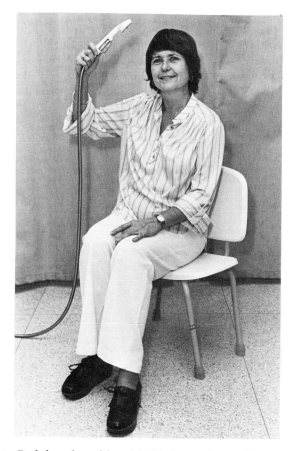

Figure 8–13 Bath bench and hand-held shower hose allow increased function, safety, and accessibility in bathing activities.

7. Washing dishes
8. Housecleaning
9. Entertaining
10. Child care

Instruction is given in each area with suggestions of alternate methods and adaptive equipment as needed. Frequent suggestions include planning a grocery list, shopping once a week or once every two weeks, stocking up on frequently used items, and purchasing manageable-size containers. Patients should also make a kitchen floor plan and rearrange items for practicality and accessibility. The patient may need to learn to stabilize a pot on the stove by placing a tea kettle behind it (Fig. 8–18), to use a spoon for pull tabs (Fig. 8–19), and to buy a dishwasher, microwave oven, or an electric can opener.

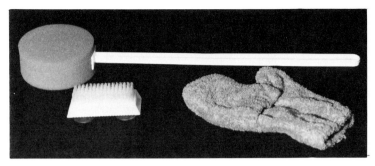

Figure 8-14 Adapted bathing equipment. *(From left to right)* Long-handled sponge allows MS patient to bathe without completely bending over to reach feet; suction brush compensates for inability to wash hands or arms; bath mitt reduces problem of dropping soap while bathing.

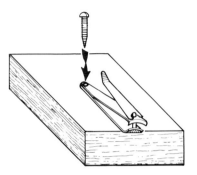

Figure 8-15 Adapted nail clipper increases MS patient's functional ability in hygiene activities.

Adaptive equipment can include plastic turntables, sliding drawers (Fig. 8-20), lid storage racks (Fig. 8-21), or can and bottle holders for the refrigerator. All are available in hardware or drug stores. A kitchen utility cart, wheelchair lap tray, adapted cutting board (Fig. 8-22), Tupperware paper-foil dispenser, or dycem or jar opener (Fig. 8-23) may be needed. Patients are taught to plan parties well in advance and to use prepared deli platters, precooked foods, paper plates, and plastic forks. The book *Mealtime Manual for the Aged and Handicapped* (see Suggested Readings) is an excellent reference for patients to obtain. House cleaning should be spread over several days and patients should learn to group tasks that require the same equipment or are located in the same area. For child care, a soft baby carrier and a baby bathtub seat (Fig. 8-24) are often a must. Homemaking is an important part of daily life and its remediation is an important aspect of the OT program for the MS patient.

(text continues on p. 127)

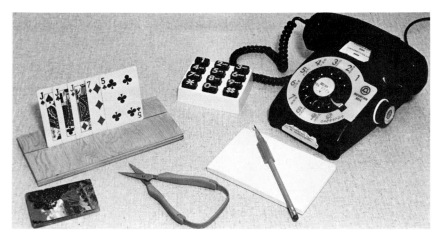

Figure 8–16 Miscellaneous adaptive equipment. *(From left to right)* Playing-card holder enables an individual to participate in a card game without holding the cards; loop scissors allows for independence in cutting when strength or coordination is impaired; pencil grip increases one's functional ability to write; phone adapters allow accuracy in dialing in those with impaired vision or coordination.

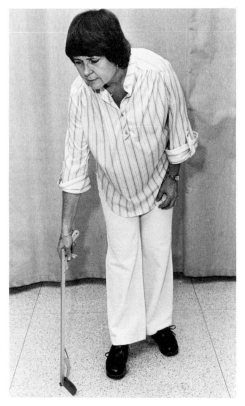

Figure 8–17 Long-handled reacher allows patients with poor balance or those confined to a wheelchair to pick up objects from the floor.

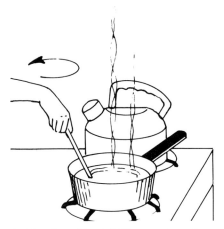

Figure 8-18 A tea kettle placed to stabilize a pot on the stove. Only one hand is then needed for stirring.

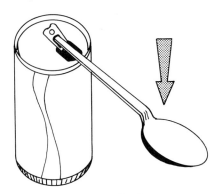

Figure 8-19 Using a spoon to open a pull tab.

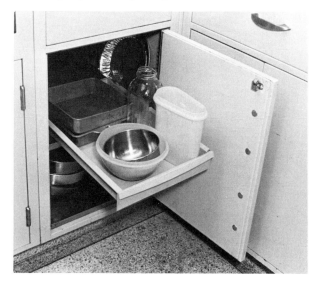

Figure 8-20 Sliding cabinet drawer increases kitchen accessibility.

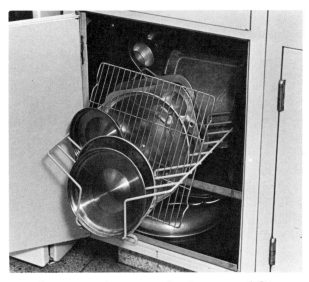

Figure 8-21   Lid storage rack increases kitchen accessibility.

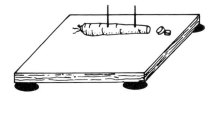

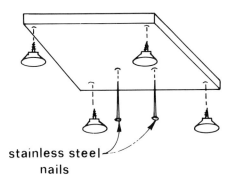

stainless steel
nails

Figure 8-22   Adaptation of a cutting board increases functional ability in cooking tasks.

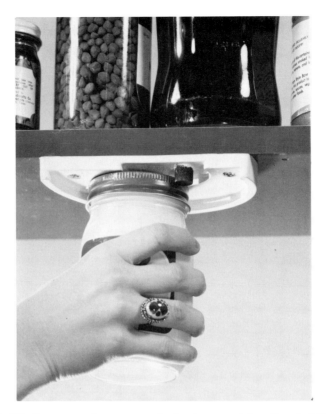

Figure 8–23 Jar opener to compensate for decreased functional ability in the upper extremities. (Courtesy of H. Hutson, Denver, Colorado)

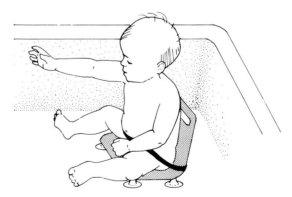

Figure 8–24 Baby bath seat allows the MS mother to bathe a baby in a tub without holding the child for an extended period of time.

Vocational Management

Many people with MS continue to work at either full-time or part-time jobs and may require assistance in adapting the work environment to suit individual needs. A major problem is the accessibility of buildings and restrooms. Reducing an MS patient's walking distance by changing parking spaces may eliminate work problems related to fatigue. On-site visits may be needed to aid the patient in positioning office furniture and supplies to the best advantage. If the patient can no longer work at a current job, an OT consultation may be helpful to the employer in placing the individual in a different position within the same company. Where adaptations are not successful, patients should be referred to vocational rehabilitation (see Chap. 28).

Wheelchairs

The use and prescription of wheelchairs and other mobility aids will be discussed in detail in Chapter 25. The MS patient must be provided with a well-fitted wheelchair, designed to meet specific needs. Three types of MS patients use wheelchairs:

Patients who are ambulatory but require a wheelchair for long distances because of fatigue

Patients who use a wheelchair for all activities

Patients who are transported by others

The requirements for a wheelchair are different in all three cases and each patient needs to be evaluated individually.

Summary

A comprehensive OT program can result in improvement in life quality for the MS patient. Patients can learn to decrease fatigue through energy-conservation and work-simplification techniques. Strength and coordination can be maintained and improved. New methods of performing activities of daily living can be learned and the use of adaptive equipment can promote independent functioning. Homemaking and vocational tasks can be simplified. Through comprehensive evaluation and an individually designed treatment program, the occupational therapist can make a positive impact on the MS patient's quality of life.

Suggested Readings

BAILEY JT: Stress and stress management: An overview. Journal of Nursing Education 19:5–7, June, 1980

DUNCAN CW: Coping with stress. Day Care and Early Education 7:18–21, Spring, 1980

HALE G (ed): Source Book for the Disabled. London, Imprint Books, 1979

GERSTEN JW, CENKOVICH FS, DINKEN H, et al: Evaluation of rehabilitation in home or clinic setting: Problems in methodology. Arch Phys Med Rehabil 47:199–203, 1966

JEBSEN RH, TRIESCHMAN R, TROTTER J, et al: An objective and standardized test of hand function. Arch Phys Med Rehabil 50:311–319, 1969

JOHNSTONE M: Restoration of Motor Function in the Stroke Patient: A Physiotherapist's Approach. New York, Churchill-Livingstone, 1978

KLINGER JL, FRIEDEN FH, SULLIVAN RA: Mealtime Manual for the Aged and Handicapped. Essanders Special Editions. New York, Simon & Schuster, 1970

WILLARD HS, SPACKMAN CS: Occupational Therapy. Philadelphia, JB Lippincott, 1963

WOLF BG,: A Guide for the Homemaker with Multiple Sclerosis, 2nd ed. Denver, University of Colorado Health Sciences Center, Department of PM&R and RMMSC, 1983

9

Nancy Ruttenberg

Assessment and Treatment of Speech and Swallowing Problems in Patients With Multiple Sclerosis

This chapter provides a comprehensive framework for the speech/language pathologist's role as a member of the Multiple Sclerosis (MS) rehabilitation team. Practical methods of evaluating, treating, and educating patients and their families are presented. These approaches are guided by the five basic principles that underlie any rehabilitation effort; early intervention, compensations, purposeful activity, self-monitoring, and motivation. Education begins during the evaluation and continues throughout treatment.

The wide spectrum of potential symptoms in patients with MS requires an eclectic approach. Because of the unpredictable course of MS, not all patients need to be seen by the speech/language pathologist. However, approximately one-third of the MS population has symptoms of dysarthria, dysphagia, or impaired cognition. These patients should be referred for evaluation regardless of the severity of their symptoms. Language disorders are rarely a feature of MS.

Assessment

The purpose of the assessment is to identify specific problems, classify the severity of symptoms, and delineate the patient's awareness and understanding in each problem area. Because remissions, exacerbations, and progression of symptoms are common in MS, the patients serve as their own baseline.

The clinical speech/swallowing and mental status assessment can be accomplished in approximately one hour. Best results are obtained with a well-rested patient. After reviewing the medical chart, a brief history from the patient and family will provide insight into their perceptions of

129

the patient's symptoms. If the patient's speech is unintelligible use questions that can be answered with a "yes" or "no" or one of the many augmentative communication systems.

An oral peripheral examination will assess the adequacy of the oral–facial structures and their functioning (Table 9–1). During testing, specific attention should be given to strength, coordination, tremor, and range and speed of motion of the observed structures. The equipment used for this examination is a flashlight, tongue blades, a tape recorder, and a stop watch.

The speech assessment includes an audio recording of (1) sustained phonation during "ah" and "e"; (2) counting on one breath; (3) reading of the "grandfather" passage; and (4) spontaneous conversation. (The latter may be obtained while taking the patient's history.) By using the audio recording, detailed and accurate assessment of the speech, vocal, temporal, and respiratory aspects of each patient's communication can be obtained. Large-print reading material with extra spaces between words and sentences is used for patients with visual deficits.

Results from the oral peripheral and swallowing assessments (see

Table 9–1 Structure and Function of the Oral Peripheral Mechanism

Structures	Functions
Mandible	Symmetry–rest/motion Alternating depression/elevation
Lips	Symmetry–rest/motion Closure/rounding/retraction Rounding with resistance Retraction with resistance Alternating rounding/retraction
Tongue	Symmetry on protrusion Protrusion with/without resistance Retraction Elevation/depression Licking lips Lateralize to corners
Palate(s) and pharynx (cough)	Observe shape Symmetry at rest/during "ah" Gag reflex/cough reflex/volitional cough
Facial (sensation)	Lower face (from nose down) Inside mouth Consistent or intermittent loss (need patients input)
Oral (diadokokinesis)	Pa-pa-pa/1 breath Ta-ta-ta/1 breath Ka-ka-ka/1 breath Pa-ta-ka/1 breath

Swallowing Assessment, below) dictate which foods should be used for the feeding evaluation. Depending on the severity of the patient's dysphagia, water, nectar, peaches, and crackers may be selectively employed. Taste evaluation is obtained on those patients with severely delayed swallowing function (see Fig. 9–3 for the recommended positioning of the patient during the evaluation).

SWALLOWING ASSESSMENT

Patient's description of swallowing problem _____
Duration _____ .
History of choking episodes: daily/weekly? _____
Current method of intake — oral vs tube feeding _____ .
Motor control
   Neck – head – mandible – lips – tongue – saliva control
   Timing of swallow reflex (delayed or not); timing of volitional swallow (delayed or not)

When administering the mental status screening (see below), observe for processing delays, impulsivity or delayed responses, need for reptition of instructions, and patient reauditorization. If language, cognitive, or memory deficits are suspected, further language or neuropsychologic testing is recommended.

MENTAL STATUS SCREENING

Orientation: Day _____ Month _____ Year _____ Place (city, state, clinic name) _____
   Clinicians Name _____
Short-term memory: 3 words in 5 minutes
                   Ability to recall a short story with details
Left/right orientation: (eyes opened) on self and others
Ability to follow commands: 1 to 4 units in length. Was sequence intact?
Proverbs: Concrete response _____ Abstract response _____

A checklist is advised for documentation of the initial findings. Patients with progressive forms of MS are reevaluated every 3 to 6 months depending on the course of their disease and the severity of symptoms. The same protocol and form should be used for successive evaluations to facilitate quick comparisons to previous results.

Clinical Problems

Frequently missed manifestations of fatigue can be a reduction in overall speech intelligibility and the magnification of existing dysarthric features, such as imprecise articulation, loudness decay, monotone, or low pitch. The probable causes are excessive exertion of the speech musculature and the inefficient use or poor coordination of the respiratory system. Prevention of avoidable fatigue will help reduce potential fear and guilt by the patient and his family. The patient should be assisted in recognizing his specific manifestations of fatigue. Offer suggestions on how a patient can more efficiently balance rest with activity related to communication and swallowing.

The goal in MS rehabilitation is to maintain function with a minimal amount of effort. Treatment should emphasize energy conservation to help minimize muscle fatigue. Abdominal breathing exercises to improve airflow is a common starting point. Applied resistance to the rib cage and abdominal wall, with care not to trigger spasticity, is helpful. Next, an audible breathy sigh is incorporated during exhalation. Words of increasing length are systematically introduced, working toward sentences. The patient is then taught to reduce phrase length and to pause between words and phrases. These techniques are beneficial in obtaining increased muscle mileage.

SPASTICITY

Dysarthria in MS may be totally or partially due to spasticity. Spastic dysarthria can involve, to varying degrees, all five processes of motor speech production: respiration, phonation, resonance, articulation, and prosody. Hypertonicity is the primary factor that interferes with speech production. Spasticity interferes with coordination and the delicate balance of the precise range of movements necessary for normal speech (Darley et al, 1975). The speech produced has a strained/strangled quality which is low pitched, harsh, and hypernasal, and accompanied by consonant imprecision. Spasticity of the respiratory and neck muscles can often be inhibited during therapy by positioning and exercise techniques. The speech/language pathologist should learn these techniques. If for any reason positioning cannot be adequately accomplished, then physical therapy should precede speech therapy. Treatment will be discussed in the Section on dysarthria, below.

ATAXIA

Ataxia, as it relates to speech and swallowing, is generally manifested by motor inaccuracy, slowness of movement, intention tremor, and hypotonia. Ataxic dysarthria, if present, may show variable features. Symptoms may include imprecise articulation, slow rate, vowel distortion, equal syllabic stress within words, or sentences accompanied by inappropriate silent intervals (scanning speech). Treatment will be discussed in the dysarthria section, below.

The normal timing and sequence of the automatic swallowing rhythm are also affected by ataxia. An intention tremor is the most obvious clinical manifestation. Medications may reduce the severity of the tremor and should be discussed with the patient's physician. Continued independent self-feeding depends on the provision of a stable body position to inhibit intention tremor.

Choking may occur secondary to muscle weakness and inappropriate motor sequencing. Aspiration can be avoided by maintaining neck flexion of at least 45 degrees. A soft cervical collar cut out at the laryngeal area to allow neck flexion can be used for neck stabilization (see Fig. 8–7).

DYSARTHRIA

Dysarthia results when damage affects the neuromuscular control of one or more of the five processes of motor speech. Dysarthric speech patterns, if present, vary in clinical presentation and severity. Although the "mixed dysarthria" frequently seen in MS may not show a consistent pattern, imprecise articulation, vocal harshness, weak phonation, inappropriate stress, and reduced speech rate are common characteristics of the dysarthria in MS, irrespective of the site of the lesion.

Therapy includes education, supportive counseling, and practical management. The goals of treatment are (1) to maintain functional verbal or nonverbal communications skills and (2) to aim therapeutic techniques toward energy conservation. Patients with relapsing/remitting MS have a greater potential for improving their dysarthric speech than do patients with chronic progressive MS for two important reasons. First, patients rarely exhibit cognitive deficits; and second, their symptoms often recover or improve.

The clinician and patient should agree on the therapeutic goals during the first treatment session. The proposed sequence of therapy and a brief background explanation of the five processes of motor speech show the patient his specific needs.

The expectations of speech therapy must be pragmatic and consider the progressive nature of MS. The greatest potential for success lies in the application of compensatory techniques in the most timely and realistic manner. Patients with minimal speech deficits may not require continuous individual therapy. Written home programs that address the specific communication needs of the patient are frequently employed. These programs are designed to be both time- and cost-efficient.

Severely unintelligible patients with poor coordination of breath control and weak phonation fatigue easily when talking. For these patients, treatment begins with the determination of a comfortable and functional number of syllables per breath cycle by tests of monosyllabic words and phrases of increasing length. Next, the techniques of phrasing and pausing to facilitate a controlled exhalation per phrase are introduced. The patient is taught to pause between phrases for 2 to 3 seconds to relax the respiratory and speech musculatures. This pause provides sufficient time for inhalation in preparation for the next utterance and gives the listener time to decipher the message.

Loss of precise articulation, a key to intelligibility, is evident with impairment of cranial nerves V, VII, and XII, which innervate the mandible, lips, and tongue. Consequently, these structures are unable to assume the appropriate phonemic position at a normal speaking rate. Therapy begins with oral exercises dependent on the type of structural impairment, reduced range of motion, or weakness of the articulating muscles. Once adequate range of motion is established, resistive force using a tongue blade may be applied to increase strength. All exercises should be done 2 separate times during each 30-minute therapy session. The patient should be instructed to do these exercises an additional 1 to 2 times daily. Next the patient is taught to develop a slow, deliberate speech rate, using optimal phrase lengths. The techniques of syllable-by-syllable separation, for example, "To-day-is-Tues-day," and overarticulation of middle and final consonants in polysyllabic words and phrases are practiced.

Impaired prosodic features such as loudness, intonation, timing, and word emphasis interfere with all elements of speech output. Once the patient has developed the ability to speak in reduced phrase lengths, impaired prosodic features are treated. Experience has shown that impaired loudness and emphasis respond more favorably to treatment than do timing and intonation.

Stress drills are employed to facilitate functional changes. Recordings and the view meter of a recorder are helpful for self-monitoring. Two or three monosyllabic words are used first. Plosives are avoided because they produce excessive laryngeal tension for severely impaired patients. Treatment progresses to functional polysyllabic words and then to practice variations of words in the same phrase. For example, "*I* am tired," "I *am* tired," and "I am *tired*." At first the intended meaning will be lost, but the patient will have the experience of producing the target behavior in all positions in a sentence. Later, key words are practiced within a sentence that readily conveys the intended meaning.

Multiple sensory feedback enhances the likelihood of success in a patient's altering his speech pattern. Sensory biofeedback equipment and oscilloscopes with colored tracings are used in some centers to assist patients.

Determination of environmental barriers that may interfere with communication should be a part of all dysarthria evaluation and treatment. The patient should be encouraged to educate his listeners to assume responsibility to ensure effective communication by (1) active listening, (2) eye contact, (3) closeness to the speaker, (4) repeating and rephrasing, and (5) elimination of background noise.

In some cases an alternative to verbal communication is necessary and can be used in conjunction with speaking. The astute speech/language pathologist should recognize the potential need for augmentation early in treatment. Presentation of the system should be in a natural progresssion working toward functional communication and should avoid connotations of failure. The MS patient with adequate vision, memory, cognition, and upper extremity function has a better prognosis for such systems as the Canon Communicator or the Vocaid. Other styles of nonverbal communication use picture, letter, and sentence communication boards (notebooks) or a combination of these. The family and patient should assist in the design of these boards. All health-care team members are encouraged to use the patient's augmentative communication system to help the patient feel more comfortable with this style of communicating.

DYSPHAGIA

Varying degrees of swallowing difficulty may occur in patients with MS. Cranial nerve damage (to nerves V, VII, IX, X, and XII), spasticity, ataxia, and muscle weakness (such as neck flexors and respiratory, lingual, and laryngeal muscles) contribute to dysphagia in MS. Remissions and exacerbations of dysphagic symptoms are common.

The principle therapy goals are the prevention of choking and aspiration, the maintenance of weight, and the facilitation of independent feeding and swallowing.

The speech/language pathologist assesses swallowing function (see Assessment, above), designs and implements the individual swallowing program, and informs the team members about the program. As treatment advances, the nursing staff and family members are taught to assume increasing responsibility for feeding with periodic program re-evaluations by the speech/language pathologist.

Normal swallowing, whether initiated reflexively or consciously, relies on an intricate, sequential coordinated, sensorimotor reflex action (Fig. 9-1). The oral stage of swallowing is volitional and begins once food has passed through the lips. The lips close while the tongue and cheek muscles manipulate the bolus of food for chewing. With the bolus on the tongue, the tongue tip raises to the alveolar ridge and then propels the bolus into the oropharynx. The soft palate elevates, barring reflex into the nasopharynx. The intricate pharyngeal stage performs two primary functions, both of which are reflexive: propulsion of the bolus toward the esophagus and protection of the airway from aspiration. Finally, the reflexive esophageal stage passes the bolus from the esophagus into the stomach through involuntary peristaltic action (Fig. 9-2A–F). Deglutition takes 5 to 10 seconds to complete. The oral and pharyngeal stages take 1 second each, whereas the esophageal stage takes 3 to 7 seconds (Dobie, 1978).

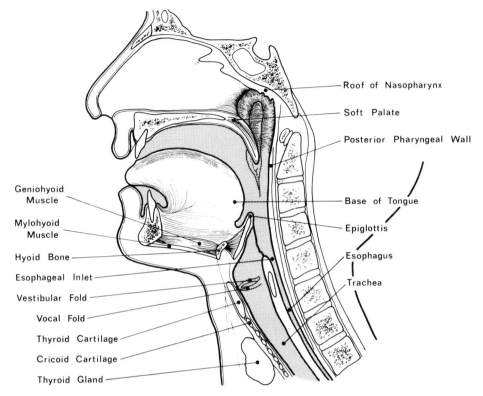

Roof of Nasopharynx

Soft Palate

Posterior Pharyngeal Wall

Base of Tongue

Epiglottis

Esophagus

Trachea

Geniohyoid Muscle

Mylohyoid Muscle

Hyoid Bone

Esophageal Inlet

Vestibular Fold

Vocal Fold

Thyroid Cartilage

Cricoid Cartilage

Thyroid Gland

Figure 9-1 Structures of swallowing. Mouth and pharynx at rest. (Redrawn from Dobie RA: Rehabilitation of swallowing disorders. Am Fam Physician, May 1978. Published by the American Academy of Family Physicians)

Treatment for dysphagia in MS focuses on the patient's environment, body position, style of eating, and types of food and liquid eaten. Treatment should begin with patient education with regard to his specific deficits and an emphasis of the concept to "think swallow." The latter encourages cortical control rather than reflexive swallowing.

The environment must be free of distractions. Patients should concentrate only on swallowing. Verbal cues are useful to facilitate cortical control.

The patient's body position is crucial, and for mild or intermittent dysphagia adjustment of body position may be the only measure required to eliminate the problem. Aspiration may be prevented if the patient is in a seated position with the head flexed. This position allows the bolus easy entry into the esophagus and the trachea is protected with the back of the tongue (Fig. 9–3). The initiation and maintenance of neck flexion is difficult for patients with intention tremors, spasticity, or neck muscle weakness. Pillows or the application of steady deep

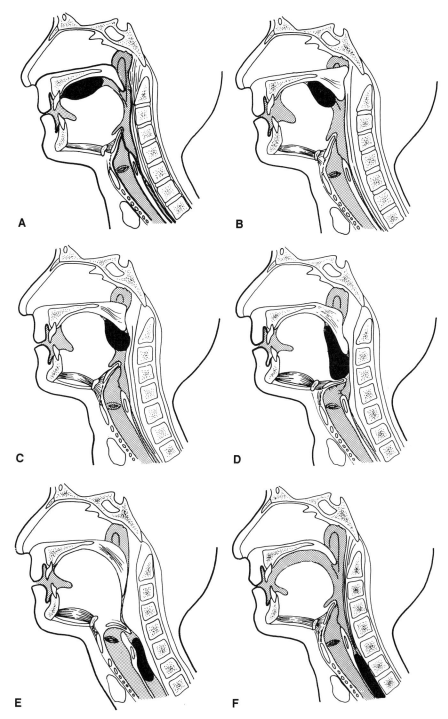

Figure 9-2 Sequence of swallowing: (A) stage 1: early oral phase; (B) stage 1: late oral phase; (C) stage 2: early pharyngeal phase; (D) stage 2: middle pharyngeal phase; (E) stage 2: late pharyngeal phase; and (F) stage 3: esophageal phase. (Redrawn from Dobie RA: Rehabilitation of swallowing disorders. Am Fam Physician, May 1978. Published by the American Academy of Family Physicians)

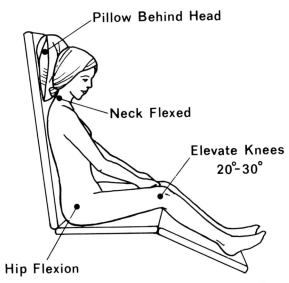

Figure 9–3 Recommended positioning for evaluation and treatment of patients with swallowing dysfunction. This can be modified according to patient's needs.

pressure to the head during flexion may stabilize the patient. Unnecessary shoulder or chest motion interferes with effective swallowing and should be avoided. Absent or diminished gag reflexes may result in aspiration of saliva. Treatment begins with the stimulation of the sucking reflex, using small amounts of water from an ice cube. Water frozen in a paper cup is more manageable than a cube. The patient is taught to swallow by consciously pocketing the liquid in his tongue, holding the liquid for 1 to 2 seconds to gain control, "think swallow," and then swallow.

Insufficient saliva is common in MS. Sucking on ice, a lemon glycerin swab, or a popsicle will stimulate saliva production. Imaging favorite foods or providing aromatic food smells may also be helpful. If excessive saliva is a problem, the patient is taught to swallow more frequently and to practice conscious swallowing every hour. Applying ice to the tongue and to the laryngeal area of the neck for 3 to 5 seconds with application of deep pressure on the neck above the thyroid notch facilitates a muscular response to encourage swallowing.

Thin liquids are very difficult to swallow. Water, juice, and mucus-producing milk products should be avoided. Tepid water is possibly the most difficult for patients to swallow because it lacks substance, taste, and texture, and slides into the pharynx too quickly for management by patients with decreased oral sensation or diminished motor responses. Thick liquids such as slushes, sherbert, nondairy creamed soup, and blended drinks should be tried first, then progressing to thin liquids.

The amount of liquid may be controlled by presenting one sip at a time from a cup or flexible straw. The conscious swallowing sequence is taught. Patients with respiratory insufficiency should use a shortened straw, ½ to ¾ inch in length, to reduce energy output.

Food selection is based on the patient's chewing, swallowing skills and fatigue level. Treatment starts with semisoft moist foods rather than pureed food. Soft food stimulates the chewing reflex, which moistens food and makes swallowing easier. Pasta, boiled chicken with gravy, moist mashed potatoes, squash, and frozen jello are rich in taste, texture, and smell. Tough, dry, stringy, sticky, or crumbly foods are difficult to chew and swallow. Progression to more challenging foods that are visually appealing and rich in taste, texture, and smell stimulates the intact nerve receptors and facilitates the swallowing reflex. All health-care team members and family should be trained in the Heimlich maneuver to dislodge food if choking occurs.

Surgical placement of feeding tubes may be indicated if a practical degree of swallowing cannot be achieved. The common surgical procedures, cervical esophagostomy, gastrostomy, and jejunostomy, are reversible. Unilateral injection of Teflon into the vocal cord may be recommended to increase cord mass and protect the airway from aspiration. Swallowing therapy should continue, with emphasis on saliva control.

Simple, but often forgotten, measures can improve mealtime. Examples are slow deliberate chewing of single bites, the use of liquids to move food to the back of the mouth, and talking between, but not during, bites. If a visitor enters while a patient is chewing, have the patient raise his hand to indicate he cannot talk until he has swallowed. This simple environmental manipulation is worth practicing in therapy. Once a new style of eating is habituated, the MS patient often finds he can enjoy a more varied diet without the fear of choking. Because fatigue is a major problem in MS, patients should eat their larger meals in the morning. Many small meals throughout the day and rest periods before meals are also advised.

IMPAIRED RESPIRATION

Respiration is the foundation for speech production. Patients with progressive forms of MS may exhibit inefficient respiration that can affect their overall communication abilities. Talking may cause fatigue and loss of speech volume. If these deficits are severe, a referral to pulmonary medicine is advised. Physical therapy is often consulted when sustained breathing resistance during treatment is needed. A corset may be recommended. Further information about respiration may be found in the discussions on fatigue and dysarthia, above.

IMPAIRED COGNITION

Symptoms of cognitive deficits range from disorientation to reduced judgment and problem-solving skills. Impaired cognition is certainly not a common manifestation of MS but its prevalence deserves attention and clinical recognition.

Nelson and associates (1982) showed that patients with relapsing/remitting MS were not significantly different from controls on measures of a broad range of cognitive and sensorimotor abilities, but 75% of the chronic/progressive patients had cognitive deficits. The greatest differences between these two groups were seen on tests requiring complex problem solving, concept formation, and sequencing tasks.

As more neurologic functions become involved, patients' overall cortical efficiency may deteriorate. Therefore, all patients should be screened for cognitive impairments (see Assessment above). Patients who do not pass the screening should be referred for neuropsychological testing. Results are shared with the interdisciplinary team and family so that cognitive expectations are uniform and realistic.

Treatment techniques must be individualized. Strategies for learning are emphasized, and impaired memory, if present, also requires attention. Compensatory measures for impaired cognition or impaired memory can be taught, such as rehearsal strategies, visual and auditory imagery, associations, list making, preplanning of daily/weekly schedules, and, most importantly, teaching people to give the patient enough time to complete simple activities.

Patients with mild to moderate deficits are seen for formal treatment in the clinic. Severely impaired patients are treated by family education and counseling. Cognitive dysfunction is reviewed in general terms and then in relation to patients' specific deficits and cognitive limitations (i.e., poor decision making and poor judgment). These patients respond best to a routine environment, without imposing pressures. The keys to a successful interaction between the patient and his family are an emphasis on the need for preplanning and providing a realistic time allotment for all, even simple, activities.

IMPAIRED MEMORY

Impairment in short-term and immediate memory may occur periodically. The neuropsychologist and speech/language pathologist work together to evaluate a patient's memory function and its three components: information registration, retention, and recall.

Patients with relapsing/remitting MS who exhibit mild to moderate memory deficits are seen for formal therapy. Treatment can range from instruction and practice in learning strategies to facilitate memory function to working with a computer. Patients with severe memory deficits also exhibit cognitive dysfunction, which requires family education and counseling. Encourage the family to provide a simple, routine environment; otherwise, the patient may encounter frustration when minimal demands are placed on him. Strategies to facilitate recall, such as word associations and imagery, and encouragement of detailed descriptions of topics have proven helpful and provide positive educational experiences.

ALTERED BEHAVIOR

Family observations about behavioral changes should be addressed during each evaluation. Questions asked are "Is the patient talking less?"; "Is the patient eating less?"; "Does the patient ever refuse social interactions that inherently involve communication?"

Organic behavioral changes in progressive MS, such as emotional lability and inappropriate and uncontrolled laughing or crying, often occur when the focus is on a patient's limitation, and they can occur in any social context. Treatment is difficult and frustrating. One way to treat lability is to first recognize it for what it is and then acknowledge it to the patient. Downplay rather than focus on the patient's lability. They should be put at ease and the labile behavior worked through. A physical maneuver such as having the patient turn his head, raising a hand, or simply a change in the topic of discussion are suggested distractors.

STRESS REACTIONS

The emotional impact of MS can be devastating to patients. The response to stress is highly individualized. Some patients may mask their emotional state by presenting signs of other problems. For example, during an instructional session patients who nod appropriately in agreement and even repeat and demonstrate tasks may forget everything by the next day. In such cases, stress rather than memory loss may be the cause. Recently diagnosed patients commonly manifest this reaction.

Summary

The speech/language pathologist working with MS patients must be optimistic and pragmatic. Understanding the individual patient's type of MS is vital for providing timely and appropriate counseling and treatment techniques. Care should be taken not to abandon efforts for improved speech intelligibility or to delay the introduction of augmentative approaches. These provide the patient with the ability to interact with others, a necessary trait for human functioning.

Dysphagic patients significantly benefit from the combined knowledge and appropriate treatment offered by the interdisciplinary rehabilitation team. Time must be taken to educate both the patient and his family toward the optimal strategies that may be utilized to improve swallowing function.

Suggested Readings

BERRY W, SANDARS S: Clinical Dysarthria. San Diego, College-Hill Press, 1983

BLOCK JM, KESTER NC: Role of rehabilitation in the management of multiple sclerosis. Modern Treatment 7:930–940, 1970

DARLEY FL, ARONSON AE, BROWN JF: Motor Speech Disorders. Philadelphia, WB Saunders, 1975

DARLEY FL, BROWN JR, GOLSTEIN NP: Dysarthria in multiple sclerosis. JSHR 15:229–245, 1972

DOBIE RA: Rehabilitation of swallowing disorders. AFP 17:84–95, 1978

FARMAKIDES MN, BOONE DR: Speech problems of patients with multiple sclerosis. JSHD 25:385–390, 1960

HARGROVE R: Feeding the severely dysphagic patient. Journal of Neurosurgical Nursing 12:102–107, 1980

LARSON GL: Rehabilitation for dysphagia paralytica. JSHD 37:187–194, 1972

NELSON LM, THOMPSON DS, HEATON RH, et al: Cognitive deficits in multiple sclerosis. Society for Neuroscience Abstract 8(2):629, 1982

NOSWORTHY SJ: A symposium on multiple sclerosis: Physiotherapy. Nursing Mirror 143:6:53–55, 1976

PERKINS WH (ed): Dysarthria and Apraxia. New York, Thieme-Stratton, 1983

SILVERMAN F: Communication for the Speechless. Englewood Cliffs, NJ, Prentice-Hall, 1983

VANDERHEIDEN G, GRILLEY K (eds): Non-Vocal Communication Techniques and Aids for the Severely Physically Handicapped. Baltimore, University Park Press, 1976

ZIMMERMAN JE, ODER LA: Swallowing dysfunction in acutely ill patients. Phys Ther 61:1755–1763, 1981

10

Emmajean Amrhein

Nursing Management
of Multiple Sclerosis

Traditionally the nurse has considered multiple sclerosis (MS) as a hopeless disease of young people. A better understanding of the disease and a working concept of the health-care team can provide the nurse with means to assist the patient with MS to effectively cope with many of the obstacles encountered during the disease process.

For each MS patient, specific nursing-care problems should be identified and a "problem solution plan" implemented within the team framework. The nurse often provides the vital link between the symptoms the patient presents to the physician and what is really bothering the patient about his disease. Although the treatment for specific symptoms may not change the natural course of the disease, the effects of MS on a patient's daily living may be even more important in the long term. The nurse can be the most effective team member in dealing with many of the practical problems of the patient's treatment.

Evaluation

Most nurses encounter the MS patient when he has been admitted to the hospital for diagnostic testing, a recent loss of function, infection, an acute exacerbation, or extensive rehabilitation. The principles of nursing management apply equally to nurses encountering the MS patient in a clinic or home situation. During the initial admission process the nurse identifies and assesses the nursing needs of the patient in the hospital and at home to develop a comprehensive nursing care plan.

The first step in defining problems is to obtain a history from the patient, family, or significant other, including the following:

1. The patient's perception of his disease and how the disease is affecting him
2. The purpose of and the results the patient expects from the hospitalization
3. The significant previous illnesses and hospitalizations, including problems the patient experienced
4. The patient's emotional status (recent changes in behavior with an understanding of the factors involved in these changes)
5. The patient's impairment of mobility (assistive devices, recent problems)
6. The activities of daily living (ADL), such as recent changes in the patient's eating pattern and habits, bladder and bowel habits, sleep patterns
7. The medications the patient is currently taking and associated problems
8. The patient's support systems (family, significant other, friends) and how the MS affects the others in the support system
9. The environmental and home situation of the patient (housing, economic conditions, involvement of any agencies)
10. The educational background and occupation of the patient and how employment has been affected by MS

The examination done by the nurse focuses on problems with cognitive and memory functioning, speech, and vision. The physical assessment provides the necessary baseline data, such as the status of skin care, measurement of vital signs, and results of a nursing neurologic examination.

After the data is gathered, a priority list of problems should be initiated, including the expected outcomes or goals. The short-term goals must be specific, realistic, and individualized to assist the patient in meeting his needs. The long-term goals need to be achievable to prevent the patient from experiencing a sense of helplessness. The goals may need to be modified later but the importance of goal setting should not be discarded because of the unpredictability of the disease.

Self-Care Dependency

The traditional role of the nurse as primarily a provider of service should be modified in the case of MS to focus on assisting the patient in developing and maintaining a productive, independent, and satisfying lifestyle. The newly diagnosed patient commonly becomes depressed or denies his disease. This period is usually temporary and should not alarm the care-givers.

The nurse must identify, confront, and deal with her own feelings about the disease before being able to give support to the patient during an adjustment period. Unnecessary misconceptions can be eliminated if the nurse takes the time to listen to the patient's concerns and frustrations.

A patient's sense of control over his life is enhanced through his participation in his own care. Positive recognition by others is essential when the patient successfully performs even the slightest exercise or task.

Fatigue

Fatigue intensifies the other symptoms related to MS and *vice versa*. Terms often used by patients to describe fatigue are "exhaustion," "weakness," "lack of energy," and "tiredness." Although the patient may initially ignore his fatigue, with disease progression the problem becomes increasingly important in the provision of care.

In the hospital, fatigue can be observed after therapy sessions, during meals, or in stressful situations. The patient should be assisted in recognizing the fatigue as it occurs.

A log kept by the patient to identify the signs and symptoms of fatigue during activities is valuable for the readjustment of activities. The patient should be encouraged to establish short, frequent rest periods within his daily lifestyle at the first sign of fatigue. Although limiting some activities may be necessary to prevent becoming overly fatigued, the patient must understand that immobility for long periods of time can cause disuse atrophy and weakness as well as medical difficulties such as decubitus ulcers, atelectasis, and edema.

Spasticity

Spasticity in MS frequently interferes with the ability to perform activities of daily living (ADL). The nurses and therapists work together to ensure that the nurse carries through the plan developed in therapy sessions and the patient independently performs the exercises correctly while in the hospital. The patient's home-care providers participate in the exercises before the patient leaves the hospital. Range-of-motion exercises to prevent contractures are performed daily in the hospital (Chap. 7).

Antispasticity medications such as baclofen (Lioresal), diazepam (Valium), and dantrolene (Dantrium) may be prescribed. The nurse should observe for any side-effects such as lethargy, weakness, dizziness, ataxia, or gastrointestinal distress and inform the physician as soon as possible if the symptoms occur. The patient and his home support system should understand the drugs prescribed, including dosage, frequency, and side-effects, in preparation for discharge. The visiting nurse should be cognizant of specifics of the home therapy and medications.

Ataxia

Assisting the ataxic or incoordinated patient to function independently can be accomplished on the nursing unit by initiating a wide-based, slow walking rate. When possible, the patient is allowed to ambulate with limited supervision. However, if the patient tends to fall or trip, the nurse should discuss the situation with the physician, therapist, and other team members.

Transfers from the bed to a wheelchair can be made easier if the wheels of the hospital bed are removed. This modification also protects the care-givers and patient from injury.

Assistive devices such as canes, walkers, or weights are necessary as tremors worsen. The patient will need help initially on the unit when using assistive devices. However, when he is able to perform specific tasks alone, the entire team should acknowledge the achievement, which will foster a sense of achievement (see Chaps. 7 and 8).

Dysarthria

Verbal communication problems can lead to overwhelming distress for the MS patient. The nurse can assume an active role in helping the patient adjust to speech problems. Specifically, the nurse should listen intently to the patient when he is trying to speak. Provision of positive reinforcement for successful communication decreases the patient's frustration.

The nurse should work closely with the speech/language pathologist to assist in implementing the therapist's program. Most patients with speech problems need to be encouraged to speak slowly and use short phrases or single words (see Chap. 9). Alphabet and language boards can be made inexpensively for more severe cases. The effectiveness of the boards depends on the patient's ability to point. Symbols for the board should be large and have an identifiable meaning for the patient.

Eye blinking for "yes" and "no" questions is another effective method used for communication. Documentation in the care plan of the number of blinks the patient uses for indicating "yes" and "no" is necessary to provide consistency among the team members.

Dysphagia

An initial evaluation by the speech/language pathologist provides the staff with information about the severity and limitations of the dysphagia. Suggestions resulting from this evaluation will help the nursing staff to teach the patient swallowing techniques (see Chap. 9).

The occupational or speech therapist initially assists the patient during mealtime. The nursing staff must understand the new program and help evaluate its effectiveness (see Chap. 8).

The dietitian, depending on the nutritional status of the patient, keeps an accurate calorie count of the food intake of the patient. These data provide necessary information in evaluating the dietary needs of the patient. If the patient is not receiving adequate nutrition, other means must be provided, such as gastrostomy feedings (see Chaps. 5 and 23).

The nursing staff may need to reinforce a variety of factors determined to be important by the therapist and dietitian.

1. The patient should be placed in an upright position (high Fowler unless contraindicated) while eating.
2. Initially all distractions should be removed, including television, noise, or high-stress environment.
3. The patient should be encouraged to eat slowly.
4. The patient must concentrate on coordinating swallowing with breathing.
5. Sufficient amounts of protein, vitamins, and fluids are necessary.

The nurse should be available initially during mealtimes to observe for any possible choking or coughing. The team should acknowledge the patient's accomplishment of independent feeding.

Impaired Respiration

When the patient becomes immobile, respiratory complications can occur unless preventive measures are taken. A daily nursing assessment includes the observation of the rate and the quality of respirations, auscultation of breath sounds, and an awareness of relevant laboratory values, such as arterial blood gases.

When undesirable changes in respiratory status occur, the patient should be turned and encouraged to cough and deep breathe at least every 2 hours. Postural drainage, with percussion and vibration, will loosen any secretions. If a hospitalized patient is unable to cough effectively, oral or nasotracheal suctioning is necessary following each treatment. If the patient requires suctioning at home, instruction should be initiated immediately (Chap. 19).

Breathing exercises can easily be done during rest periods to promote relaxation. Mechanical breathing devices are available to stimulate deep breathing. The incentive spirometer is the most effective mechanical device because it encourages the patient to use his inspiratory muscles (Chap. 19). The patient and care-givers must be taught the rationale and techniques of respiratory therapy for home-care purposes.

Visual Impairment

Diplopia, nystagmus, and blurred vision often occur early in the course of the disease and are frequently the primary presenting symptom. The cranial nerves most often affected are the oculomotor and optic nerves.

The patient can prevent diplopia by alternating eye patches every 4 hours during waking hours. The nurse should discuss the problem of decreased depth perception before instituting the unilateral eye patch regimen. Fatigue frequently increases visual problems. Therefore, short rest periods incorporated into the daily schedule can be beneficial. For some visual problems, patients are advised to use magnifying glasses, "talking books," and large-type reading materials that can be obtained in libraries, bookstores, or through the local multiple sclerosis agency.

Decubitus Ulcers

Proper skin care is emphasized in the prevention of pressure sores. Skin care includes not only the alleviation of pressure over bony prominences (Fig. 10–1) but also the avoidance of subsequent damage from friction on or shearing of the skin surfaces. This shearing effect and subsequent rupture of capillaries determines the size of a pressure sore. Unfortunately, the tissue impairment from shearing can occur with or without pressure. Once the damage occurs no treatment can prevent the damage caused by clotting and stasis of the blood supply. Prophylactically, therefore, the care-giver should use turn sheets, heel pads, and a trapeze to prevent skin damage when patients are moved up or down or across a bed or chair.

There are four basic rules for treating decubitus ulcers:

1. Remove the potential causes (friction, pressure, moisture, chemical damage).
2. Debridement. All necrotic tissue or eschar must be removed before healing can occur.
3. Eradicate infection. Most pressure sores are contaminated but rarely infected.
4. Protect healthy tissue, and hydrate. This aspect is probably the most

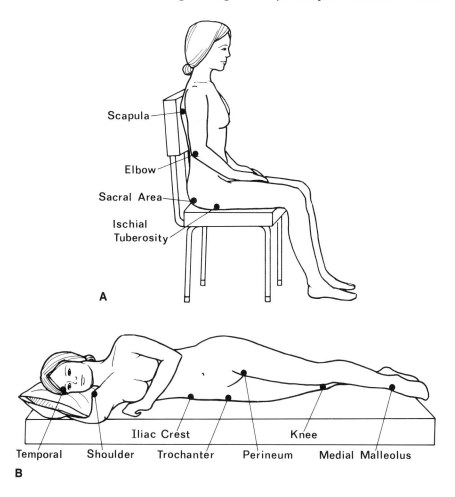

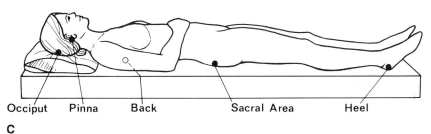

Figure 10–1 (A) Potential pressure areas in a sitting position; (B) potential pressure areas in a lateral position; and (C) potential pressure areas in a supine position.

important in promoting the healing process. An environment as close to normal conditions as possible must be maintained. Heat lamps and antacids are not always appropriate.

Among the many treatments that can be used are

Gelatin dressings
Film dressing
Ointments
Moist gauze (not "wet to dry")
Polyethylene oxide and water

Consistency in the treatment is important for long-term value. If the patient returns home before the pressure sores are completely healed, home nursing services are helpful in reinforcing the plan of care initiated in the hospital.

Although healing time cannot be accelerated, impediments to healing can be removed to enhance the healing process. The following can hinder healing:

Infection
Necrosis
Indiscriminatory "wet to dry" dressings
Excessive inflammation
Medications (steroids, wound detergents)
Hypoxia
Vascular insufficiency
Protein depletion
Concurrent illness
Malnutrition
Lack of moisture

All of these factors must be considered when initiating or evaluating the care plan.

Bladder Dysfunction

Frequency, urgency, retention, and incontinence are common urinary tract symptoms. A urologic nursing treatment plan is initiated, often in conjunction with the urologist's evaluation, with emphasis on specific patient needs and prevention of infection (see Chap. 4).

Incontinence, if not treated properly, leads to major nursing-care problems, such as skin irritation and breakdown. A bedpan or urinal offered at least every 2 hours can eliminate some problems. External condoms for males and incontinent pads for females are used effectively to prevent embarrassment for the patient. The perineal area and bedding must be kept clean and dry.

Urinary tract infections are common in patients with urinary incontinence and must be treated appropriately to prevent recurrence and possible septicemia. The physician faces a major challenge in the judicious use of antibiotics.

Several voiding aids are used to help a patient with bladder frequency and urgency. Methods to stimulate bladder contractions includes Credé massage, pulling of pubic hair, digital stimulation, and pressure applied to the lower abdomen. The patient is then taught to void at timed intervals. To regulate the intervals, intake and output are documented carefully. The patient is encouraged to drink at least 3000 ml of fluids every 24 hours. More fluid intake during the day and less toward evening may prevent nocturnal incontinence.

The residual urine should be measured after the patient has voided. If there is no residual urine, timed voiding, if done consistently, is appropriate.

If urinary retention persists, neuropharmacologic agents specific to bladder dysfunctions may assist voiding. Eventually patients may need to learn intermittent self-catheterization. If the patient is physically unable to perform the procedure, a motivated member of his home support group can be taught the technique of catheterization.

Catheterizations are usually done at 4-hour intervals, but can be done up to every 6 hours. If done just before bedtime the procedure can be eliminated during sleep when there is no oral fluid intake.

The patient is given a step-by-step instruction sheet prior to being taught the actual procedure. For females, the nurse reviews the anatomical arrangement of the perineal area. The proper angle to hold the penis is reviewed with the male patient.

The equipment necessary for self-catheterization can be obtained inexpensively and includes

"Soft Soap" liquid, or a bar of mild soap, or towelettes (three for each catheterization)

Mentor female, male, or pediatric self-catheters are kept in a clean plastic bag, toothbrush holder, or clean container. (If the patient uses a plastic bag, it should be replaced daily. Containers such as toothbrush holders should be washed with soap and water daily)

Water-soluble lubricant

After the equipment is obtained, the patient is instructed to wash his hands and follow procedures:

1. The female patient is instructed to visualize, palpate, or feel her urethra. Once palpated, a finger is left in place at the urethra. Using her dominant hand, she is instructed to hold the catheter ½ inch from its tip and to insert the catheter straight into the urethra, next to her finger. (If the catheter enters the vagina, she has probably held the catheter too far away from its tip.) The catheter is inserted until urine flows (Fig. 10–2).

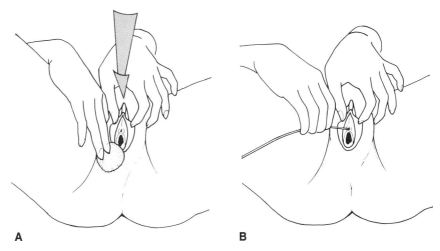

A   **B**

Figure 10-2   (A) Perineal area cleansing. The motion is downward from the urethral meatus toward the rectum in female patients to prevent bacterial contamination. (B) Proper positioning for catheter insertion in a female patient.

2. The male patient is instructed to lubricate his catheter (the last 2 inches from its tip) and then to insert the catheter into the urethra, using steady, gentle pressure, holding his penis erect to straighten the urethra. If resistance is met after partially inserting the catheter, continued gentle but firm pressure is used until the sphincter muscle relaxes and urine flows (Fig. 10-3).
3. Credé massage, straining, or changing position may increase urine flow.
4. The catheter is then removed slowly, stopping any time urine flows to ensure complete emptying of the bladder.
5. The patient then cleans and dries the perineal area with toilet paper or soap and water.
6. The catheter is then washed with soap-lathered hands, coiling the catheter between the hands. The catheter is rinsed with tap water, inside and out, dried, and stored in a plastic bag or other container.

The patient must understand that the procedure is considered a clean but not sterile technique. The educational process is not complete until the patient can perform the procedure successfully without assistance.

Bowel Dysfunction

Commonly, the MS patient experiences impairment of bowel function. Constipation and, less frequently, incontinence may occur as the disease progresses. Therefore, a bowel program should be implemented early in the course of the disease.

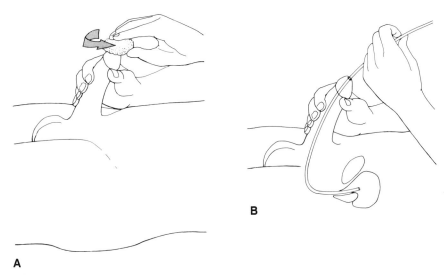

Figure 10 – 3   (A) Circular motion used to cleanse urethral meatus. (B) Proper positioning for catheter insertion in a male patient.

Questions in history taking range from the frequency of bowel movement to the time of day that bowel evacuation is more convenient. Additional assessment of dietary habits helps determine needed changes in fluid and roughage intake (see Chap. 5).

The characteristics of the stools are determined during the initial assessment. Observing whether the stools are hard or loose, have an unusual odor, or contain blood or mucus helps determine the most suitable bowel program.

Factors essential for proper bowel functioning are a well-balanced diet, an adequate fluid intake, and exercise. The nurse participates in meal planning with the patient to include foods that promote adequate bowel elimination.

The patient may receive oral or rectal laxatives depending on the elimination problems. To prevent chronic abuse, medications should not be considered until all other measures have been expended.

The nurse should help the patient establish a time for bowel elimination according to his lifestyle needs. The ideal time for most patients is usually just after breakfast or before bedtime. Enough time must be allowed to prevent the patient from being hurried. To prevent embarrassment, privacy must be provided in the hospital. If the patient is unable to use the bathroom, a commode chair next to the bed is sufficient. Proper positioning, with both feet on the floor, the knees bent, and body leaning forward, will be helpful (see Chap. 5).

If the stool becomes too hard because of a poor diet, insufficient fluid intake, and inadequate exercises, fecal impaction can occur. The nurse may need to provide manual stimulation or extraction of the stool from the rectum. The patient and those involved in the home support system should be taught this procedure.

Due to the loss of sensation or sphincter control, incontinence of stool may occur. The patient needs to be aware that every effort will be made to provide him some control of bowel functioning.

Whatever bowel program is appropriate, the nurse must work with the patient to ensure consistent follow-through. The visiting nurse can then implement the plan in the home setting.

Stress Reactions

The patient's psychological mechanism for dealing with physical and emotional disruptions in his life need to be understood.

The grieving process is likely to ensue when the diagnosis is discussed. Emotional support begins with the team allowing the patient to verbalize his feelings. The nurse must use effective communication skills, including active, attentive listening techniques. Through comfortable expression of his concerns and future goals, a patient is helped to form realistic goals in a positive manner.

The stresses that the MS patient experiences are similar to those of patients with other chronic diseases. Fear of the future is realistic. False reassurance must be discouraged, but pointing out improvements in function is helpful.

Family and others close to the patient should be encouraged to verbalize concerns. They can only help the patient when they are able to understand and accept the disease. If the patient's problems are not dealt with effectively by his home support system, isolation occurs.

A psychiatrist, psychologist, or social worker is often helpful in sorting out feelings associated with MS. The psychological support person can also provide valuable suggestions to the nursing staff caring for the patient (see Chaps. 11 and 21).

Hospital Discharge Planning

Proper hospital discharge planning is critical for the patient's successful transition to the home. The discharge process is often coordinated by the nurse in the health-care team. Conferences on patient care should be initiated well in advance to solve any problem issues the patient may have concerning going home. Home visits by the visiting nurse, therapists, and social worker before discharge often relieves the patient's fears concerning safety issues.

Patient education checklists ensure that information about MS is provided to the patient. The nurse ensures that medication information, a dietary plan, bowel and bladder regimens, and home therapy are

University of Colorado Health Sciences Center
University Hospital
Department of Nursing Service

Teaching Standards

Multiple Sclerosis

Pt. = Patient

Date initiated   9/4/83 SJ

S.O. = Significant other
  * = Refer to pre-op & post-op standards of care for routine pre-op & post-op
      care.

Date & initial

Patient outcome criteria		Instructed Pt.	Instructed S.O.	Assess learning	Understands Pt.	Understands S.O.
I. Pt./S.O. has some basic knowledge of multiple sclerosis (M.S.).						
A. Verbalizes that he/she has MS	A	9/4	9/4	9/5 verbalizes depression	9/10	9/10
B. Verbalizes MS is considered a chronic illness with exacerbation and remission.	B	9/4	9/4	9/5	9/10	9/10
C. Verbalizes an awareness of major complications and understands basic management:						
1. Fatigue	1	9/4	9/4	9/5	9/10	9/10
2. Weakness	2	9/4	9/4	9/5	9/10	9/10
3. Spasticity, ataxia	3	9/4	9/4	9/5	9/10	9/10
4. Gait abnormalities	4	9/4	9/4	9/5	9/10	9/10
5. Dysarthria, dysphagia	5	9/4	9/4	9/5	9/10	9/10
6. Impaired respiration	6	9/4	9/4	9/5	9/10	9/10
7. Visual impairment	7	9/4	9/4	9/5	9/10	9/10
8. Ducubitis ulcers	8	9/4	9/4	9/5	9/10	9/10
9. Bladder dysfunction	9	9/4	9/4	9/5	9/10	9/10
10. Bowel dysfunction	10	9/4	9/4	9/5	9/10	9/10
11. Impaired cognition, memory	11	9/4	9/4	9/5	9/10	9/10
12. Altered behavior	12	9/4	9/4	9/5	9/10	9/10
13. Stress reactions	13	9/4	9/4	9/5	9/10	9/10
II. Pt./S.O. has understanding of management of MS:						
A. Verbalizes needed life-style changes he/she should make:						
1. Exercise	1	9/6	9/6		9/10	9/10
2. Lower stress	2	9/6	9/6		9/10	9/10
3. Diet	3	9/6	9/6		9/10	9/10
4. Occupation	4	9/6	9/6		9/10	9/10
5. Rest periods	5	9/6	9/6		9/10	9/10
B. Verbalizes knowledge of medications; to include name, side-effects, administration instruction. Name of Medication:						
1. _____	1	9/9	9/9		9/10	9/10
2. _____	2	9/9	9/9		9/10	9/10
3. _____	3	9/9	9/9		9/10	9/10
4. _____	4					
5. _____	5					
III. Pt./S.O. understands home care:						
A. Has scheduled follow-up appointment with physician.	A	9/9	9/9		9/10	9/10
B. Has scheduled follow-up with physical therapy, occupational therapy, and/or speech language pathologist.	B	9/9	9/9	Will come to hospital for therapy Mon, Wed	9/10	9/10
C. Accepts visiting nurse referral and/or evaluation.	C	9/9	9/9	Weekly visit	9/10	9/10
D. Verbalizes signs and symptoms of exacerbation.	D	9/9	9/9		9/10	9/10
E. Verbalizes knowledge of prescribed level of activity.	E	9/9	9/9		9/10	9/10

Name	Init	Name	Init	Name	Init
Jane Doe	JD				
Sally James	SJ				

Figure 10–4   Teaching standards used by a nursing service for discharge planning instruction for patients with MS. (Used by permission. University of Colorado Health Sciences Center. All rights reserved.)

155

understood by the patient, his home support system, and the visiting nurse before discharge (Fig. 10–4). The patient should be aware of the services available in the community such as the local MS society.

Summary

The nurse should have an ongoing basic knowledge of MS whether employed in an acute-care setting, rehabilitation center, nursing home, clinic, or in the community. An effective and creative care plan must be developed and individualized for each patient. The ability to coordinate the nursing process and the use of the health-care team will assist the nurse to help the MS patient sustain a level of optimal independence.

Suggested Readings

BRUNNER L, SUDDARTH D: The Lippincott Manual of Nursing Practice, 2nd ed, pp 931–934. Philadelphia, JB Lippincott, 1978

CATANZARO M: Multiple sclerosis: Exploding myths that compromise patient care. RN 40:42–47, 1977

CATANZARO M: Nursing care of the MS patient. Am J Nurs 2:273–302, 1980

CHRISTOPHERSON V, et al: Rehabilitation Nursing: Perspectives and Implications. New York, McGraw-Hill, 1974

DILLAN A: Nursing Care of the Patient with M.S. Nurs Clin North Am 8:656–664, 1973

DOLAN B: Multiple sclerosis. J Neurosurg Nurs 11:83–91, 1979

HICKEY J: The Clinical Practice of Neurological and Neurosurgical Nursing, pp 452–455. Philadelphia, JB Lippincott, 1981

KINLEY A: MS—From shock to acceptance. Am J Nurs 2:274–275, 1980

LEWIS S, LEWIS U: Multiple sclerosis: Does the mystery remain? J Neurosurg Nurs 11(3):176–181, 1979

McDONNELL M, et al: MS—Problem-oriented nursing care plans. Am J Nurs 2:292–297, 1980

PRICE G: MS—The challenge to the family. Am J Nurs 2:283–287, 1980

SLATER R, YEARWOOD A: MS—Facts, faith, and hope. Am J Nurs 2:176–181, 1980

SNYDER M: A Guide to Neurological and Neurosurgical Nursing. New York, John Wiley & Sons, 1983

11   Laura L. Knutson

Understanding and Managing
the Psychosocial Aspects
of Multiple Sclerosis

Psychosocial aspects of multiple sclerosis (MS) are vital components to be considered by all members of the interdisciplinary health-care team in assessing and planning effective treatment for the MS patient. Attention to the emotional and behavioral reactions of the patient to MS will help to avoid noncompliance with treatment recommendations or lack of understanding or ability on the patient's part to carry out specific instructions of the team. Often, an MS patient will not be assertive enough or will be too upset to clarify confusing aspects of the disease or instructions that are given. Taking the time to be supportive, listening to the patient, and making sure the patient understands MS and the reasons for specific treatment recommendations are crucial to the therapeutic process.

This chapter will provide specific guidelines to help members of the health-care team identify and assess the problems presented by MS. Any member of the health-care team can successfully help the patient with psychological or social problems. However, it may be necessary to consult with or refer the patient to a psychotherapist if problems continue to interfere with effective treatment or realistic adjustment to the disease.

A differentiation between the patient who is newly diagnosed or has mild symptoms and the patient who has moderate to severe disability will be made because each presents a different set of problems. The characteristics of a profile of a patient with MS who has made a good adjustment are presented in the summary at the end of this chapter.

General Aspects of Multiple Sclerosis

DIAGNOSIS AND UNPREDICTABILITY

The person diagnosed as having MS has likely experienced a long period of apprehension during which physicians were unable to determine the problem. A diagnosis of MS is often made after suspicion of other neurologic diseases or psychiatric conditions (Eisen et al, 1979). Once a diagnosis is established, ambiguity surrounds the course of the disease. Will the disease be the relapsing/remitting type or will it be progressive? How much disability will the patient face? At diagnosis, the patient will be told that there is no cure and that little is known about what the patient can do to influence the course of the disease. Uncertainty and potential loss of control are issues all humans face, but for the MS patient, these issues are exaggerated and pervasive on a daily basis.

INTERFERENCE WITH LIFE PLANS

Patients diagnosed as having MS are most often between the ages of 20 and 40. They are young and in the prime of establishing careers and family. The unpredictability of MS becomes a major stress factor. Planning for the future is difficult and necessitates developing alternative plans to already-established goals.

Redetermining a productive and contributing role in society despite the reality of the disease is a difficult issue to resolve.

EARLY STAGES OF MULTIPLE SCLEROSIS

In the early or mild stages of MS, the patient may experience fatigue, weakness, or numbness without visible signs of disability. Physical limitations may require adjustments, but the need for these adjustments is difficult for the patient and others to acknowledge when the patient feels and appears quite healthy (Eisen et al, 1979; Hartings et al, 1976; Pavlou et al, 1979).

LATER STAGES OF MULTIPLE SCLEROSIS

More visible signs of disability create problems of negative reactions from others and increased dependency on the part of the patient. Changes occur in established relationships (employer, spouse, family, and friends). The patient will require more assistance and will not be able to perform tasks as usual or continue in set roles. Renegotiation of these roles and requests for assistance become necessary.

STRESS AND CHANGE IN RELATIONSHIPS

Stress management, effective communication, and a belief system that serves short-range and long-range goals are important to all humans. For the MS patient, deficits in these areas of psychological and interpersonal competence become especially problematic.

Inability to manage stress may influence the progression of the disease; inability to communicate effectively will make negotiating change with others difficult; and a belief system that causes constant emotional upset or self-defeating behavior will prevent the successful integration of the effects of the disease into the whole of the patient's life.

SOCIAL REACTION TO DISEASE AND DISABILITY

A person having a chronic disease and potential or real disability requires an adjustment to others' reactions of fear, pity, avoidance, and frustration with the helplessness they experience. Therapists and doctors may react with insensitivity or may withdraw because of frustration with the lack of a cure. The patient's spouse, family, and friends may withdraw from or reject the patient because of their discomfort with disease and disability or their unwillingness to play the role of care-giver (Horenstein, 1976). In the early stages of MS others may not take the patient seriously because there is no obvious sign of illness. In later stages, others will discriminate against the obvious disability of the patient. The MS patient struggles with being viewed as a burden or as "abnormal" and must learn to live with rejection and disapproval.

REACTION OF THE FAMILY TO THE PATIENT WITH MULTIPLE SCLEROSIS

The effect of MS on the entire family of the patient must be addressed by the health-care team. Family members of the MS patient experience anxiety, guilt, depression, or anger, both at the time of diagnosis of the disease and as symptoms worsen (Block and Kester, 1970). They must reevaluate their commitment to the patient and adjust to the real and potential impact of MS on their lives. As with the patient, uncertainty and unpredictability become a daily concern, and life plans and goals must be reassessed. In addition, family members are faced with the possibility of the patient's increasing dependence and need for assistance, which may require a change in work schedules or limit recreational activities. Educating, supporting, and facilitating the negotiation of role changes in the family can greatly increase the likelihood that the family can remain together with a positive adjustment to MS (Pavlou et al, 1979; Vas, 1969).

MS patients who are parents are concerned about the impact the disease and disability will have on their children. Will the children have difficulty developing normally or adjusting to life as adults? Will the children experience shame or embarrassment about having a "disabled" parent? Will the children experience deprivation or lack of involvement with the parent that will affect their emotional well-being? A good adjustment to MS by the parents will most likely lead to development of alternative parenting methods and plans, and children will respond accordingly with little difficulty.

SEXUAL FUNCTIONING

MS may affect normal sexual functioning because of a diminished or heightened sensitivity in the genital area, changes in intensity of orgasm, inability to achieve or maintain an erection, or the inability to achieve "sexual readiness" (Comfort, 1978; Lillius et al, 1976; Robmault, 1978). In a culture where there is a pervasive belief that sexual performance determines one's adequacy as a person, the MS patient faces the difficult task of developing a view of self-acceptance and worthiness despite impaired sexual functioning. A change in the ability to achieve sexual pleasure in the usual manner is a great loss, and alternative means for sensual and sexual pleasure must be determined (Carrera and Kelly, 1979). In addition, the emotional reactions and tendency to withdraw from sexual partners become as much the problem as the physical limitations imposed by MS.

The person with MS who experiences changes in his or her usual sexual response must be open to a different, more expanded view of sexuality. For example, a shift from the usual focus on genital sex, intercourse, and orgasms to a focus on experimentation to discover various means to derive sexual pleasures from the whole body could be essential. At a workshop on sexuality, I drew a picture of a human body and asked participants to put an "X" on those parts of the body that are erogenous or potentially sexually stimulating. There was no part of the body that was omitted. Since the effects of MS are unpredictable and always changing, an openness to experience sexual pleasure in a variety of ways becomes crucial. Ideally, the person with MS will have a partner with whom he or she is comfortable to communicate during this process of experimentation and exploration. Communication and sexual assertiveness will continue to be a vital aspect of the sexual relationship as the sexual response changes for the MS patient. A more detailed discussion of emotional blocks that affect assertiveness, communication, and involvement with otl.ers follows later in this chapter.

Emotional and Behavioral Reactions to Multiple Sclerosis

The cognitive-behaviorists offer a useful framework in dealing with the MS patient. A precise system whereby human problems can be understood is presented by Ellis in *Reason and Emotion in Psychotherapy* and *Humanistic Psychotherapy* and by Walen and co-authors in *A Practitioner's Guide to Rational–Emotive Therapy*. These authors believe that emotional disturbance and self-defeating behavior are caused not by the events in one's life but by the view one takes of these events (Epictetus, 1970). Therefore, if MS, with all of its unpredictability, incurability, variety of symptoms, and social consequences, is an event, then the attitudes or beliefs concerning the event will determine the patient's emotional and behavioral adjustment. As therapists, we are faced with the fact that MS, the event, cannot be cured. Our goal is the facilitation of a good adjustment and attitude toward MS.

STAGES OF GRIEF

As an overall perspective of emotional and behavioral reactions to MS, the grief process as described by Elizabeth Kübler-Ross in *On Death and Dying* can be helpful. The grief process is described in the following stages: (1) shock, (2) denial, (3) bargaining, (4) anger, (5) depression, and (6) acceptance. MS patients react to their disease with all the components of grief, not only at the time of diagnosis but also with each exacerbation of the disease or worsening of symptoms. The patient should be helped to understand that although emotional upset is caused by beliefs and attitudes, the reaction with all the stages of grief is natural and "human." Adjustment to the disease is blocked only when the patient remains in a stage for too long a time or with too great intensity (Gallineck and Kalinowsky, 1958; Hartings et al, 1976).

For the purposes of this chapter, the focus will be on four common emotional reactions to MS. The discussion will encompass the stages of grief and provide strategies for resolution. The four emotions discussed are anxiety, anger, guilt, and depression. Each will be presented with its cognitive and behavioral components.

Anxiety

Anxiety is the most basic emotional reaction to both the diagnosis of MS and to the progression of the disease on its unpredictable course (Lawrence and Lawrence, 1979; Leech, 1976). Predicting or worrying about the future is an inevitable reaction. Possible future events are imaged and evaluated as awful or catastrophic, with resultant anxiety.

Common predictions made by the patient are "All aspects of my life will always be bad," "I will be absolutely and totally disabled," "I will be completely alone and unable to take care of myself," "No one will help me," "I will never succeed at anything," "People will reject and abandon me," and "My lifestyle will change completely." These thoughts are self-defeating when they represent overgeneralization and absolute thinking (Burns, 1980). However, it is possible that the predicted events will occur, at least in part. Disputing the overgeneralizations or absolute thinking will provide only a temporary solution to the anxiety. Anxiety is created not by the images of future events but by the evaluation of these events as awful, catastrophic, or terrible (Ellis, 1962). To avoid being overwhelmed with anxiety and worry, the patient can "de-awfulize" the disease and its consequences and more realistically view MS as an unfortunate event or difficult problem to solve. Greater attention can be directed to the problems of the present as possible future events are "de-awfulized."

Another set of beliefs that lead to anxiety is "demand" statements such as "I have to . . . ," "I must . . . ," "I should . . . ," or "I ought to . . . ." Demands do not allow for human error or the physical limitations imposed by MS. Anxiety results when the patient is not able to perform or function 100% of the time. Examples are "I must perform well at all times despite the fact that I have MS," "My body should function better," "I have to get this task done today," and "I have to be perfect at all things at all times." With decreased ability to function, perfectionism or the tendency toward self-demands in the MS patient results in intense anxiety. The goal of treatment is to facilitate a less demanding belief system so that acceptance and adjustment to imposed limits can occur. Striving for perfection gives meaning to life; demanding perfection leads to emotional disturbance.

Common behaviors that accompany anxiety are avoidance, passivity, withdrawal, reactiveness, dependency, overextension, and "giving-up." Worry or "awfulizing" about the future course of the disease leads to immobilization. Demands or perfectionism will lead to overextending or denying the realities of the limits imposed by MS. The role of the therapist is to dispute the beliefs that lead to these behaviors. In addition, homework assignments that encourage a more active, risk-taking outlook despite the limits of MS can be very helpful. Anxiety may increase temporarily as new behaviors and confrontation of the fears are attempted, but the patient will discover that projected or possible outcomes are not "awful."

Anger

Most patients feel anger when diagnosed as having MS and as new symptoms or external consequences occur. This anger may be covert or clearly acknowledged by the patient and expressed verbally and behaviorally. Beliefs that are present with anger are "It is unfair that I have MS," "Life should be fair," "Doctors should be able to help me," "My body should function better," "Others should understand and care about me," and "There should be a solution."

Anger is directed at those on whom the patient relies for support and assistance (Schwartz and Pierron, 1972). When the support or assistance is not available, anger is expressed in response to the fear of being alone at the same time as dependency and the need for assistance increase.

Behaviors that are commonly exhibited when patients are angry are aggression, passivity, reactiveness, noncompliance to medical recommendations, blaming others, verbal explosions, withdrawal, and irritability. Anger is usually based in vulnerability and fear and tends to dissipate as the patient resolves issues about aloneness and self-care. The role of the therapist is to facilitate acceptance that life is not fair and that the choices that others make are often beyond our control. Acknowledgment of anger is important, but continued expression or creation of anger will only add internal stress to already existing problems. Suppression of anger is not advised. Resolution of the beliefs that cause anger will help the patient to solve problems more objectively.

Guilt

Whereas anger stems from "shoulds" placed on others or the universe, guilt is caused by "shoulds" placed on one's self. Guilt or self-blame for having a chronic disease is a frequent reaction at both the mild and more severe stages of MS. A sense of responsibility for one's health is important; however, it is self-defeating to produce guilt by thinking that "I should have acted better," "MS is a punishment for wrongdoing," "Since this has happened to me, I am a bad person," or "I would not have this disease if I had lived my life better." Guilt is also produced in relation to social, family, and employment roles. Self-defeating statements related to changes in these roles are "I should work as much and as well as I have in the past," "I should perform my usual duties," "I should give to others as in the past," "I should give others what they want," "I have no right to set limits or say no," and "I must never hurt or disappoint others when they have expectations of me."

Guilt will result in behaviors such as being overly apologetic, overcompensating, passive and nonassertive, self-degrading, and overextending. Reduction of guilt and behavioral change are accomplished when the above statements are replaced by statements like "Having MS makes no statement about my worth or goodness as a person," "Others are responsible for themselves and, although it is good to give to others and perform well, I had better accept that I may not always be able to do so," "I have the right to say no and set limits," and "I had better accept that I cannot ever be perfect as a human being; to demand that I be perfect will only make me suffer more." Assertiveness training based on the premise that the patient has the right to say no or make requests for assistance and that others are responsible for their emotions and well-being can be very helpful.

Depression

Depression is not to be confused with the fatigue or periods of low energy that most MS patients experience. Depression that is psychologically based is often present, however, and is usually distinguishable from fatigue by more chronic symptoms of lethargy, sluggishness, low energy, and a sense of worthlessness. Fatigue and low energy caused by MS are usually of shorter duration, occur at certain times of the day, and are not accompanied by statements of a self-degrading or hopeless nature.

The MS patient who is depressed is usually reacting to the loss of ability to function and the interference of MS with established life goals and purpose (Leech, 1976). In addition, discrimination and rejection by others increase as the ability to function decreases. Loss is experienced in almost every aspect of the patient's life. The MS patient tends to withdraw and become passive. Suicidal tendencies are often present (Langworthy, 1948; Surridge, 1969; Weinstein, 1970). Life is perceived as having no meaning or hope. Alternatives to the accustomed lifestyle appear nonexistent, and, in general, life is viewed as "all bad."

The MS patient is depressed because of two self-defeating beliefs: (1) that one must be productive and perform well to be a worthwhile person, and (2) that one needs the approval of others to be happy and worthwhile. Until these beliefs are changed, there will be little motivation to develop alternative plans and goals or to become actively involved with others. In his book, *Feeling Good,* Burns describes in more detail the cognitive and behavioral components of depression with excellent strategies for resolution. The therapist's role is to help the patient determine alternative means for productivity with a focus on what can be done, despite physical limits, instead of on what cannot be done. More importantly, disputation of the beliefs that the patient's worth is contingent on others' approval or ability to function is vital to reduction of the depression. Homework that promotes activity as opposed to passivity is very important and therapeutic.

The use of antidepressants or tranquilizers is advised only if the patient is so greatly disturbed that therapy is difficult. Mood elevation or reduction of anxiety with the use of medication can enhance the therapeutic process but should not be relied on as a sole method of treatment. Patients often experience greater emotional disturbance while facing difficult issues; medication may interfere with the availability of these emotions and block resolution.

Therapeutic Approaches

The psychological issues and circumstances presented by individual patients vary greatly. Not only does the course of MS vary greatly from patient to patient, but the coping patterns, attitudes, and life difficulties present before a diagnosis of MS are important to determine therapeutic strategies or approaches to treatment. Individual, group, couples, or family therapy may be appropriate and may be used in conjunction with each other. Many MS patients avoid MS groups because they fear exposure to others with greater disability; yet other MS patients enjoy the supportive environment of a group where they can share information and can experience being understood.

Couples or family therapy is encouraged whenever possible. Family members can be educated about the nature of MS and can be helped to understand suggested plans for therapy or rehabilitation. Disregard of "significant others" in the patient's life may result in noncompliance with recommendations because of ignorance, lack of appreciation or acknowledgment of important factors related to treatment, or resistance to assisting the patient in ways that would be helpful. A support network that can be flexible and adjust to the realities that MS presents to the patient is crucial. The therapist can facilitate communication and help others in the patient's life adjust to the disease.

At times, a listening or supportive role by the therapist is most desirable. MS patients tend not to communicate frequently with others because they fear they will be a burden or will be viewed as "complaining." The therapist can be very helpful simply by allowing the patient to communicate about MS. As the relationship with the patient develops and a therapeutic contract is established, it is recommended that a more active and direct approach to therapy be used. The goal of therapy is to change self-defeating beliefs, which can be accomplished best by actively challenging and disputing these beliefs.

Attitude of the Therapist

When faced with a person who has MS, therapists may experience fear, pity, guilt, or a strong urge to avoid the patient, which are natural and human reactions to the patient's story about how MS has not only affected his health and physical functioning but has precipitated loss and unpleasant change in every aspect of his life. Often, a patient will wonder how the therapist can "understand" him without the therapist having MS himself. The best response is to state that probably the therapist cannot completely know what it is like to have MS; however, this does not mean he cannot still be helpful.

The therapist's attitudes and beliefs can greatly interfere with the therapeutic process. If the therapist believes that disease and disability are awful or catastrophic, he will find it difficult to dispute this belief for the patient. Empathy can be supportive and indicate understanding; fear and pity will serve to reinforce the patient's self-defeating beliefs about the effects of MS. If the therapist believes that one must be productive and achieve to be a worthwhile person, he will not be able to challenge this belief for the patient. In the same way, believing that one's worth is dependent on the love and approval of others will be detrimental as the patient experiences rejection from others.

The belief that may interfere most with the therapeutic process if held by the therapist is "I should be able to make this problem go away!" If the therapist cannot accept and admit to the patient that little can be done about the disease or the losses, he may not respond to the patient's questions or listen to concerns in a helpful manner. The most frequent complaint heard from MS patients is that members of the health-care team did not explain the disease sufficiently or did not appear supportive or empathetic to their situation. Although we may not be able to solve the problem, we can be of great help by attending to and responding to the patient's reactions.

Summary

In summary, the patient who has made a good adjustment to MS will exhibit the following characteristics:

1. The patient will have developed new approaches to recreation or enjoyment, work, and interpersonal involvement.
2. The patient will be actively pursuing newly determined life goals.
3. MS will not be the focus of the patient's life.
4. The patient's focus will be on what can be done, not on what cannot be done.
5. There will be a realistic, yet hopeful, attitude about the future.
6. The patient will be self-accepting despite physical limitations.
7. A readiness will be demonstrated for either a mild course or future progression of the disease.
8. The patient's fears about the future will not be overwhelming.
9. The patient will not be a burden to others but will be able to ask for help as needed.
10. The patient will exercise control over the view or perspective held about MS and the manner in which MS will be integrated into his life.

Suggested Readings

BLOCK JM, KESTER NC: Role of rehabilitation in the management of multiple sclerosis. Modern Treatment 7:930–940, 1970

BURNS DD: Feeling Good. New York, Morrow, 1980

CARRERA MA, KELLY S: Multiple sclerosis: The right to a sexual life. MS Quarterly pp 4–18, Summer, 1979

COMFORT A: Sexual Consequences of Disability, pp 19–60. Philadelphia, Stickley, 1978

EISEN A, STEWART J, NUDLEMAN K, et al: Short latency somatosensory responses in multiple sclerosis. Neurology 29:827–834, 1979

ELLIS A: Reason and Emotion in Psychotherapy. New York, Lyle Stuart, 1962

ELLIS A: Humanistic Psychotherapy. New York, Crown Publishers, 1973

EPICTETUS: Enchiridion. Indianapolis, Bobbs-Merrill, 1970

GALLINECK A, KALINOWSKY LB: Psychiatric aspects of multiple sclerosis. Diseases of the Nervous System 19:77–80, 1958

HARTINGS MF, PAVLOU MM, DAVID FA: Group counseling of MS patients in a program of comprehensive care. J Chronic Dis 29:65–73, 1976

HORENSTEIN S: The management of sexual disorders in multiple sclerosis. Medical Aspects of Human Sexuality 10:103–104, 1976

KÜBLER-ROSS E: On Death and Dying. New York, Macmillan, 1969

LANGWORTHY OR: Relation of personality problems to onset and progress of multiple sclerosis. Arch Neurol Psychiatr 59:13, 1948

LAWRENCE SA, LAWRENCE RM: A model of adaptation to the stress of chronic illness. Nurs Forum 18:32–42, 1979

LEECH P: Emotional responses in the newly disabled adult: Clinical considerations. Unpublished manuscript. Santa Rosa, California, 1976

LILLIUS HG, VALTONEN EJ, WIKSTROM J: Sexual problems in patients suffering from multiple sclerosis. J Chronic Dis 29:643–647, 1976

PAVLOU M, SCHAUF C, STEFOSKI S, et al: Variety and possibility in multiple sclerosis. In Pavlou M (ed): A Training Syllabus for the Vocational Professional. Chicago, Rush-Presbyterian St. Luke's Medical Center, 1979

ROBMAULT ID: Sex, Society and the Disabled, pp 133–139. Hagerstown, Harper & Row, 1978

SCHWARTZ ML, PIERRON M: Suicide and fatal accidents in multiple sclerosis. Omega 3:291: 293, 1972

SURRIDGE D: An investigation into some aspects of multiple sclerosis. Br J Psychiatry 115:749–764, 1969

VAS CJ: Sexual impotence and some autonomic disturbances in men with multiple sclerosis. Acta Neurol Scand 45:166–182, 1969

WALEN SR, DiGIUSEPPE R, WESSLER RL: A Practitioner's Guide to Rational–Emotive Therapy. New York, Oxford, 1980

WEINSTEIN EA: Behavioral aspects of multiple sclerosis. Modern Treatment 7:961–968, 1970

Part III

**REHABILITATION OF PATIENTS WITH
MUSCULAR DYSTROPHIES**

Steven P. Ringel
William H. Cooper

12

Classification of Neuromuscular Disorders

Motor disorders are readily divided into those that primarily affect either the central nervous system (CNS) or peripheral nervous system (PNS). The functional unit of the PNS is the motor unit, which includes the anterior horn cell, its axon, the neuromuscular junction, and all the muscle fibers innervated by that axon (Fig. 12–1). Because more than 40 neuromuscular diseases affect some part of the motor unit (see Lower Motor Neuron Disorders, listed below), a comprehensive review of all of these illnesses would be bewildering and exhausting to any reader exposed only occasionally to patients with neuromuscular diseases. In this chapter, therefore, major consideration is given to the more common neuromuscular disorders seen for chronic rehabilitative care. For greater detail, the reader may wish to refer to any of several more comprehensive texts listed under Suggested Readings at the end of this chapter.

Because PNS diseases share certain features, including diminished tone and reflexes, and weakness and atrophy in the distribution of the affected motor neurons or muscles, the diagnosis and treatment for this group of disorders are quite similar regardless of localization of the lesion in the PNS. In large part, the problems these patients face depend more on the degree of disability than on the disease that produces the dysfunction. Common treatment issues, including correction of deformities, exercise and stretching, ambulation, adaptive aids, respiratory therapy, and psychotherapy, are covered only briefly because other chapters are devoted to each of these subjects. Treatment issues and complications unique to individual disorders are emphasized so that the reader can anticipate and prevent complications while maximizing the patient's function.

The initial diagnosis of patients with neuromuscular symptoms re-

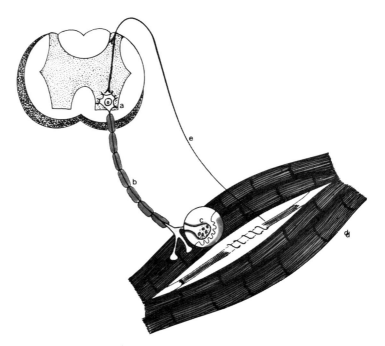

Figure 12 – 1   Anatomy of the neuromuscular system. The efferent limb (motor unit) includes the anterior horn cell (*a*), its axon (*b*) the neuromuscular junction (*c*), and the muscle fibers (*d*). Afferent fibers (*e*) that arise from the muscle spindle provide a feedback loop for monitoring muscle tension and length. (Wiederholt WC [ed]: Neurology for Non-Neurologists. New York, Academic Press, 1982)

quires a complete neurologic examination and, frequently, comprehensive electrophysiologic investigations, and muscle and nerve biopsy (see Chap. 13). Undiagnosed patients with PNS signs and symptoms can have a free comprehensive evaluation at one of the more than 200 muscular dystrophy clinics in the United States.

Diseases of the Lower Motor Neuron

Diseases affecting the lower motor neuron include the inherited spinal muscular atrophies (SMAs), amyotrophic lateral sclerosis (ALS), and poliomyelitis.

LOWER MOTOR NEURON DISORDERS

1. Spinal muscular atrophies (SMAs)
      Infantile SMA (Werdnig-Hoffmann, type I SMA)
      Intermediate SMA (type II SMA)
      Juvenile SMA (Kugelberg-Welander, type III SMA)

2. Amyotrophic lateral sclerosis (motor neuron disease)
   Progressive bulbar atrophy
   Progressive muscular atrophy
   Primary lateral sclerosis
3. Poliomyelitis

SPINAL MUSCULAR ATROPHIES

The spinal muscular atrophies are a heterogeneous group of hereditofamilial disorders in which pathologically there is degeneration of anterior horn cells (and brain stem motor nuclei) without corticospinal or sensory tract involvement. Changes of denervation and reinnervation are seen with both electromyogram (EMG) and muscle biopsy. The inheritance pattern is usually autosomal recessive, although X-linked recessive or dominant transmission occurs in 10% of cases. Several authors have suggested that SMA represents a clinical continuum between its most acute (infantile SMA) and its more chronic forms (chronic infantile and juvenile SMA). Others have separated each clinical variety, which include the more uncommon facioscapulohumeral, scapuloperoneal, and late-onset varieties.

The three most common SMAs are classified according to the age of onset and severity of involvement. In the *infantile form* (SMA I; Werdnig-Hoffmann disease), babies are either hypotonic and weak at birth or become weak within the first few months of life. The infantile form occurs once in approximately every 20,000 births; the affected infants have a weak cry and a poor respiratory effort and frequently aspirate when fed. Treatment involves careful monitoring of nutrition to avoid aspiration and early recognition and treatment of pneumonia. These children rarely live beyond the age of 1 to 2 years.

An intermediate form (SMA II) becomes apparent in children who fail to achieve normal motor milestones. Many children affected with this form of SMA can sit unsupported and occasionally some stand, but they rarely walk. Contractures and scoliosis are major complications. Proper wheelchair positioning, the use of body jackets or molded seat inserts, and, in selected cases, spinal fusion will delay progressive spinal collapse. Although these patients may survive into the second and third decades of life, many succumb to sudden respiratory failure. Aggressive respiratory therapy, including postural drainage and antibiotics, should be started at the first signs of respiratory infection and decompensation.

The juvenile form of SMA (Kugelberg-Welander) begins between the ages 5 to 15 years. Clinical features include slowly progressive proximal weakness, prominent lordosis, fasciculations (50%), and diminished deep tendon reflexes. Because of progressive difficulty in walking, many patients require a wheelchair within 5 to 10 years of the onset of symptoms. Stretching of extremity contractures, as with all progressive neuromuscular diseases, will often prolong ambulation. With aggressive management of progressive kyphoscoliosis and respiratory infections, many patients live well beyond the third decade.

MOTOR NEURON DISEASE (AMYOTROPHIC LATERAL SCLEROSIS)

In this sporadic disorder (5% – 10% are inherited), patients develop progressive weakness, wasting, and spasticity of bulbar and extremity musculature. Bulbar motor neurons, anterior horn cells, or corticospinal tracts may be primarily affected so that the terms *progressive bulbar palsy, progressive muscular atrophy,* and *primary lateral sclerosis* have been used. As the disease progresses, involvement of bulbar, lower, and upper motor neurons is usually seen so that the inclusive term *amyotrophic lateral sclerosis* (ALS) is applied.

The disease, more common in men, may begin any time during adulthood, especially in later years. Common presentations include weakness and clumsiness of a limb (Fig. 12 – 2) and difficulty in speaking and swallowing. Loss of corticobulbar pathways produces pseudobulbar symptoms such as a hyperactive cough reflex, spastic dysphagia, and inappropriate bursts of laughter or crying.

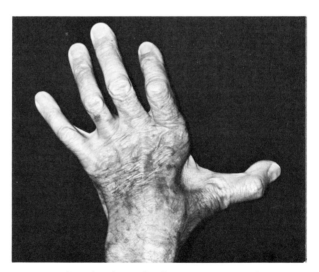

Figure 12 – 2 Amyothrophic lateral sclerosis (ALS). Striking hand atrophy is seen particularly involving the first dorsal interosseus muscle between the thumb and first finger. The hand has a claw-like configuration. (Handbook of Clinical Neurology, vol 40. Amsterdam, Elsevier/North Holland Biomedical Press, 1979)

Examination reveals asymmetrical weakness, atrophy, fasciculations of tongue and limb muscles, and a mixture of hypoactive and hyperactive stretch reflexes. Electrodiagnostic studies are helpful by demonstrating changes of denervation in weak as well as clinically unaffected muscles.

Treatment of this usually progressive disorder is entirely symptomatic because its cause remains unknown. Aside from providing exercises, stretching, braces, adaptive equipment, and respiratory care, the patient's chronic bulbar dysfunction should be monitored to avoid malnutrition, recurrent aspiration, and choking. Liquid nutritional supplements are often useful to prevent rapid weight loss. Surgical section of the nerves to the major salivary glands on one side (chorda tympani and Jacobsen's nerve) prevents saliva from choking the patient when supine. Injection of a vocal cord with a Teflon substance strengthens the patient's cough and reduces the risk of aspiration. Cricopharyngeal myotomy may further improve esophageal transport. If these procedures are insufficient, placement of a pharyngostomy or gastrostomy tube may be necessary to allow for adequate intake and to lessen the risk of choking.

In patients who become severely dysarthric or mute, every effort should be made to help them communicate. Unable to write or talk, a patient will feel isolated from his environment and can become hopelessly depressed. A variety of electronic devices are now available to assist the patient in maintaining this important language contact.

About 80% of patients succumb to intercurrent infection 2 to 3 years after the onset of symptoms. Respiratory complications due to aspiration pneumonia are reversible and must be treated if the general quality of life is still acceptable. Terminally, low-flow oxygen may provide symptomatic relief for respiratory insufficiency. The use and indications for ventilatory assistance are discussed in Chapter 14. About 25% of patients have a more benign course with prolonged survival, particularly those with few bulbar and upper motor neuron signs. Infrequently, in patients with widespread disease, the progression of symptoms ceases unexplainably.

POLIOMYELITIS

Although the widespread use of immunizations against the polio virus has markedly reduced the frequency of new cases, there still remain many older patients with residual weakness from polio who are followed by rehabilitation specialists. After many years of static deficit, progressive weakness may develop, which sometimes is caused by unrecognized nerve compression in a flaccid, weakened extremity. In other patients, the cause of the progression is obscure and may be the result of superimposed dropout of anterior horn cells with normal aging.

Diseases of Peripheral Nerve

Peripheral nerve disorders include mononeuropathies, multiple mononeuropathies (mononeuritis multiplex), plexopathies, and polyneuropathies (peripheral neuropathies):

PERIPHEAL NERVE DISORDERS

1. Mononeuropathies (including entrapment neuropathies)
   Median (carpal tunnel)
   Ulnar (at elbow)
   Radial (Saturday night palsy)
   Peroneal
   Posterior tibial
   Mononeuritis multiplex
2. Plexopathies
   Acute brachial neuritis
   Lumbosacral plexitis
   Thoracic outlet syndrome
3. Polyneuropathies
   Axonal neuropathies
     Diabetes
     Alcohol related
     Uremia
     Hypothyroidism
     Sarcoidosis
     Collagen vascular diseases
       Systemic lupus erythematosus
       Rheumatoid arthritis
       Wegener's granulomatosis
     Paraproteinemias
     Drugs
       Isoniazid
       Hydralazine
       Nitrofurantoin
       Vincristine
     Heavy Metals
       Lead
       Arsenic
       Mercury
       Thallium
     Industrial toxins
       N-hexane
       N-butylketone
       Acrylamide
       Organophosphates

Amyloidosis
Carcinoma (remote effect)
Tick paralysis
Demyelinating neuropathies
Guillain-Barre syndrome
Chronic inflammatory polyradiculoneuropathy
Diphtheria
Porphyria

MONONEUROPATHY AND MONONEURITIS MULTIPLEX

The most common cause of damage to a single peripheral nerve is compression and traction. Common causes of mononeuropathies include compression of the median nerve in the carpal tunnel at the wrist; injury of the ulnar nerve in the ulnar groove at the elbow; compression of the radial nerve in the spinal groove of the humerus; and compression of the peroneal nerve as it crosses below the fibular head. When two or more isolated peripheral nerves are damaged (mononeuritis multiplex), the cause is more likely to be diabetes, collagen vascular diseases, sarcoidosis, or ischemic vascular disease.

PLEXOPATHY

Several distinct syndromes of the brachial and lumbosacral plexus are recognized in addition to trauma, infection, or tumorous invasion of the plexus. In idiopathic brachial neuritis, patients develop pain in the shoulder followed within several weeks by atrophy and weakness of the upper arm (Fig. 12–3). A history of antecedent trauma, infection, or

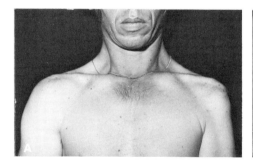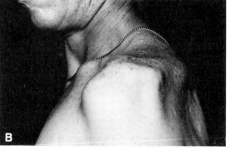

Figure 12–3 Brachial neuritis. (A) The left deltoid muscle is severely wasted, resulting in a loss of the normal round contour of the shoulder. (B) Bony prominences are readily seen because of atrophy of the left deltoid, supraspinatus, and infraspinatus muscles. (Handbook of Clinical Neurology, vol 40. Amsterdam, Elsevier/North Holland Biomedical Press, 1979)

immunization is often present. Patients usually recover completely as the damaged nerve slowly regenerates.

Lumbosacral plexopathy may occur from vascular infarction in diabetes and can be difficult to distinguish from a femoral ischemic neuropathy (diabetic amyotrophy). With a femoral neuropathy, patients develop severe, persistent pain in the thigh, followed within several weeks by weakness and atrophy of femoral innervated thigh muscles. When the entire plexus is involved, weakness and atrophy develop in muscles of the buttocks and the posterior and lower leg, in addition to the femoral innervated muscles. Pain tends to slowly subside and strength returns, often incompletely, over the course of a year or more.

POLYNEUROPATHY

Peripheral or polyneuropathy is the condition in which progressive distal sensory loss (stocking–glove distribution) and weakness develop in the legs and arms in a symmetrical fashion. Patients have difficulty with fine coordinated hand movements, such as buttoning a shirt, and with grip. With weakness in the legs, patients walk with a characteristic "steppage" or slapping gait and frequently twist an ankle or trip over small objects (Fig. 12–4). Early absence of deep tendon reflexes and complaints of paresthesias or numbness in hands and feet point toward a neuropathy, although some neuropathies may result in extreme weakness without any apparent sensory loss. Occasionally, impotence, sweating disturbances, and impaired bowel and bladder function are also present.

The clinical picture of acquired polyneuropathies is conveniently divided into axonal neuropathies, in which the nerve fiber (axon) is damaged, and demyelinating neuropathies, in which the covering of myelin is stripped away. Axonal polyneuropathies, which are encountered more frequently, have a wide variety of toxic and metabolic causes, of which diabetes and alcohol abuse are the most common. Chronic exposure to heavy metals, industrial toxins, household solvents, or medications should always be looked for, and in older patients an occult malignancy should be considered because many of these neuropathies will reverse with appropriate treatment.

Perforating ulcers and arthropathy can develop from chronic injury to painless extremities; therefore, hands and feet should be protected and wounds kept clean. In patients with severe, burning pain, phenytoin, carbamazepine, prolixin, or amytriptyline occasionally provide relief. A polypropylene ankle–foot orthosis (AFO) reduces the footdrop.

In contrast to the axonal neuropathies, acquired demyelinating polyneuropathies are more rapidly progressive and involve motor weakness more than sensory loss. In acute infectious polyradiculoneuropathy (Guillain-Barre syndrome) evanescent paresthesias of the extremities

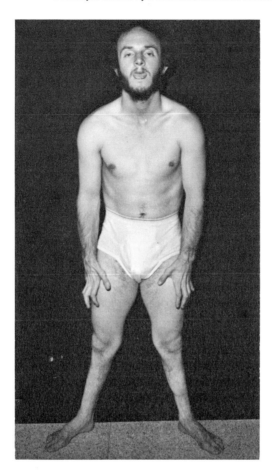

Figure 12–4   Charcot-Marie-Tooth disease. Distal wasting of the leg muscles produces a stork-leg appearance. The hands have a claw-like appearance, and there are prominent grooves on the dorsal surface because of interosseus muscle-wasting. (Handbook of Clinical Neurology, vol 40. Amsterdam, Elsevier/ North Holland Biomedical Press, 1979)

are followed by rapidly ascending weakness and arreflexia, first in the legs and then in the arms. In 50% of patients, there is a history of infection, immunization, surgery, or trauma several weeks before the onset of symptoms. Weakness reaches its peak within 1 to 3 weeks, at which point the patient may be totally paralyzed, requiring respiratory assistance. Transient autonomic disturbances (arrhythmias, hypotension, and hypertension) and inappropriate antidiuretic hormone secretion may occur. Cranial nerve muscles are often affected, resulting in facial weakness, dysphagia, and, rarely, impaired eye movements and pupillary responses (Miller-Fisher variant).

Nerve conduction velocities are usually markedly slowed, confirming demyelination, and cerebrospinal fluid protein is often increased above 100 mg/dl with a normal cell count (albuminocytologic dissociation).

The physician should be particularly alert for aspiration pneumonia from bulbar dysfunction and for respiratory failure. Intubation or tracheostomy is necessary when vital capacity falls to less than 30% of that predicted. Corticosteroids and plasmapheresis have been used in treatment but are generally felt not to be beneficial. Fortunately, with good supportive care, most patients improve within several months and 90% recover without significant residual disability.

Both axonal (neuronal) and demyelinating (hypertrophic) inherited sensorimotor neuropathies have been characterized as Charcot-Marie-Tooth disease. The clinical expression is variable, but it usually is milder in dominantly inherited forms and more severe with recessive forms. Patients often benefit from ankle–foot orthoses and occasionally from hand splints. Tendon transfers or joint fusions, or both, should be considered in patients who do not improve with these orthotic aids (see Chap. 18).

Diseases of the Neuromuscular Junction

Disturbances of the neuromuscular junction may result from disorders that interfere with release of acetylcholine from the presynaptic membrane (botulism, Eaton-Lambert syndrome), that disrupt the postsynaptic membrane (myasthenia gravis), or that interfere with inactivation of acetylcholine (organophosphate poisoning). In all cases, rapid onset of life-threatening weakness may develop because of interference with neuromuscular transmission. Because these disorders are reversible with proper medical treatment, complete supportive care, including ventilatory assistance, should be provided. It can be particularly rewarding to manage these patients, since, unlike in most other neuromuscular diseases, recovery is often complete.

NEUROMUSCULAR JUNCTION DISORDERS

Myasthenia gravis
Botulism
Eaton-Lambert syndrome
Pseudocholinesterase deficiency
Organophosphate intoxication

MYASTHENIA GRAVIS

Myasthenia gravis (MG) is an autoimmune disorder in which acetylcholine receptor antibodies (ACHRab) bind to the postsynaptic membrane, interfering with neuromuscular transmission. A majority of patients have thymic hyperplasia, while 10% harbor thymic tumors. A concomitant autoimmune disease, particularly of the thyroid, is present in 15% of cases.

MG occurs in all age groups, but is most frequent in women between 20 and 30 years of age. It may also occur as a transient disturbance in infants born to myasthenic mothers (neonatal myasthenia). Symptoms fluctuate throughout the day and are worse in frequently used muscles or after sustained activity. Typically, symptoms affect cranial muscles and include ptosis, diplopia, nasal or slurred speech, and difficulty chewing and swallowing. Arms and legs are often weak but to a lesser extent. Examination usually reveals significant facial (Fig. 12–5A) and neck muscle weakness as well.

The diagnosis is confirmed by the production of a decrement in the compound muscle action potential following repetitive stimulation, by improvement in strength (Fig. 12–5B); and in the amplitude of repetitive action potentials following intravenous edrophonium (Tensilon test), or by detection of ACHRab (see Chap. 13).

Although the onset and progression of weakness in MG is usually insidious and occasionally limited to the eye muscles (ocular MG), patients may experience sudden deterioration with life-threatening dysphagia and aspiration or severe respiratory compromise. This sudden decline is often precipitated by an infection, hypokalemia, emotional

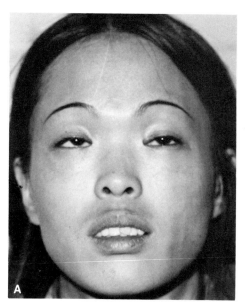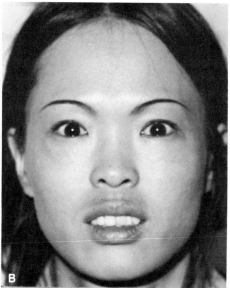

Figure 12–5   Myasthenia gravis. (A) Ptosis and facial weakness and (B) reversal after 10 mg edrophonium (Tensilon) IV. (Handbook of Clinical Neurology, vol 40. Amsterdam, Elsevier/North Holland Biomedical Press, 1979)

stress, or unrecognized thyroid dysfunction, or with the administration of medications known to potentiate neuromuscular blockade, including several antibiotics (neomycin, streptomycin), antiarrhythmics (propranolol, procainamide, phenytoin), quinine, and curare.

In the past, the mainstay of treatment in MG was cholinesterase inhibitors (pyridostigmine, neostigmine), which prolong the activity of acetylcholine at the neuromuscular junction. More recently, concurrent with the recognition of the autoimmune nature of MG, corticosteroids and other immunosuppressive drugs have been used increasingly. Although side-effects of these medications are few during the first months of therapy, chronic administration may be associated with numerous iatrogenic complications. Thymectomy is routinely employed in adults under the age of 65 years with generalized symptoms. Plasmapheresis can be lifesaving by providing temporary (2 – 3 weeks) improvement for patients who deteriorate acutely.

Patients with predominantly ocular symptoms have the best prognosis, although 40% will progress to have generalized symptoms within 2 years. Childhood MG is treated conservatively because aggressive treatment can adversely affect the child's growth.

Diseases of Muscle

A diverse array of disorders may affect voluntary skeletal muscles, including the dystrophies, myotonic disorders, inflammatory myopathies, metabolic, toxic, and endocrine myopathies, and several congenital myopathies. This section focuses on the more common, chronic disorders, highlighting distinguishing features and therapeutic management.

DISORDERS OF MUSCLE

1. Muscular dystrophies
     X-linked (Duchenne, Becker)
     Facioscapulohumeral (FSH)
     Scapuloperoneal (SP)
     Limb girdle (LG)
     Progressive external ophthalmoplegias
     Myotonic disorders
        Myotonia congenita
        Myotonic dystrophy (MYD)
2. Inflammatory myopathies
     Infectious (viral, bacterial, parasitic)
     Immune mediated
        Polymyositis

Dermatomyositis
Myositis associated with other connective tissue disorders (systemic lupus, polyarteritis nodosa, Sjögren's, rheumatoid arthritis, scleroderma)
3. Endocrine myopathies
   Hyper-/hypothyroidism
   Hyper-/hypocalcemia
   Hyper-/hypoadrenalism
4. Toxic myopathies
   Alcohol
   Amphotericin B
   Vincristine
   Chloroquine
   Steroid
5. Inherited metabolic myopathies
   Glycogen storage disorders (McArdle's, phosphofructokinase and acid maltase deficiency)
   Lipid myopathies (carnitine and carnitine palmityl transferase deficiency)
   Periodic paralyses (hypo-/hyper-/normokalemic)
   Malignant hyperthermia
6. Congenital myopathies

X-LINKED DYSTROPHIES

Duchenne muscular dystrophy (DMD), an X-linked recessive disorder with a high incidence (2–3/10,000), begins insidiously, with walking usually noted to be clumsy by the age of 4 to 6 years. Pseudohypertrophy of the calves, macroglossia, a lordotic posture, and toe-walking are characteristic. As the child loses strength in hip girdle muscles, he resorts to his arms to arise from the floor (Gower's sign; Fig. 12–6). By the age 9 to 12, frequent falls and increasing proximal weakness make independent walking impossible. Once in a wheelchair, contractures of extremities increase, the feet invert (equinovarus deformity), and progressive kyphoscoliosis develops. These children become totally immobile, requiring complete care for all activities of daily living. The combination of respiratory muscle weakness plus scoliosis predisposes to pulmonary infection and failure, and patients often succumb to pneumonia or congestive heart failure by the late teens or early twenties.

Confirmatory laboratory tests include striking elevation of serum creatine phosphokinase (CPK) (70 to 100 times normal), myopathic EMG, a necrotic, fibrotic muscle biopsy, and electrocardiographic changes.

A competent rehabilitative team can do much to ease discomfort in this incurable disease. Stretching of contractures, particularly of the

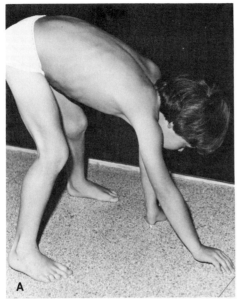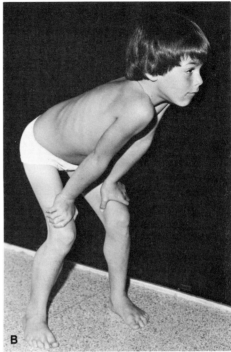

Figure 12-6 Duchenne muscular dystrophy (DMD). *(A)* In arising from the floor, the child elevates his buttocks high into the air, supporting his weight on both hands and feet. *(B)* He straightens his upper torso by "walking" up his legs with his hands. (Handbook of Clinical Neurology, vol 40. Amsterdam, Elsevier/North Holland Biomedical Press, 1979)

Achilles tendon and iliotibial band, prolongs ambulation (see Chap. 16). Long leg braces can further prolong independent walking for several years, although surgical release of contractures may initially be necessary to fit the braces. When confined to a wheelchair, the development of scoliosis can be retarded with proper positioning, a body jacket, scoliosis pads, or a molded seat insert (see Chap. 17). Increasingly, spinal fusion is being recommended, but it has not gained popularity because of the poor prognosis of these patients (see Chap. 18). Chronic respiratory management, including early recognition and treatment of infection, can prolong life. Ventilatory assistance is discussed in Chapter 14.

Genetic counseling depends on identification of all potential female carriers (mother, sister, and other females on maternal side of the family). The most practical and useful test is serum CPK, which is mildly elevated (2 to 3 times) in 70% of known female carriers.

Approximately 10% of males with X-linked muscular dystrophy have a more slowly progressive disease called Becker's dystrophy (Fig.

12 – 7), in which age of onset is later than for Duchenne's dystrophy and ambulation continues until the late teens or early twenties. Unfortunately, early in the disease it is virtually impossible to distinguish children with Duchenne's dystrophy from those with Becker's form. A similarly affected older sibling may help in differentiating between these disorders because they are relatively homogeneous within a single family.

FACIOSCAPULOHUMERAL AND SCAPULOPERONEAL DYSTROPHIES

Facioscapulohumeral (FSH) and scapuloperoneal (SP) dystrophies are dominantly inherited disorders characterized by slowly progressive weakness beginning in the first two decades of life and with predomi-

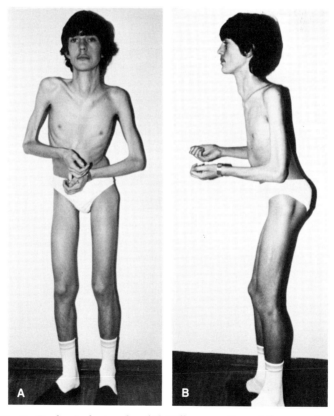

Figure 12 – 7   Becker's dystrophy. (A) Diffuse wasting of the muscles and lateral scoliosis can prominently be seen. (B) The forearms and knees cannot be fully extended because of contractures. A rigid spine further impairs mobility.

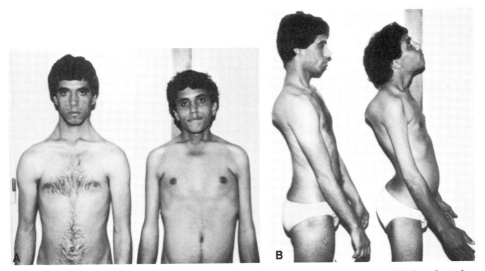

Figure 12-8 Facioscapulohumeral (FSH) dystrophy in two brothers. *(A)* the clavicles slope downward and a deep anterior axillary crease caused by internal rotation of weakened shoulder muscles can be seen. *(B)* Winging of the scapulae and compensatory lordosis are evident. The boy on the right is more severely affected.

nant involvement of scapular suspension muscles, and variable amounts of facial (FSH) and peroneal (SP) muscle weakness. A variety of clinical expressions may appear within the same family, sometimes limited to insignificant facial weakness (forme fruste). In most patients, the shoulders sag and rotate forward, causing the clavicles to slope downward and appear more prominently (Fig. 12-8A). The scapulae, having lost their fixation, push the trapezius up medially and wing out posteriorly (Fig. 12-8B). Few patients lose the ability to ambulate, although footdrop may be prominent. A rarer infantile variety is characterized by more extensive weakness, bulbar dysfunction, and striking lumbar lordosis.

The majority of patients have EMG and muscle biopsy evidence of a myopathy (i.e., FSH dystrophy), although other cases with an identical clinical syndrome have laboratory evidence of peripheral nerve or anterior horn cell disease (i.e., FSH atrophy). Surgical fixation of the scapula to the thoracic wall may help a patient to elevate his arm over his head, but often this procedure is unsuccessful. Life span is not usually reduced in these mildly affected patients.

LIMB GIRDLE DYSTROPHY

The term *limb girdle* (LG) *dystrophy* is often incorrectly applied to a number of disorders that cause progressive proximal weakness and wasting of all four extremities. Careful laboratory assessment is necessary to distinguish true LG dystrophy from toxic, metabolic, endocrine, and inflammatory myopathies, or from spinal muscular atrophy.

The most common form of LG dystrophy is recessively inherited, with onset during the second or third decades of life. Progressive weakness results in loss of ambulation 5 to 20 years after onset. Those patients with respiratory muscle involvement are susceptible to pneumonia and respiratory failure.

MYOTONIC DISORDERS

Myotonia is an abnormality of the excitable muscle membrane that results in difficulty in initiating an activity or in relaxing muscles after forceful contraction. Electrodiagnostic studies reveal increased irritability to mechanical stimulation and repetitive discharges of muscle action potentials (dive-bomber pattern). Myotonia may be diffuse and not associated with weakness (myotonia congenita) or an almost incidental finding compared with associated weakness (myotonic dystrophy).

Myotonia Congenita

Either autosomally dominant or recessively inherited, patients with myotonia congenita complain of stiffness of muscles, particularly after rest and less with continual exercise. Because of repeated muscle contraction, muscle hypertrophy is frequent and occasionally gives the patient a Herculean appearance. Medications that reduce myotonia include phenytoin, procainamide, quinine, and carbamazepine.

Myotonic Dystrophy

Myotonic dystrophy (MyD) is a multisystemic disorder with an autosomal dominant inheritance. Ptosis, temporalis and masseter wasting, pouting of the lower lip, and thinning of the sternocleidomastoid muscles give a characteristic appearance (Fig. 12–9). The speech is often dysarthric and extremity weakness is either distal or diffuse.

The onset of symptoms occurs insidiously in the second to third decades of life, but milder forms are typical, so that numerous members of a family may be unaware that they are affected (Fig. 12–10). Non-neuromuscular symptoms can predominate, including early cataracts, endocrine dysfunction, intellectual deficits, hypersomnolence, and gastrointestinal disturbances (dysphagia, gallstones, diarrhea). Potentially life-threatening problems include cardiac conduction defects and hypoventilation. Serial electrocardiograms should be performed to identify those patients that require pacemakers to protect against sudden

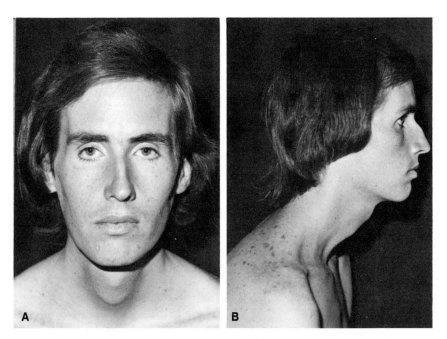

Figure 12-9 Myotonic dystrophy (MyD). *(A)* Wasting of the temporalis muscle, an elongated face, and ptosis are prominent. *(B)* Weakness and wasting of the sternocleidomastoid and other neck muscles result in a "swan neck" appearance. (Handbook of Clinical Neurology, vol 40. Amsterdam, Elsevier/North Holland Biomedical Press, 1979)

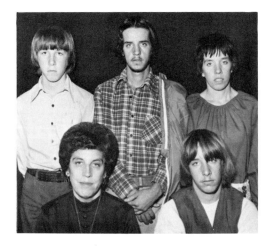

Figure 12-10 Myotonic dystrophy (MyD). A mother and her four children were unaware that they had myotonic dystrophy until the boy in the center sought help for hand-cramping. Typical facial features of this disorder are apparent in all family members. (Handbook of Clinical Neurology, vol 40. Amsterdam, Elsevier/North Holland Biomedical Press, 1979)

death. Pulmonary insufficiency may result from muscle weakness, aspiration, or respiratory center dysfunction.

Treatment of myotonia is usually unnecessary since patients rarely find it to be troublesome as compared to their major complaint of hand and foot muscle weakness. Footdrop may be helped by posterior polypropylene AFOs. General anesthesia should be given with caution, since these patients are unduly sensitive to barbiturates and other medications that depress ventilatory drive.

A severe but rare form of myotonic dystrophy may present at birth, with hypotonia, facial diplegia, profound mental retardation, and recurrent aspiration pneumonia. Although unexplained, in almost all cases the affected relative carrier is the patient's mother rather than the patient's father.

INFLAMMATORY MYOPATHIES

Muscle may be the site of infections (viral, bacterial, parasitic) or immune-mediated inflammatory reactions. Although viral myositis is usually mild and self-limited, immunologic disorders of muscle are more chronic and can produce profound weakness. The latter forms of myositis may be confined to muscle (polymyositis), be associated with a skin rash (dermatomyositis), or develop in association with other connective tissue disorders such as systemic lupus erythematosus, polyarteritis nodosa, rheumatoid arthritis, and scleroderma.

The inflammatory myopathies can occur at any age but are most common in childhood or in the fifth and sixth decades of life. Initially, patients may complain of systemic symptoms including fever, arthralgias, Raynaud's phenomenon, and myalgias. Weakness may begin precipitously, but more commonly there is subacute progression of proximal weakness that is not readily distinguishable from other limb girdle syndromes. The rash of dermatomyositis usually appears as a heliotrope discoloration of the upper eyelids along with an erythematous, thickened, scaling discoloration over joint extensor surfaces. When present, muscle pain, neck flexor weakness, and dysphagia further aid in the diagnosis.

In addition to an inflammatory muscle biopsy, other typical laboratory features include elevated CPK and the presence of antinuclear antibodies, rheumatoid factor, or an elevated sedimentation rate. Myopathic units and spontaneous activity are typically noted with EMG.

Treatment is with corticosteroids (prednisone) or other immunosuppressive drugs (azathioprine, cyclophosphamide, methotrexate). The disease has a variable course; some patients recover completely from an isolated episode, while others demonstrate a more relapsing, remitting course with incomplete recovery between episodes. In a third variety, progression is chronic and indolent and responds poorly to treatment.

Overall mortality is 15%, usually from infection, cardiopulmonary complications, or an associated malignancy.

METABOLIC, TOXIC, AND ENDOCRINE MYOPATHIES

A host of metabolic disturbances and toxic agents can produce acute weakness, muscle pain and cramps, or rhabdomyolysis with myoglobinuria. Since many of these disorders are reversible with proper treatment, a physician should carefully consider each of them in the differential diagnosis of patients with unexplained neuromuscular dysfunction. Because these rare disorders are infrequently seen by a rehabilitation specialist, the reader wishing specific details of any of the illnesses listed under Disorders of Muscle (above) should refer to more comprehensive reviews.

CONGENITAL MYOPATHIES

The term *congenital myopathy* evolved historically to include a group of diseases that are frequently inherited and nonprogressive or slowly progressive, and have characteristic alterations on muscle biopsy (see Chap. 13). Occasionally, symptoms begin later in life or progress more rapidly. There is also evidence that altered neural influence contributes to the patient's weakness.

Clinically, the diseases are frequently indistinguishable, presenting as a hypotonic (floppy) infant or in later childhood with delayed motor milestones. Weakness may be proximal or diffuse and often includes the facial muscles, producing an elongated face with a high-arched palate. Skeletal deformities such as a clubfoot, hip dislocation, or scoliosis are frequent.

The diagnosis, based on morphologic grounds, allows accurate genetic counseling, since autosomal dominant, recessive, and X-linked varieties occur. Treatment is entirely symptomatic and includes exercise, stretching, correction of deformities, and the use of bracing or other assistive devices.

Suggested Readings

BROOKE MH: A Clinician's View of Neuromuscular Disease. Baltimore, Williams & Wilkins, 1977

DUBOWITZ V: Muscle Disorders in Childhood. Philadelphia, WB Saunders, 1977

GRIGGS RC, MOXLEY RT: Treatment of neuromuscular diseases. Adv Neurol 17, 1977

MULDER DW: The Diagnosis and Treatment of Amyotrophic Lateral Sclerosis. Boston, Houghton Mifflin, 1980

ROWLAND LP: Human motor neuron diseases. Adv Neurol 36, 1982

SCHAUMBURG HH, SPENCER PS, THOMAS PK: Disorders of Peripheral Nerve. Philadelphia, FA Davis, 1983

SWAIMAN KF, WRIGHT FS: Pediatric Neuromuscular Diseases. St Louis, CV Mosby, 1979

VINKEN PJ, BRUYN GW, RINGEL SP: Diseases of Muscle. Handbook of Clinical Neurology, vols 40–41. Amsterdam, North Holland, 1979

WALTON J: Disorders of Voluntary Muscle, 4th ed. New York, Churchill Livingstone, 1981

Hans E. Neville
Marc Mitchell Treihaft

13

Tests Used in the Diagnosis of Muscle and Peripheral Nerve Disorders

Patients with nerve or muscle diseases may have a wide variety of clinical complaints (see Chap. 12). After obtaining a careful history and performing a complete examination, experienced physicians can usually determine that the peripheral nervous system is impaired, but special tests are needed to define the exact level of involvement (anterior horn cell, peripheral nerve, neuromuscular junction, or muscle). These tests fall into four categories: (1) blood tests, (2) electrical studies, (3) muscle and nerve biopsy, and (4) miscellaneous studies. The following sections outline available tests and the reasons for obtaining them.

Blood Tests

CREATINE KINASE LEVEL

Creatine kinase (CPK or CK) phosphorylates adenosine diphosphate (ADP) to adenosine triphosphate (ATP), the basic repository of cellular energy in muscle. Under normal conditions muscle contains high concentrations of CK with only low levels of the enzyme detectable in blood. When skeletal muscle is damaged or diseased, the limiting cell membrane becomes permeable to many intracellular proteins, including CK, which may rise to very high levels in the blood. CK is a convenient marker of muscle cell breakdown and, although extremely sensitive, is relatively nonspecific for muscle disease. The following outlines the many conditions in which elevation of serum CK occurs:

1. *Transient elevation*
     Minor muscle trauma
        Intramuscular injection

Electromyogram (EMG)
Surgery
Exercise
Rhabdomyolysis
Nonneuromuscular causes
Myocardial necrosis
Acute neurologic disorders
Acute pulmonary disease
Acute psychosis
2. *Persistent elevation*
Mildly elevated (or normal)
Myotonic dystrophy
Facioscapulohumeral syndromes
Scapuloperoneal syndromes
Oculopharyngeal dystrophy
Ocular "myopathies"
Metabolic and endocrine myopathy
Spinal muscular atrophies
Motor neuron disease
Peripheral neuropathies
Duchenne and Becker dystrophy carrier
Malignant hyperpyrexia
Moderate, very elevated
Duchenne and Becker dystrophy
Limb girdle dystrophy
Inflammatory myopathies
Hypothyroidism

(Ringel SP: Clinical presentations in neuromuscular disease. In Handbook of Clinical Neurology, vol 40, Diseases of Muscle, pp 338–344. New York, North Holland Publishing, 1979)

Serum CK is primarily useful as a screening procedure because it is virtually always elevated in primary muscle diseases and in some neuropathic diseases as well. When the CK level is normal, certain muscle disorders, such as Duchenne muscular dystrophy in which CK levels are always elevated to levels usually in excess of 5000 units, can be excluded. Unfortunately, many muscle disorders produce values in the 100s or low 1000s and are not differentiated by this test alone.

THYROID, POTASSIUM, AND CALCIUM LEVELS

Endocrine gland dysfunction can lead to diffuse muscle weakness, a feature common to almost any neuromuscular disease. Table 13–1 lists the various clinical conditions, special diagnostic features, and associated serum abnormalities of the endocrine myopathies.

Table 13-1   Endocrine Myopathies

Condition	Symptoms and Signs	Blood Test
Hyperthyroidism	Proximal weakness	T3, T4 elevated
Hypothyroidism	Cramps and aches	T3, T4 low
Periodic paralysis	Episodic weakness that is often severe	Potassium level high, low, or normal
Hypoparathyroidism	Cramps, tetany	Calcium level low
Hyperparathyroidism	Aching, hoarseness; tongue fasciculations	Calcium level high

STUDIES TO DETECT COLLAGEN-VASCULAR DISEASE

The collagen–vascular disorders, including polymyositis, dermato-myositis, scleroderma, and some overlap syndromes, may demonstrate a variety of serologic abnormalities. Elevations of sedimentation rate, a positive antinuclear antibody (ANA), and a positive rheumatoid factor (RF) can occur in these disorders, although weakly positive or even negative results are occasionally seen in the presence of active disease.

ACETYLCHOLINE RECEPTOR ANTIBODY LEVELS

The term *acetylcholine receptor antibody* (ACHRab) is applied to a heterogenous group of abnormal antibodies found in the blood of patients with myasthenia gravis. One or more of these antibodies bind to the receptor proteins of the neuromuscular junction, interfere with the normal action of acetylcholine, and create irreversible morphologic changes in the receptor over time. The test to detect ACHRab is quite specific for myasthenia gravis, the only false-positive having been reported in patients receiving the drug penicillamine. Despite its great specificity, the test is positive in only about 90% of patients with myasthenia gravis so that a negative test does not totally exclude the diagnosis.

Electrodiagnostic Studies

Electrodiagnostic studies play an important role in the evaluation of neuromuscular disorders. Based on Galvani's original nerve–muscle stimulation experiments in 1780, they require active participation and cooperation of the patient and on-line interpretation by an experienced electromyographer. Since these procedures are accompanied by some degree of discomfort, results are more readily obtained if the patient is placed in a quiet room and the procedure is carefully explained to reduce pretest anxiety.

Although specialized electromyographic (EMG) techniques may shed light on central neurologic disorders such as tremor (central EMG), this chapter focuses only on electrodiagnostic abnormalities of the motor unit. The motor unit of the peripheral nervous system is composed of an anterior horn cell and its axis cylinder (alpha motor neuron); a Schwann cell, which contributes the myelin sheath surrounding the axon; a neuromuscular junction; and an end-organ, the muscle fiber (see Fig. 12 – 1).

NERVE CONDUCTION STUDIES

Nerve conduction velocities (NCV) are determined by stimulating a peripheral nerve proximally and recording a muscle action potential from distal musculature. Median and ulnar nerves in the arm and posterior tibial and peroneal nerves in the leg are the four nerves most commonly studied, although any major peripheral nerve can be investigated. A square wave direct current (DC) stimulus is applied transcutaneously to a peripheral nerve. If threshold is achieved, a nerve depolrization occurs (details of ionic shifts and electrochemical gradients are beyond the scope of this text; the reader is referred to a standard textbook of EMG or electrophysiology for additional information). The depolrization wave propagates along the myelin sheath to the nerve terminal; releases acetylcholine, which traverses the synaptic cleft; binds to receptor protein; and causes muscle membrane depolarization. This membrane change induces filament contraction and a mechanical twitch of the muscle. With recording electrodes placed over the muscle belly, the twitch is recorded as a muscle action potential, or M response, which is amplified and exhibited on a cathode ray oscilloscope. For example, the median conduction studies are obtained by stimulating the median nerve both at the wrist and at the anticubital fossa, with recording electrodes placed over the abductor pollicis brevis (Fig. 13 – 1). The conduction velocity (CV) of the nerve is determined by dividing the difference in latency (L) of the M responses by the distance between the stimulation sites.

$$CV = \frac{(L_{prox} - L_{dist})}{D}$$

Absolute latency measurements, useful in the evaluation of distal entrapments (i.e., carpal tunnel syndrome; tarsal tunnel syndrome), may also be obtained by stimulating a nerve closely situated to the muscle. For more accurate nerve conduction studies, needle electrodes may be used for either recording or stimulating purposes.

Sensory conduction studies are performed by placing stimulating

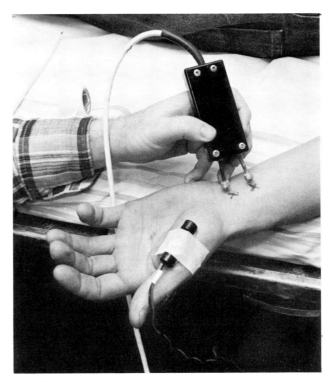

Figure 13–1   The standard equipment used for determining distal latency and nerve conduction velocity. The recording electrode is placed on the thumb over the abductor pollicis brevis muscle. The median nerve is stimulated transcutaneously at the wrist (*x marks*), and the time required for the stimulus to pass from the wrist to the thumb is recorded on an oscilloscope. This is the *distal latency* (L_{dist}). For determining *nerve conduction velocity*, a second latency (L_{prox}) is recorded by stimulating the nerve at the anticubital fossa. See text for conduction velocity calculations.

electrodes distally (as on a finger) and recording electrodes further proximally along a cutaneous sensory or mixed sensory–motor nerve. When the nerve is stimulated distally, an antidromic response is generated and the time required for passage to the recording electrode (the latency) is recorded. Sensory studies require increased amplification and averaging devices because of the small size of the sensory action potentials (less than 20 μV). Late waves (F and H responses) can also be identified and are considered to be depolarization waves that have traveled antidromically up the spinal nerves to the spinal cord and returned orthodromically down the stimulated peripheral nerve. In some cases, these waves provide additional information regarding proximal nerve segments and roots.

ELECTROMYOGRAPHY

Standard electromyography (EMG) uses the same amplifying equipment as nerve conduction studies. A concentric needle or monopolar needle is inserted into a muscle belly so that electrical activity may be amplified and displayed on a cathode ray oscilloscope and a loudspeaker. Muscle activity, both seen and heard by the examiner, is evaluated at rest (normally it is silent) and in degrees of graded exercise. Abnormal spontaneous activity in the form of fibrillation potentials, positive sharp waves, bizarre high-frequency waves, and myotonic discharges are seen with a variety of neuropathic and myopathic disorders. Insertional activity produced by brief small movements of the needle demonstrates the muscle fibers' response to mechanical damage. By asking the patient to minimally contract the muscle, the electrical activity of several motor units may be seen on the screen and measured in terms of duration, amplitude, and configuration. Normal motor units are biphasic or triphasic, but may occasionally contain four phases or five baseline crossings (Fig. 13–2). Abnormal motor unit potentials with five or more phases are termed *polyphasic*. Long-duration, high-amplitude polyphasic potentials are frequently seen with neuropathies, whereas short-duration, low-amplitude polyphasic potentials usually indicate a myopathy (Fig. 13–2). Estimates of polyphasic potentials in normal muscle range from 3% to 12%.

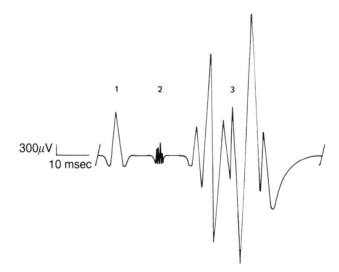

Figure 13–2 Comparison of representative electromyographic potentials. *(1)* Normal motor unit; *(2)* short duration, low-amplitude potential (characteristic of myopathy); and *(3)* large polyphasic potential (typical finding in motor neuron disease).

As the force of contraction increases, motor units fire with increasing frequency and additional units are recruited. Specific recruitment patterns of normal muscle are quite different from those seen in myopathies or neurogenic or upper motor neuron disorders.

The following is a discussion of nerve conduction studies and EMG in representative neuromuscular disorders.

Peripheral Nerve Diseases

Peripheral nerve diseases result from defects in or loss of the myelin sheath or from abnormalities of the axon, or both.

Demyelinating Neuropathies Prolonged conduction velocities or delayed distal latencies are the hallmark of the hereditary neuropathies. The dominantly inherited Charcot-Marie-Tooth disease, (hereditary sensory motor neuropathy type I) is the prototype disorder, and conduction velocities are often 50% of normal or less. NCVs vary considerably among affected individuals in a given family. Other demyelinating neuropathies with extremely slow conduction velocities include Dejerine-Sottas disease, Refsum's disease, metachromatic leukodystrophy, and Krabbe's leukodystrophy.

A group of acquired demyelinating neuropathies that often improve with treatment includes the acute inflammatory polyradiculoneuropathies (Guillain-Barre syndrome) and the relapsing or chronic progressive polyradiculoneuropathies. NCVs are variable, with some parts of a peripheral nerve conducting normally and other segments showing patchy slowing, dispersion of potentials, and prolongation of H and F wave latencies.

In a third group of demyelinating neuropathies, a segment of peripheral nerve is trapped by a tight fascial band, such as at the wrist (carpal tunnel syndrome), ankle (cubital tunnel syndrome), or lateral upper femoral head (peroneal entrapment). Focal demyelination at the site of entrapment causes a delay of conduction at the point. Such a focal block may also develop in any peripheral nerve where vascular inflammation (vasculitis) or infarction (diabetes) has occurred. Multiple blocks are collectively termed *mononeuritis multiplex*.

Axonal Neuropathies The most common of all neuropathies affect the axon and result from a variety of toxic – metabolic disturbances, including alcoholism, heavy metal intoxication, diabetes, solvent exposure, and uremia. Less commonly, an axonal neuropathy develops with vitamin B_{12} deficiency, porphyria, lead poisoning, and in Friedreich's ataxia. Since there is a loss of functional axons due to a "dying back" of terminal positions in peripheral nerves, evoked amplitudes are significantly reduced whereas NCVs remain normal. This reduction in amplitude is the hallmark of an axonal neuropathy. In some diseases, such as porphyria, the reduction in amplitudes of motor nerves is much greater than for sensory nerves, whereas in carcinomatous neuropathy and Friedreich's ataxia, sensory nerves are more severely involved. In diabetes mellitus a mixture of axonal and demyelinating features are seen. There may be focal or segmental slowing superimposed on these diffuse changes, producing a mononeuritis multiplex.

Anterior Horn Cell Disease

When anterior horn cells in the spinal cord degenerate, axons innervating skeletal muscle are simultaneously lost. Denervated muscle fibers may be reinnervated by nerve sprouts from adjacent healthy axons, but the repair process is often incomplete so that progressive loss of muscle strength develops.

EMG of patients with anterior horn cell degeneration may demonstrate electrical abnormalities similar to axonal neuropathies but usually to a greater degree. With placement of the EMG needle there is an increase in insertional activity. At rest the muscle is quite active with fibrillations, fasciculations, positive sharp waves, and bizarre high-frequency activity. On voluntary contraction giant (high-amplitude, increased-duration) polyphasic potentials occur and are considered to result from reinnervation. Low-amplitude, short-duration polyphasic potentials, more commonly seen in myopathies, occur infrequently.

As the force of voluntary contraction is increased, the surviving motor units fire at increasing rates. Due to dropout of neurons, a decreased interference pattern is seen with surviving units firing at an increased recruitment frequency. Neuronal loss results in reduced amplitude of compound muscle action potentials, and in severe cases motor NCVs may also be slightly reduced. Electrodiagnostic findings are similar in all anterior horn cell degenerations (i.e., amyotrophic lateral sclerosis, poliomyelitis, spinal muscular atrophies). With chronic nerve root compression, the findings are similar but occur only in muscles supplied by the affected spinal cord root.

Myopathies

Electrical abnormalities are widespread and varied in muscle affected by dystrophic changes, inflammation, metabolic abnormalities, abnormal stored material, or toxins. Muscle cell necrosis and fiber splitting in any of these conditions produce increased insertional activity, bizarre high-frequency potentials, fibrillations, positive sharp waves, and increased numbers of short-duration, low-amplitude polyphasic potentials. Since involvement may be patchy, it is common to find portions of a muscle heavily involved while an adjacent area is spared entirely.

It is usually impossible to define the type of muscle disease by needle EMG sampling alone. For example, although short-amplitude, short-duration polyphasia is a frequent finding in Duchenne dystrophy, it also occurs in facioscapulohumeral and limb girdle dystrophy. In addition, giant polyphasic potentials, usually suggestive of denervation, may occasionally be seen in facioscapulohumeral dystrophy. Probably the only relatively specific finding for a myopathy is the "dive-bomber"-like action potentials commonly observed in myotonic dystrophy and myotonia congenita.

Neuromuscular Junction Disorders

The neuromuscular junction defects in myasthenia gravis, clinically manifested by muscle fatigue, are best evaluated by electrical testing. If a series of supramaximal stimuli are applied to a nerve at slow rates (2 Hz – 5 Hz), the compound muscle action potential amplitude remains constant. In myasthenia gravis, the amplitude drops slightly with each successive stimulus, a phenomenon termed *decrement* (Fig. 13 – 3). Excluding artifact, a "decremental" response of greater than 10% between the first and fifth responses is diagnostic of a neuromuscular junction defect.

In our laboratory, additional information is obtained by stimulating first with the muscle at rest and then 30 seconds and 1, 2, 3, and 4

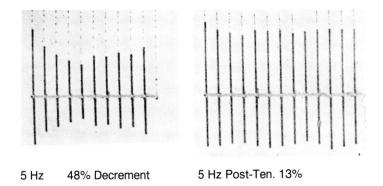

5 Hz   48% Decrement   5 Hz Post-Ten. 13%

Figure 13 – 3 Stimulating and recording electrodes are set up as shown in Figure 13 – 1. A series of five per second stimuli (5 Hz) are applied to the median nerve; the response is received by the recording electrode and registered on an oscilloscope screen as thin vertical lines. In normal circumstances, each stimulus is followed by a response of constant amplitude. In myasthenia gravis *(left)*, the first response is of normal amplitude but successive responses are reduced in a decremental manner. After giving the patient 10 mg edrophonium chloride IV *(right — Post-Ten.)*, the decrement is "repaired" and each successive stimulus produces a response with an amplitude that is nearly equal to the initial response.

minutes after a 30-second period of voluntary tetanic contraction. Immediately after exercise a brief period of postexercise facilitation may be seen, followed by postexercise exhaustion decrement of the compound muscle action potentials. The diagnostic yield on repetitive studies may also be enhanced by specialized procedures such as warming the limb, ischemia, regional curare testing, and evaluation of proximal as well as distal musculature.

Similar to myasthenia gravis, patients with the Eaton Lambert syndrome may show a decrement at low stimulation rates (less than 10 Hz). However, at higher rates of stimulation or following tetanic exercise, the presynaptic defect results in a paradoxical augmentation of the compound muscle action potential. Other abnormalities that affect the presynaptic site include botulism, hypocalcemia, and neomycin.

Single-fiber EMG may also be useful in evaluating neuromuscular junction disorders. Variability of firing between two or more fibers in a motor unit, termed *jitter*, occurs with neuromuscular junction dysfunction.

ELECTROCARDIOGRAM

An electrocardiogram (ECG) should be routinely obtained in neuromuscular disorders because cardiac conduction disturbances can occur early or late in the disease. In Duchenne dystrophy, the disease process involves the heart muscle and leads to heart failure and characteristic electrical changes. Potentially fatal conduction delays may be detected early in myotonic dystrophy and, if severe enough, may indicate the need for placement of a cardiac pacemaker. Similar conduction defects may occur in the syndrome of "ophthalmoplegia plus," some of the mitochondrial myopathies, and in Friedreich's ataxia.

Muscle and Nerve Biopsy

Direct examination of diseased tissue is an invaluable diagnostic procedure for use by clinicians. In myopathies, muscle biopsy can be carried out using local anesthesia. The muscle selected for biopsy should be moderately weak, but one frequently studied, such as the quadriceps or biceps. The skin overlying the affected muscle is anesthetized and incised, exposing the muscle, and a small cylinder ¼ inch by ¾ inch is removed. The muscle is quickly frozen in isopentane–nitrogen and 10-μm thick sections are cut and mounted on glass coverslips. The sections are then processed with various stains or reactions and examined under a standard light microscope. Full details of the procedure can be found in the text by Dubowitz and Brooke (1973).

Muscle fibers are conventionally examined in transverse section where they appear as round–oval or slightly irregular profiles (Figs. 13–4 and 13–5). Individual fibers possess unique biochemical and physiologic characteristics that determine their morphologic appearance with each stain or reaction. When muscle is diseased, there appears to be only a limited number of pathologic reactions that the muscle cell can undergo. When correlated with the patient's clinical complaints, the muscle biopsy often provides a definitive diagnosis.

Examples of pathologic change in muscle are shown in the accompanying illustrations, which demonstrate typical abnormalities occurring in human neuromuscular disorders. An early and common abnormality is widely differing sizes of muscle fibers. Such variability (Fig. 13–6) is the hallmark of any of the dystrophies and may be particularly prominent in Duchenne dystrophy. When accompanied by an excess of connective tissue (Fig. 13–6) between fascicles and between individual muscle fibers, the diagnosis of dystrophy is almost certain. A second type of size variation is that best demonstrated by histochemical studies (Fig. 13–7) in which all light-reacting fibers (type 1) are of a uniformly small size and the darker fibers (type 2) are significantly larger. This unique constellation is diagnostic of congenital fiber-type disproportion. Finally, a kind of size variation may occur in which large clusters of

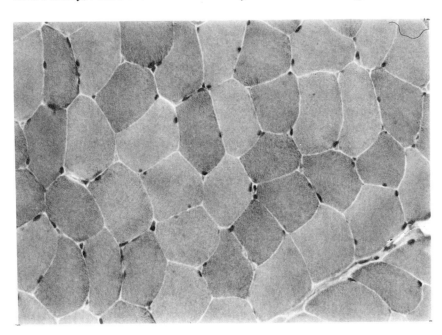

Figure 13–4   Normal adult muscle. Muscle fibers are cut in a plane transverse to their long axis and appear as round, oval, or slightly irregular profiles. One or more darkly stained nuclei are seen at the edge of most fibers. (Trichrome, ×300)

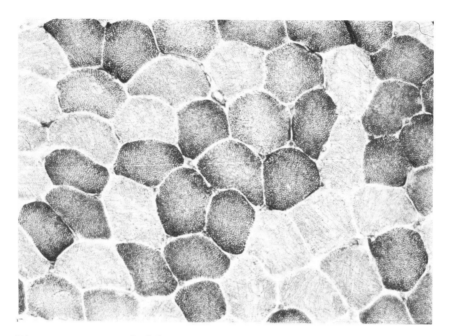

Figure 13–5 Normal adult muscle. The histochemical reaction carried out on these muscle cells demonstrates oxidative enzyme activity. Darker type 1 fibers contain more enzyme compared with lighter-reacting type 2 fibers. (NADH-TR, ×300)

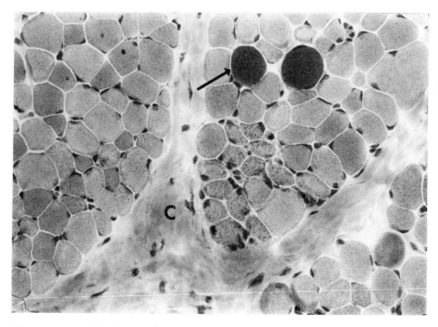

Figure 13–6 Duchenne dystrophy. Compare these fibers to normal muscle (Fig. 13–4). Dystrophic changes include a marked variability in fiber size; dark, "opaque" fibers (*arrow*); and abnormal quantities of fibrous connective tissue (C). (Trichrome, ×300)

very small fibers are seen adjacent to normal-size fibers (Fig. 13–8), typical of spinal muscular atrophy.

The inflammatory myopathies are associated with large numbers of cells, primarily lymphocytes, infiltrating the muscle (Fig. 13–9). A complex antigen–antibody response may trigger this striking pathologic change, which can be associated with varying degrees of cell necrosis. Except for the findings of eosinophilic infiltrates in some of the rarer autoimmune muscle disorders, the common finding in all these disorders is the rather widespread mononuclear cell inflammatory response.

In the so-called congenital myopathies, a prominent abnormality of muscle morphology may be the only finding on biopsy. For example, in myotubular myopathy (Fig. 13–10) a distinctive, centrally placed nucleus is seen in most of the small fibers. In central core disease, the oxidative histochemical reactions reveal central zones totally lacking in oxidative activity (Fig. 13–11) while the fibers appear normal with other stains.

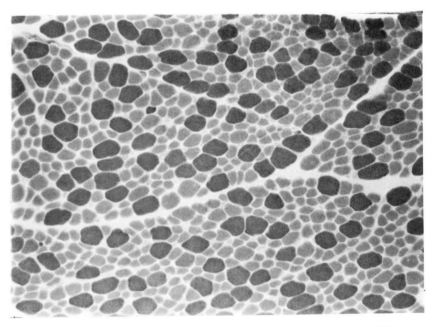

Figure 13–7   Congenital fiber-type dysproportion. The enzyme ATPase reveals a typical "checkerboard" pattern consisting of type 1 (light-reacting) and type 2 (dark-reacting) fibers. Unlike normal biopsies, in which all fibers are generally of the same size, the type 1 fibers shown here are much smaller than the dark type 2 fibers. The overall smallness of all fibers, compared with the normals (Figs. 13–4 and 13–5) is expected because this biopsy is from a 2-year-old child. Muscle fiber size increases with age, with typical fibers averaging 10 to 20 μ at birth compared with 50 to 60 μ in adults. (ATPase pH 9.4, $\times$300)

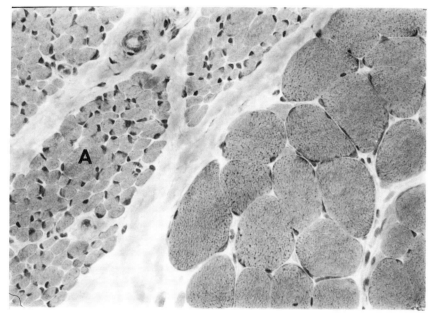

Figure 13–8 Spinal muscular atrophy. The atrophied fibers (A), averaging 15 to 25 μ, are denervated as a result of anterior horn cell death. The fibers at the right are actually larger than normal for the patient's age. This combination of groups of atrophied and hypertrophied fibers is typical of motor neuron diseases that occur in infancy and childhood. (Trichrome, ×300)

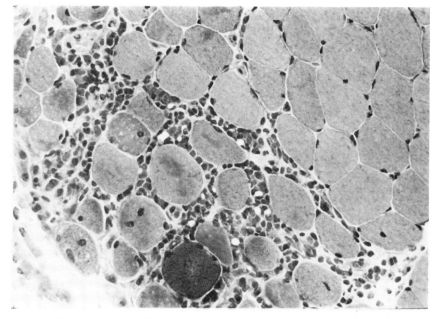

Figure 13–9 Polymyositis, showing a prominent infiltrate of inflammatory cells lying between muscle fibers. The dark cell at bottom left of center is undergoing degeneration. (Trichrome, ×300)

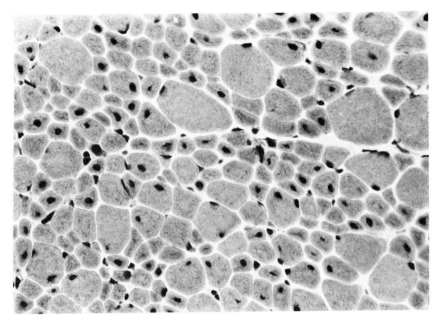

Figure 13-10 Myotubular myopathy, showing a marked variability in fiber size. In most of the smaller fibers, a dark, centrally placed nucleus is evident, suggesting that muscle cell development has been arrested in an embryonic stage. (H & E, ×473)

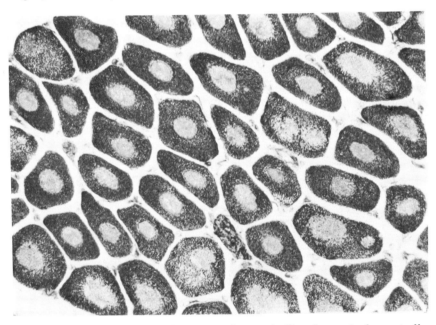

Figure 13-11 Central core disease. Each muscle fiber has a single centrally located area in which there is little or no oxidative enzyme activity. When examined by electron microscopy, such enzyme-deficient areas may be structurally normal (structured cores) or may have a marked disruption of contractile protein (unstructured cores). (NADH-TR, ×300)

A peripheral nerve may also be biopsied under local anesthesia. The sural nerve, located low in the leg, is often chosen because it is entirely sensory. A 2-cm specimen is removed under local anesthesia, cut into three pieces, and processed. One specimen is frozen, cut and stained much like muscle, and examined. A second portion is generally fixed in formaldehyde, paraffin-embedded, and stained with a variety of agents to demonstrate myelin, axons, connective tissue, and inflammatory cells. A third piece is fixed in glutaraldehyde, plastic-embedded, cut at 1-μm thickness for light microscopic examination, and, in selected instances, further processed for electron microscopy. Sural nerve biopsy is particularly useful in confirming inflammatory disorders (Fig. 13–12), amyloid deposition (Fig. 13–13), or hereditary diseases such as Charcot-Marie-Tooth disease (Fig. 13–14).

Miscellaneous Studies

Tests of pulmonary and swallowing function and spine x-ray films are often helpful in establishing the cause of patient complaints (e.g., swallowing dysfunction in amyotrophic lateral sclerosis, shortness of breath

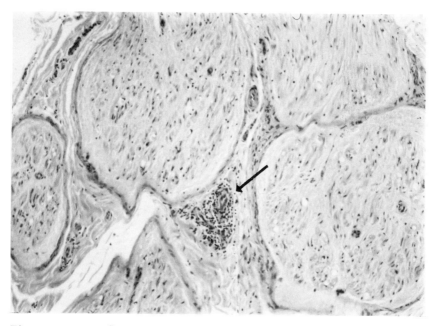

Figure 13–12 Inflammatory polyradiculoneuropathy in sural nerve. In this field, there are five nerve fascicles cut transversely. Each contains a slightly reduced number of myelinated nerve fibers (difficult to resolve at this low magnification). The prominant abnormality here is the deposition of inflammatory cells (*arrow*), involving a single vessel and its walls. (H & E stain of formalin-fixed, paraffin-embedded nerve, ×116)

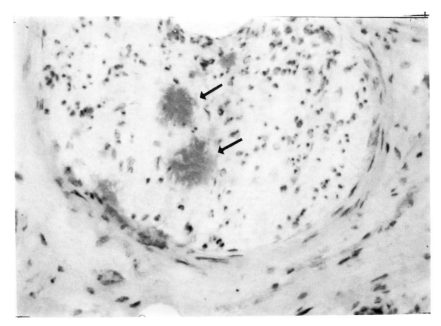

Figure 13–13   Amyloid deposit in sural nerve. The single nerve fascicle shown contains two prominent deposits *(arrows)* of orange-red material that, under polarized light, appear an apple green color (typical of amyloid). This fascicle contains numerous nuclei of Schwann cells and fibroblasts, but all myelinated fibers have been lost. (Congo Red stain of formalin-fixed, paraffin-embedded nerve, ×300)

in Duchenne dystrophy, back pain from a pathologic fracture of an osteoporotic spine of the polymyositis patient receiving chronic steroid therapy). Such tests are rarely useful in pinpointing the exact neuro-muscular disease but are important in helping the clinician better understand and effectively treat respiratory symptoms.

Muscle biochemistry tests are quite specialized and perform only in specific instances. For example, in patients suspected of abnormal glycogen storage in muscle (as in McArdle's disease), an ischemic exercise test is performed. This can be carried out easily on out-patients to determine if lactic acid accumulates in the blood after exercise of forearm muscles. Other tests for biochemical dysfunction are more complicated and are performed on muscle biopsy specimens to detect carnitine deficiency, acid maltase deficiency, or carnitine palmityl transferase defi-

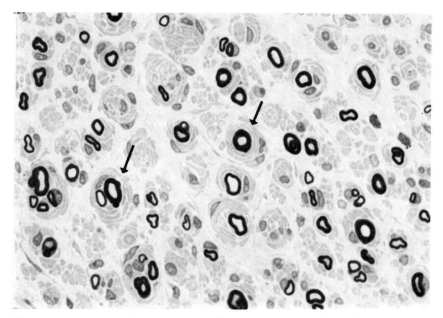

Figure 13–14 Hereditary motor and sensory neuropathy (Charcot-Marie-Tooth disease). High-power view showing "onion bulb" profiles. Myelinated fibers appear as black ovals or circles. Many are surrounded by concentrically applied layers of lighter-staining material (*arrows*), resembling the cut surface of an onion. These layers formed of cell cytoplasm represent defective remyelination attempts by Schwann cells. The number of myelinated fibers is reduced by about 50%. (Toluidine blue stained, plastic-embedded nerve, ×756)

ciency. Because of technical difficulties, these latter studies are performed by special arrangement in only a few laboratories in the United States.

Summary

A wide variety of special tests are available for the diagnosis of neuromuscular disorders. These studies do not stand alone and should be considered as an extension of the clinical examination. None should be ordered until the patient is examined by a physician familiar with the clinical manifestations of neuromuscular diseases. Selected studies are then obtained to confirm a clinical impression. With this approach, the majority of nerve and muscle disorders can be diagnosed, effective therapy started, and appropriate counselling undertaken with the patient and family.

Suggested Readings

ASBURY AK, JOHNSON PC: Pathology of Peripheral Nerve. Philadelphia, WB Saunders, 1978

BROOKE MH: A Clinician's View of Neuromuscular Disease. Baltimore, Williams & Wilkins, 1977

DUBOWITZ V: Muscle Disorders of Childhood. Philadelphia, WB Saunders, 1978

DUBOWITZ V, BROOKE MH: Muscle Biopsy: A Modern Approach. Philadelphia, WB Saunders, 1973

KIMURA J: Electrodiagnosis in Diseases of Nerve and Muscle: Principles and Practice. Philadelphia, FA Davis, 1983

RINGEL SP: Clinical Presentations in Neuromuscular Disease. Handbook of Clinical Neurology, vol 40, Diseases of Muscle, pp 338–344. New York, North Holland Publishing, 1979

GOODGOLD J, EBERSTEN A: Electrodiagnosis of Neuromuscular Disorders. Baltimore, Williams & Wilkins, 1983

Steven P. Ringel
Richard J. Martin

14

Respiratory Complications and Their Management in Neuromuscular Disorders

Patients with neuromuscular diseases are at risk for life-threatening pulmonary complications at any stage of their illness, whether awake or during sleep. The unwary physician or therapist who overlooks mild, nonspecific symptoms of respiratory distress will be both startled and unprepared when a "mildly weakened" patient suddenly develops respiratory failure. At the other end of the continuum, rehabilitation therapists must daily anticipate and treat pulmonary complications in the totally paralyzed patient who is unable to adequately ventilate the lungs. Such a patient is compromised not only by weakened muscles of respiration, but also by recurrent aspiration, an insufficient cough reflex, and shrinking pulmonary reserve from progressive scoliosis. Even for this unfortunate individual, many respiratory complications are reversible and should be treated if the general quality of life is still acceptable to the patient and family.

This chapter discusses the diagnosis and treatment of the aforementioned pulmonary complications in patients with neuromuscular disorders. As a framework, a brief review of the physiology of respiratory failure is provided, including the laboratory assessment of pulmonary function. Management of the ventilator-dependent patient is reviewed, including choices of equipment and ethical concerns, since it is currently feasible, although quite difficult, to provide long-term ventilatory assistance.

Physiology of Respiratory Failure

Respiratory failure can be defined on the basis of ventilation or oxygenation. As ventilatory failure occurs, the carbon dioxide (CO_2) level increases. In the patient with a neuromuscular disorder without primary lung disease, ventilatory failure can be secondary to either central nervous system dysfunction or respiratory muscle weakness. Although the diaphragm is the principle muscle of inspiration, the intercostals and accessory muscles of respiration may become the primary inspiratory muscles and sustain ventilation without leading to respiratory failure. Figure 14–1 illustrates how a recumbent position can play a major role in producing hypoventilation by taking away the beneficial effects of gravity on the diaphragm. As a patient with muscular dystrophy reclines, spirometry and minute ventilation decrease.

Inadequate oxygenation (hypoxemia) can occur in four ways. (1) Ventilation-to-perfusion mismatching occurs where there is obstruction to air flow, as in asthma. In neuromuscular patients, such mismatching comes into play if a patient has bronchospasm or narrowing of the airways due to poor inspiratory effort from weakened musculature. (2) A shunt occurs when blood flow continues through areas of the lung but no ventilation is present to these areas. Because some neuromuscular patients do not have either the neural input to the respiratory muscles or the strength to fully open all the airways, microatelectasis or radiographically visible collapse develops and produces a shunt. (3) Hypoventilation, as discussed above, is a major cause of hypoxemia in neuromuscular patients. (4) Diffusion abnormalities, which develop when there is a block in the transfer of oxygen from the alveoli to the red blood cells, are rarely a problem in neuromuscular patients. Carefully selected treatment can improve the condition of the patient with inadequate oxygenation or ventilatory failure.

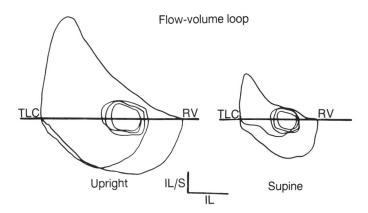

Figure 14–1 Flow-volume loop measures flow on the vertical axis and volume on the horizontal axis. Initially, the patient breathes normally (inner circles); then he takes a deep inspiration (downward deflection) to total lung capacity (TLC) and blows out (upward deflection) as hard and fast as possible to residual volume (RV). Finally, he breathes in rapidly back to TLC. In this patient with muscular dystrophy, the flow and volume are significantly better in the upright position than in the supine position because of the effect of gravity and better diaphragmatic expansion and contraction while upright.

Pulmonary Function Tests

A restrictive pattern seen by pulmonary function tests is most common in neuromuscular patients with respiratory impairment; that is, the patients have difficulty expanding their lungs completely so that small lung volumes and decreased flows are recorded. A simple test to detect respiratory impairment is spirometry, in which a forced expiratory maneuver is measured against time (Fig. 14–2). With a restrictive pattern, the vital capacity (VC) and, to a lesser extent, the forced expiratory volume in 1 second (FEV_1) may decrease below 80% of predicted (mild reduction, 70%–79%; moderate reduction, 60%–69%; severe reduction, 50%–59%; very severe, less than 50%). Since an obstructive pattern (indicative of diseases such as asthma, bronchitis, emphysema) has a greater decrease in FEV_1 and a normal or mildly decreased VC, the FEV_1/VC ratio is used to distinguish patterns. A ratio greater than 75% in the presence of a reduced VC denotes a restrictive pattern, whereas a ratio less than 75% with a decreased FEV_1 is indicative of an obstructive pattern. More formal testing, such as measurement of other lung volumes and airway resistance, should be performed in the neuromuscular patient with a reduced FEV_1 because there may be a concomitant, treatable obstructive process.

An alternate means of measuring pulmonary function is a flow–volume curve where volume is plotted against flow instead of time. Figure 14–1 shows these loops in a patient with muscular dystrophy in

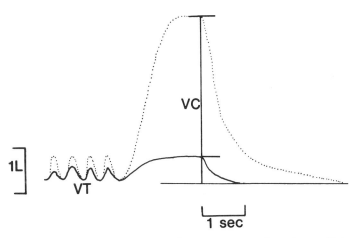

Figure 14–2 Spirometric tracing of a patient with poliomyelitis (*solid line* = patient values; *dotted line* = predicted values; *vertical axis* = volume; and *horizontal axis* = time). The patient's tidal volume (*VT*) is much smaller than would be expected, owing to a restrictive pattern that is typical of neuromuscular patients. The vital capacity (maximum inspiration) of this patient is severely reduced compared with that predicted. A decreased amount of flow compared with that predicted is also seen during forced expiration.

the upright and supine positions. Note that when the helpful gravitational forces are eliminated by recumbency, the flow and volumes decrease markedly. By simply elevating the head of a patient's bed with blocks, gravity will assist the patient in respiration.

Maximal inspiratory and expiratory muscle force is a measurement of muscle strength. Using nose clips and a pressure manometer at the mouth, occlusion on inspiration following a full expiration gives the inspiratory pressure, and the occlusion pressure on expiration following a maximal inspiration defines the expiratory strength. Since the range of normal values for these pressures is wide, sequential measurements are more important for following improvement or worsening in individual patients. Usually a mouthpiece is used, but if facial weakness is present, a tight-fitting mask should be substituted.

Acute Muscle Weakness

Diseases that produce acute paralysis (see list, below) are life-threatening when there is accompanying respiratory muscle paralysis. As a physician hastens to determine the cause of the weakness, he must simultaneously anticipate and treat acute respiratory dysfunction. Although some patients with respiratory failure will experience clinical signs of respiratory distress, including intercostal and suprasternal retraction, flaring of the nasal alae, and cyanosis, other patients, because weakness masks these signs, may only appear confused, restless, or drowsy, or may complain of a headache. Given the nonspecificity of these latter signs and symptoms, all patients with acute weakness should be closely monitored in an intensive care unit with serial arterial blood gases. If the patient develops any rapid elevation of arterial partial pressure of carbon dioxide (pCO_2), intubation and mechanical ventilation is usually necessary. A prepared medical and nursing team that anticipates tracheal intubation in advance of an emergent situation will avoid unnecessary complications from hasty decisions. Following is a list of diseases producing acute paralysis:

1. Lower motor neuron disorder
      Poliomyelitis
2. Peripheral nerve disorders
      Guillain-Barre syndrome
      Tick paralysis
      Diphtheria
      Porphyria
3. Neuromuscular junction disorders
      Myasthenia gravis
      Botulism

Organophosphate poisoning
4. Muscle disorders
Inflammatory myopathy
Periodic paralysis
Rhabdomyolysis

After immediate measures are taken to ensure stable cardiorespiratory function, a rapid, sequential diagnostic evaluation should be pursued, since prompt and specific treatment can reverse weakness and avoid prolonged ventilatory assistance. For example, the signs and symptoms of myasthenia gravis will respond to cholinesterase inhibitors, immunosuppression, and plasmapheresis. Weakness from organophosphate poisoning will reverse with atropine, and patients with tick paralysis will generally improve within hours of removal of the female *Dermacentor andersoni*, or North American tick. Diseases of the anterior horn cell, peripheral nerve, neuromuscular junction, or muscle that can produce acute weakness are reviewed in Chapter 12.

In the ventilator-dependent patient, arterial blood gases are monitored frequently to reverse hypercapnia or hypoxemia. Inspired air is humidified to prevent drying of bronchial secretions. The patient's position is changed regularly to allow for gravity drainage of the bronchial tree. Chest percussion additionally aids the removal of secretions (see Chap. 19). Tracheobronchial aspiration using sterile catheters and gloves is performed both to obtain cultures and to clear secretions. Compliant, low-pressure endotracheal tube cuffs avoid pressure necrosis of the tracheal mucosa and can be used for several weeks. Tracheostomy is preferable if prolonged ventilation is required or if secretions cannot be adequately suctioned through the endotracheal tube.

Importantly, if complications are avoided, the survival rate in patients with acute respiratory failure from neuromuscular disease is much higher than in patients with primary pulmonary disease. Accordingly, the medical team should anticipate and aggressively treat respiratory and urinary tract infections, decubitus ulcers, thrombophlebitis, pulmonary emboli, and malnutrition. Early feeding by nasogastric tube will prevent excessive protein catabolism and hasten recovery of strength (see Chap. 23). Patients should be fed small volumes in an upright position to prevent gastroesophageal reflux and aspiration (see Chap. 19). When the patient resumes oral feedings, physicians and nurses must still be alert for aspiration. All too often a patient recovering from acute paralysis can have a life-threatening relapse caused by unrecognized, recurrent aspiration. Swallowing may be impaired, yet the patient will be eager to take nourishment by mouth to avoid the nasogastric tube. In the tracheotomized patient it is helpful to initially use small sips of water colored with food dye, because the dye will be recovered during tracheal suctioning if the patient is aspirating.

Chronic Muscle Weakness

Apart from respiratory muscle weakness, patients with neuromuscular disease also develop pulmonary complications from dysphagia with recurrent aspiration, and from scoliosis, which further reduces pulmonary reserve. Sudden respiratory failure may also occur in patients who do not have end-stage respiratory muscle weakness either from superimposed diaphragmatic paralysis or from central hypoventilation. Several respiratory complications are more significant during sleep, yet often are not recognized. Since all of these complications are, in part, reversible, early recognition and aggressive therapy should be instituted prior to irreversible changes.

PROGRESSIVE DYSPHAGIA

Progressive dysphagia or recurrent aspiration is often prominent in amyotrophic lateral sclerosis, X-linked spinal muscular atrophy, myasthenia gravis, and oculopharyngeal dystrophy, but can also occur in a variety of other neuromuscular diseases. Aspiration occasionally develops without overt signs of dysphagia. A barium swallow with cine radiography should not just be reserved for patients who complain of dysphagia but should also be performed to demonstrate aspiration in any patient who coughs while eating or who develops unexplained recurrent pneumonia.

Patients initially have difficulty swallowing hard solids, but with time, liquids become more difficult. A dietitian can be helpful at this point to monitor caloric intake and to instruct the patient in preparing foods that can be more easily swallowed. A speech therapist can also reinforce proper swallowing technique at this time (see Chap. 9).

Several surgical procedures have been developed that temporarily improve swallowing function. Injection of Teflon into a vocal cord, by making the glottis more competent, allows a stronger cough for expelling tracheobronchial secretions and aspirated material. In a patient who pools food and fluid in the hypopharynx, a cricopharyngeal myotomy has been used to improve pharyngeal transport. Surgical section of the nerves to the major salivary glands on one side (chorda tympani and Jacobsen's nerves) through a small incision in the tympanic membrane will reduce saliva without the side-effects of atropinelike medications. Alternatively, salivary glands can be irradiated if a patient is not a good surgical risk.

With continual weight loss, feeding through a nasogastric tube will temporarily maintain nutrition, although this method is not satisfactory for long-term management because of irritation and ulceration of the nasal mucosa and pharynx. Placement of a cervical esophagostomy or gastrostomy tube may ultimately be necessary to maintain nutrition in patients with severe pharyngeal dysfunction. Proper care of a feeding tube is discussed in Chapter 19 and the content of tube feedings is reviewed in Chapter 24. No tubes completely prevent aspiration of oral secretions or regurgitation of foods into the trachea. A cuffed tracheotomy during feeding minimizes aspiration but only surgical closure of the glottis is foolproof. This procedure is rarely used, however, since it deprives the patient of all vocalizing.

All families should be instructed as to what to do if the patient suddenly develops obstruction of the respiratory pathway. The Heimlich maneuver (Fig. 14–3), or abdominal hug of life, can be lifesaving. The patient is bent forward over a chair or the rescuer's arm so that his head is lower than his chest. The rescuer stands behind the patient, encircling him with his arms, hands interlocked, and presses forcefully upward in the upper abdomen. This sudden pressure forces the diaphragm up, expelling residual air from the chest cavity and thus dislodging the foreign body.

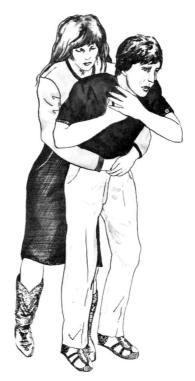

Figure 14–3 Heimlich maneuver (hug of life). When a rescuer presses forcefully upward on the upper abdomen, air is expelled from the chest and will dislodge a foreign body obstructing the airway. See text for full explanation. (Wiederholt WC [ed]: Neurology for Non-Neurologists. New York, Academic Press, 1982)

PROGRESSIVE SCOLIOSIS

In progressive scoliosis (see also Chaps. 16 to 18), as paraspinal muscles weaken, the spine collapses, producing an unequal matching of ventilation to lung perfusion, an increased physiologic dead space, and reduction in both vital capacity and total lung capacity. The amount of abnormality is directly proportional to the degree of scoliosis, so that a concerted effort should be made to prevent progressive deformity.

A properly fitted wheelchair that uses pads or a molded seat insert to maintain an erect spine is helpful. A polypropylene thoracolumbar body jacket is additionally useful in young children who cannot be properly positioned in a wheelchair. Forced vital capacity and maximum voluntary ventilations are often mildly reduced when the patient is wearing the jacket. Therefore, the body jacket should be removed with an acute infection to allow the patient to take advantage of his full pulmonary reserve.

One author has proposed that severe scoliosis can be prevented if the spine is maintained hyperextended, locking the posterior facet joints and preventing lateral collapse. Such hyperextension can be maintained with a brace or body jacket or with a modified wheelchair that accentuates hyperextension. The chair should not be too wide, so that the child does not accentuate scoliosis by leaning to the side to gain arm support.

Early spinal fusion is advocated by many in the treatment of scoliosis because the risk of further pulmonary decompensation increases when surgery is postposed (see Chap. 18). In considering surgery, the physician must take into account the natural history of the disease as well as the patient's level of disability. Few recommend surgery in Duchenne dystrophy because the prognosis is so poor. On the other hand, patients with a static deficit (poliomyelitis) or with slow progression (intermediate and juvenile spinal muscular atrophy) are better candidates for fusion. In general, patients with vital capacities greater than 70% of normal tolerate surgery well. In patients with vital capacities below 30% of predicted, a period of postoperative mechanical ventilation should be anticipated.

It is advantageous to have a pulmonary physical therapist treat the patient before surgery, since training the patient to use accessory muscles of respiration preoperatively can enhance pulmonary function after surgery. A patient can also be taught how to adequately cough and the positions for postural drainage. It is imperative that the patient be made fully aware that he might require an endotracheal tube postoperatively so that he is not alarmed when he awakens from general anesthesia and is unable to talk. The physical therapist can visit the patient in the recovery room and start intensive chest physical therapy. Weaning from ventilatory support is not undertaken until the patient is stabilized.

SUDDEN RESPIRATORY FAILURE

Sudden respiratory failure has been reported in patients with a variety of neuromuscular diseases (myotonic dystrophy, congenital myopathies, ocular myopathies, acid maltase deficiency, poliomyelitis) in which sufficient weakness is not present to account for the respiratory embarrassment. A diminished ventilatory response to decreased oxygen tension or increased CO_2 tension has been noted, suggesting that these patients have the muscle power to ventilate but lack central chemoreceptor responsiveness. This hyporesponsiveness either to hypoxemia or hypercapnia may account for neuromuscular patients who develop respiratory failure following general anesthesia or exposure to depressant drugs.

Occasionally a patient with only mild weakness of accessory muscles of respiration develops acute respiratory failure from dominant diaphragmatic weakness. With paralysis of the diaphragm, abdominal muscles can assist in respiratory function but only when the patient is upright. If a patient complains of increasing shortness of breath when reclining and his vital capacity is less than when upright, diaphragm weakness should be suspected. The patient may also be unable to sniff, a predominantly diaphragmatic function. Fluoroscopy is often inadequate to assess diaphragmatic function, but the measurement of transdiaphragmatic pressure is more sensitive.

Phrenic nerve pacing is rarely successful in neuromuscular patients with diaphragmatic weakness. Nocturnally, a cuirass ventilator or rocking chair device is more useful.

RESPIRATORY DISORDERS DURING SLEEP

Disordered breathing patterns, oxygen desaturation, hypercapnia, and cardiac arrhythmias occur more commonly than usually expected in neuromuscular patients during sleep. It is important that the therapist working with neuromuscular patients be aware of certain signs and symptoms that point to periodic breathing during sleep. The following can occur to any degree in the neuromuscular patient: daytime somnolence, morning headaches, restless sleep, loud snoring, decreased mental alertness, personality change, systemic hypertension, erythrocytosis, congestive heart failure, pulmonary hypertension, or enuresis. If any of these symptoms or signs are unexplained by other causes, a polysonographic study should be done to document nocturnal disorders (Fig. 14–4). Since simple therapeutic daytime interventions such as respiratory muscle training can dramatically improve the nocturnal respiratory pattern and oxygen level, the quality of life can be improved and future morbidity or mortality due to respiratory complications prevented.

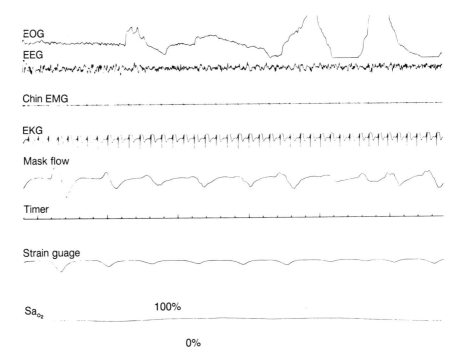

EOG

EEG

Chin EMG

EKG

Mask flow

Timer

Strain guage

Sa_{O_2} 100%

0%

Figure 14–4   Sleep tracing in a patient with MD. The patient is in rapid eye movement (REM) sleep, which is defined by the first three panels: The electro-culogram (EOG), the electroencephalogram (EEG), and the electromyogram (EMG). Note the large fast swings on the EOG trace typical of REM sleep. The fourth panel, the electrocardiogram (EKG), shows a regular rhythm. The patient has diminished air movement as shown on mask flow panel and decreased amount of effort shown on the strain gauge panel. This hypopneic breathing produces oxygen desaturation to approximately 64%, as shown on the last panel marked, Sa_{O_2}. This type of breathing can cause marked oxygen desaturation during sleep in neuromuscular patients.

Disordered nocturnal breathing that causes hypoxemia can take the form of apnea (mechanical upper airway obstruction or central cessation of neural output to the respiratory muscles), hypoventilation (elevation of carbon dioxide), hypopnea (small irregular breaths), or ventilation-to-perfusion mismatching. Although discussion of the specific medical or surgical therapeutic interventions is not within the scope of this chapter, it is important for the therapist to recognize any undiagnosed problem and channel this information back to the physician. Since excessive secretions and aspiration (Fig. 14–5) develop in many neuromuscular patients during sleep, the family should be instructed in postural drainage and percussion if nocturnal breathing distress is

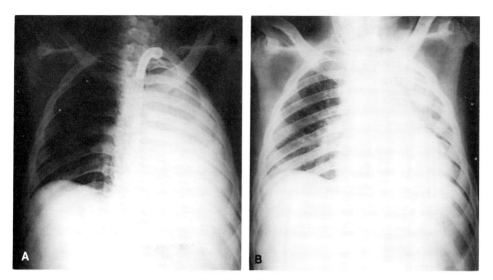

Figure 14–5 These chest x-ray films show the importance of postural drainage and percussion in neuromuscular patients. Atelectasis *(A)* clears with good postural drainage and percussion *(B)*.

present. Elevation of the head allows gravity to further assist in inspiration.

CHRONIC RESPIRATORY FAILURE

The efficacy of respiratory therapy in neuromuscular disease without accompanying pulmonary disease is not clearly established. Several groups have demonstrated a modest increase in maximum voluntary ventilation in Duchenne dystrophy patients using positive-pressure breathing, and another group found similar improvement in Duchenne dystrophy boys taught diaphragmatic breathing. Recently, we demonstrated reversal in both waking and sleeping respiratory insufficiency in a patient with acid maltase deficiency, using inspiratory muscle training (Fig. 14–6). The training was accomplished by having the patient breath against inspiratory resistors for 15 minutes twice a day. Although there is still no evidence that an increase in pulmonary function alters prognosis, inspiratory muscle training may prove valuable for symptomatic relief in patients with respiratory muscle weakness. Rather than using conventional incentive spirometers (see Chap. 19), inhaling against progressively harder inspiratory resistors appears more efficacious.

In an ambulatory neuromuscular patient, a respiratory infection can

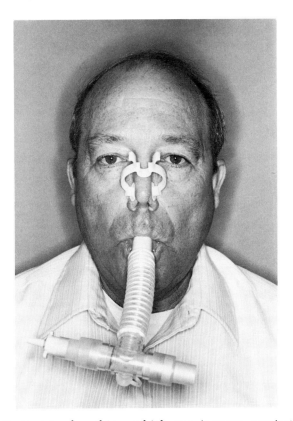

Figure 14-6 Resistor breathing, which can improve respiratory muscle strength, is easily accomplished by a series of one-way valves and a narrow inspiratory lumen.

frequently be managed on an outpatient basis since pulmonary function remains good. The diagnosis of pneumonia can be overlooked in a weak, wheelchair-dependent patient, so that a chest radiograph is mandatory if respiratory secretion problems develop. In such severely, compromised individuals, a respiratory infection causing any difficulty in breathing is a medical emergency and requires prompt hospitalization.

After obtaining a Gram's stain and cultures, antibiotics should be begun immediately if the patient has a pulmonary infiltrate. The most frequently found bacterial organisms are *Hemophilus influenzae* and *Streptococcus pneumoniae*. Postural drainage, pharyngeal suctioning, and percussion of the chest are best done by a trained nurse or physical therapist. Beta-agonists by aerosol or oral aminophylline accelerate mucociliary transport and relieve bronchospasm. Low-flow oxygen provides symptomatic relief from dyspnea.

Prophylactic immunization for influenza and *Pneumococcus* is recommended for all debilitated patients.

Mechanical Ventilation

There are three types of ventilatory support systems: positive-pressure units, negative-pressure units, and units that use gravity. If a neuromuscular patient needs the use of ventilation until an acute reversible process resolves, a positive-pressure ventilator is used with an endotracheal tube. If irreversible ventilatory failure develops and long-term ventilatory assistance is planned, the advantages and disadvantages of the different systems need to be considered in more detail.

The simplest form of ventilatory support is a rocking bed (Fig. 14–7), which uses gravitational forces to lower and raise the diaphragm to bring in and force out air, respectively. As the bed rocks (feet down–head up for inspiration and return to the neutral position for expiration), the abdominal contents are pulled away from the diaphragm or pushed toward the diaphragm to produce air movement. Respiratory rate is controlled by the speed of the rocking. If a patient can tolerate the continual motion, the rocking bed is particularly useful for a patient who can ventilate on his own during the day but needs support when asleep. A major advantage of this system is that there is nothing attached to the patient so he can sleep in any position. The only support is a foot board to prevent the patient from sliding off the bed. With advanced

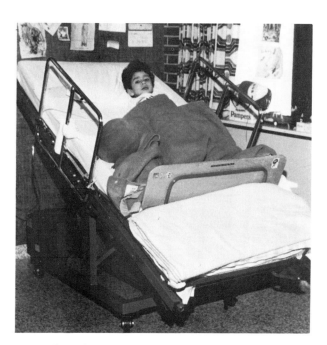

Figure 14–7 Rocking bed used to assist ventilation in neuromuscular patients. See text for full description.

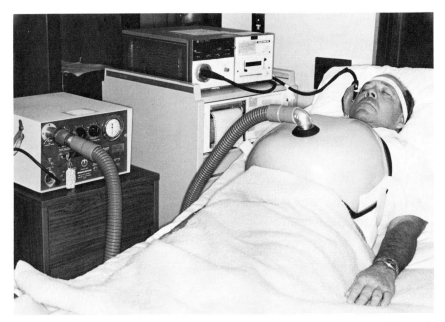

Figure 14–8 Chest cuirass, a negative pressure ventilator that tightly seals around a patient's chest and can adequately ventilate many neuromuscular patients. (See text for full description.) Attached to the patient's ear is an ear oximeter, a noninvasive monitoring technique that measures oxygen saturation continuously.

neuromuscular weakness, this mode of ventilation is usually not forceful enough to produce the desired effects.

A negative-pressure ventilator produces an external negative force around the chest wall to "pull" air into the lungs (Fig. 14–8). When the negative pressure cycles off, air is expelled passively by the elastic recoil of the lungs. The rate and amount of inspiratory force can be controlled to produce the appropriate amount of ventilation measured by an arterial carbon dioxide level. Advantages of negative-pressure ventilators such as the chest cuirass and the "iron lung" are that there is better control than with a rocking bed and that an endotracheal or tracheostomy tube is not required. Drawbacks include difficulty in getting a good seal, particularly if the patient is obese, and that the patient must remain supine.

Positive-pressure units include volume-controlled and pressure-controlled respirators (Fig. 14–9). The more versatile and accurate (therefore the most expensive) is the volume-controlled unit, where the exact volume and rate are set and delivered to the patient. A pressure pop-off valve protects the patient against high pressure. A pressure ventilator sets the amount of pressure delivered and the rate, while the

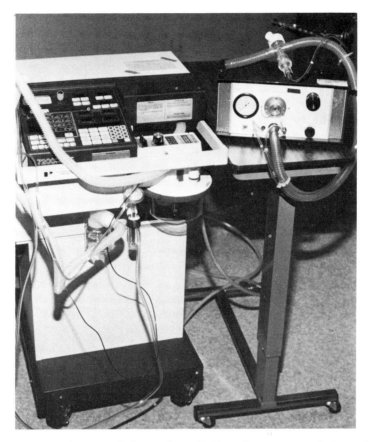

Figure 14-9 Volume-cycled ventilator *(left)*, and pressure-cycled ventilator *(right)*. Although accuracy of the volume ventilator is much greater than that for the pressure ventilator, the smaller pressure unit is more mobile for patient use.

tidal volume is indirectly set by the amount of pressure used. Most neuromuscular patients on long-term ventilatory support, especially if at home, can do well on the markedly less expensive pressure system. If a ventilator is used chronically, a tracheostomy is essential for long-term comfort, better suctioning, and more ease in oral hygiene. Certain positive-pressure units allow patient mobility because they are portable and readily attached to power wheelchairs (Fig. 14-10).

Final Considerations

In all patients with neuromuscular disease, respiratory complications should be anticipated and assessed for potentially reversible causes. Above all, the rehabilitation specialist must be sensitive to the patient's

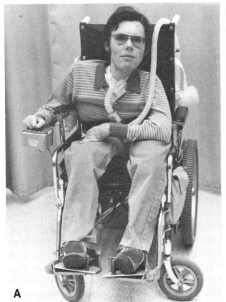
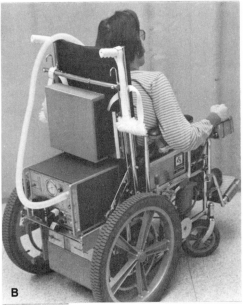
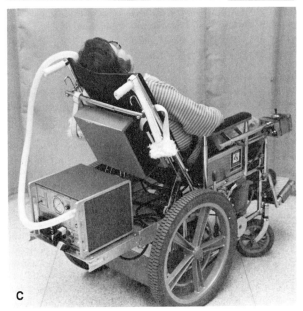

Figure 14-10 Front (A) and back (B) views of electric wheelchair with attached pressure-cycled ventilator. The patient must charge the battery every 24 hours but is otherwise free to move about using a hand control drive that requires minimal strength. (C) A reclining back is possible if the ventilator is placed on an extendable tray.

wishes. Understandably, some patients will chose not to undergo "extraordinary" procedures because life has lost meaning for them under these circumstances. The doctor's and therapist's emotional support at this difficult time can be more valuable to the patient than the prolongation of his life.

Rarely, a patient with a severe neuromuscular disease requests mechanical ventilatory support even if there is no prospect for future unassisted ventilation. Currently, few extended-care facilities will accept ventilator-dependent patients, and most medical assistance programs (private and government) will not pay for expenses related to long-term ventilatory support. Whenever possible, these issues should be addressed openly and honestly with the patient and his family in advance of impending respiratory failure, since momentary decisions can commit a patient and family to unanticipated suffering and expense. Assurance that the patient's comfort is of prime concern should be conveyed throughout the course of a progressive neuromuscular disease.

Suggested Readings

ALEXANDER MA, JOHNSON EW, PETTY J, et al: Mechanical ventilation of patients with late stage Duchenne muscular dystrophy: Management in the home. Arch Phys Med Rehabil 60:289–292, 1979

BLACK LF, HYATT RE: Maximal respiratory pressure: Normal values in relationship to age and sex. Am Rev Respir Dis 99:696–702, 1969

CHERNIACK RM: Pulmonary Function Testing. Philadelphia, WB Saunders, 1977

DERENNE J, MACKLEM PT, ROUSSOS CH: The respiratory muscles: Mechanics, control and pathophysiology. Part 3. Am Rev Respir Dis 118:581–601, 1978

GORSS D, LADD WH, RILEY EJ, et al: The effect of training on strength and endurance on the diaphragm in quadriplegia. Am J Med 68:27–35, 1980

MARTIN RJ: Cardiorespiratory disorders during sleep. New York, Futura, 1984

MARTIN RJ, SUFIT RL, RINGEL SP, et al: Respiratory improvement by muscle training in adult onset acid maltase deficiency. Muscle and Nerve 6:201–203, 1983

RIDEAU Y, JANKOWSKI LW, GRELLET J: Respiratory function in the muscular dystrophies. Muscle and Nerve 4:155–164, 1981

RINGEL SP, CARROLL JE: Respiratory complications of neuromuscular disease. In Weiner WJ (ed): Respiratory Dysfunction in Neurologic Disease, pp 113–156. New York, Futura, 1980

ROCHESTER DF, BRAUN NMT: The respiratory muscles. Resp Care 23:616–621, 1978

ROUSSOS C, MACKLEM PT: The respiratory muscles. N Engl J Med 307:786–796, 1982

SHAPIRO BJ: Pulmonary rehabilitation of the neuromuscular patient. In Kaplan PE, Materson RS (eds): The Practice of Rehabilitation Medicine, pp 148–185. Springfield, Illinois, Charles C Thomas, 1982

Nancy D. Cobble
F. Patrick Maloney

15

Effects of Exercise on Neuromuscular Disease

A comprehensive rehabilitation program for neuromuscular patients seeks to prolong function as long as possible. Improving strength and endurance is fundamental to the goal of optimizing function. Improvement can involve increasing strength and endurance, but in progressive disorders it can also mean maintaining or even slowing the rate of loss. Improved strength also helps function by preventing or slowing the development of complications such as contractures, cardiovascular deconditioning, and disuse atrophy.

Since there is no cure for many neuromuscular disorders, improved function is most often achieved by physical methods, including a carefully prescribed and supervised exercise program. Although vigorous exercise training markedly improves strength and endurance in a normal individual, its effects are less dramatic in a patient with neuromuscular disease. Evidence in the medical literature suggests that exercise in neuromuscular disorders can help improve function when prescribed within safe and effective guidelines.

Effects of Exercise in Normal Muscle

The potential for exercise programs to increase function in impaired muscle is based on the known effects of exercise in normal muscle.

Exercise has powerful effects that can increase muscle strength and endurance, and even reverse certain experimental muscle wasting conditions. For example, starved mice with generalized muscle wasting still develop hypertrophy of specifically exercised muscles, and exercise will reverse the catabolic effects of administered glucocorticoids. Hypertrophy also develops following exercise in the absence of the hormones required for normal muscle growth and maturation (growth hormone, insulin, and thyroid hormone).

Exercise has specific effects (i.e., different types of exercise cause different adaptations in exercised muscle). Strengthening exercise (high tension, low repetition, which stresses the contractile apparatus) causes increased contractile protein synthesis, decreased protein degradation, and muscle fiber hypertrophy. Contractile protein also increases because of muscle fiber hyperplasia secondary to muscle fiber splitting. Other factors that improve strength but do not cause morphologic changes in the muscle include better synchronization and more effective recruitment of motor units during exercise and the learning or practice that occurs as a person trains. Endurance exercise (low tension, high repetition, which stresses the muscle's metabolic system), produces increased and more effective muscle oxidative enzymes in the absence of significant hypertrophy.

Exercise has limited effects; even a normal muscle cannot be trained beyond a certain maximal response. A vigorous training program shortens the time required to reach the maximal response, but it does not increase the limit (Fig. 15–1). A less intense training program prolongs the time required to reach the limit.

A muscle responds in a graded fashion to varying exercise stress. With increasing amounts of exercise, muscle responses are disuse atrophy, the maintenance of strength training, an upper limit plateau, and, if extreme, overwork damage (Fig. 15–2). Although the precise demarcations of muscle responses along this continuum are not clearly established for all muscle groups or for most disease states, inferences can be

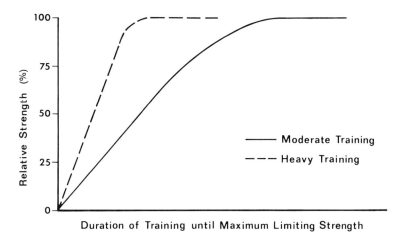

Figure 15–1　Relative time needed to attain maximum strength with different levels of exercise. (Modified from Krusen FH, Kottke FJ, Ellwood PM: Handbook of Physical Medicine and Rehabilitation, 2nd ed. Philadelphia, WB Saunders, 1971)

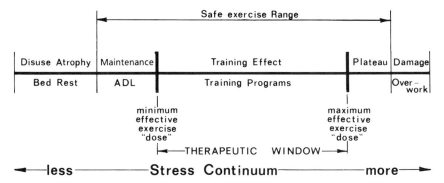

Figure 15–2 Therapeutic window for exercise as part of a stress continuum.

drawn from known evidence. Disuse atrophy develops with insufficient activity when muscle contractions are less than approximately 20% of the total tension a muscle is capable of producing. As contractile proteins are lost, the muscle weakens at a rate of 3% per day. Strength is maintained with contractions producing 20% to 35% of maximal tension. Many activities of daily living are at this maintenance level. No matter how frequently activities are repeated at this tension level, strengthening does not occur.

If strengthening is to be achieved, tension must be greater than 35% of maximal. Improvement continues until an upper limit is reached (plateau), beyond which exercise no longer increases strength. Overwork damage can occur with training that is too near the maximal attainable tension. The actual point of damage is difficult to define and may vary with different muscle groups. Muscle tissue breakdown (rhabdomyolysis) with fiber necrosis, release of muscle enzymes, and progressive weakness occurs in previously untrained individuals during forced exercise, such as in boot camp, marathon runs, or during survival mountain climbing. Recovery may be prolonged and incomplete.

Accordingly, even in individuals with normal muscles, exercise should be prescribed and administered in safe and effective amounts. The figures cited above are approximate and vary from muscle group to muscle group, but the trend remains the same, and similar principles can be used to prescribe safe and effective exercise. Exercise is safe if activity is greater than the amount required to prevent disuse atrophy but less than the amount that causes overwork damage. Within this safe range is the effective range wherein training (progressive improvement in strength and endurance) occurs. Exercise must be greater than maintenance activities (minimum effective "dose"), but does not need to be any greater than the amount that stimulates maximal response (maximum effective "dose"). This effective training range is a therapeutic window for exercise prescription (see Fig. 15–2). With activity below or above the effective "dose," no training occurs. Within the therapeutic window, the larger the dose of exercise, the faster the improvement.

These same training concepts are important in prescribing exercise for individuals with diseased muscle. When there is significant damaged or destroyed motor units, the safe range for exercise is reduced. A weak muscle is more susceptible to overwork damage because it is already functioning closer to its maximal limit. Therefore, exercise must be prescribed and carefully supervised to avoid overwork. Since the therapeutic window, or effective training range, is only slightly narrowed in milder and earlier diseases, moderate exercise can be prescribed to prevent disuse atrophy, to improve muscle performance, and to counteract progressive weakness. With more severely diseased muscles, the therapeutic window may be narrow or closed. Because the severely weakened muscles are already functioning maximally, attempts to train may prove fruitless and other aspects of the rehabilitation program can be more profitably emphasized.

Effect of Exercise in Nonprogressive Disorders

Nonprogressive neuromuscular disorders, such as poliomyelitis, incomplete spinal cord injury, and central core disease, provide a simple model of the response of impaired muscles to exercise. In these disorders, a fixed number of motor units are lost or damaged. Muscles respond to exercise, but the maximal response is lowered proportional to the amount of remaining muscle. Also, to achieve a given tension with fewer than normal motor units, each motor unit must work harder and is more susceptible to overwork.

For example, in early studies of recovered polio patients, resistive or isometric exercises strengthened paretic muscles. If 60% or more of the motor neurons were destroyed, maximal response of the muscle to training was reached before the muscle gained normal or even functional strength. In practical terms, because weakness cannot be detected by manual muscle testing until 30% to 35% of motor units are absent, a muscle with less than antigravity strength before exercising is unlikely to become functional with exercise even though limited improvement can occur (Fig. 15–3).

In a single subject with central core disease who underwent endurance training, Hagberg and associates (1980) found that exercise endurance capacity increased by 50%, but no higher, even with prolonged training. These authors concluded that the limited response in this nonprogressive myopathy may have been due to the absence of motor units that respond to intense prolonged exercise.

Several reports demonstrate that partially innervated muscle can be overworked. In humans, the evidence involves the effects of exercise in

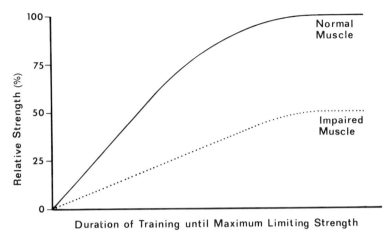

Figure 15-3 Response of impaired muscle to stress compared with that of normal muscle. (Modified from Krusen FH, Kottke FJ, Ellwood PM: Handbook of Physical Medicine and Rehabilitation, 2nd ed. Philadelphia, WB Saunders, 1971).

nerve damage during early recovery, and also from continued stress on partially innervated muscle. In patients with polio or incomplete spinal cord injury, progressive weakness of paretic muscles develops if daily, repetitive, strenuous exercise of the paretic muscles is performed in early recovery. The late decompensation of paretic muscles after 30 to 40 years of functional use has been attributed to chronic overwork. Myopathic changes noted in partially denervated muscles of chronic neuropathies suggest that chronic overwork may be a factor in producing the necrosis.

In animals, the evidence of the effects of exercise on partial innervation is derived from nerve injury and muscle resection experiments. Herbison and co-workers (1983), investigating the effect of exercise on rat muscle following nerve injury, found a loss of contractile proteins during early reinnervation when there were few functioning motor units. The same amount of exercise resulted in muscle hypertrophy after reinnervation was complete. Reitsma (1969), by removing healthy muscle and then strenuously exercising rats, found that exercise damaged remaining muscle if less than one-third of motor units remained. When more than one-third remained, the same intensity of exercise produced muscle hypertrophy.

The detailed cellular mechanisms for exercise-induced injury are incompletely defined. Theories on the mechanisms of damage include mechanical overstress of the contractile apparatus and inflammatory response, edema pressure, circulatory overload, activation of lysosomal enzymes, and increased muscle membrane permeability.

Thus, special attention must be paid to prescribing exercise in non-

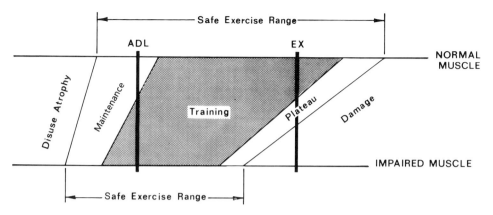

Figure 15–4 Safe exercise range and therapeutic window narrow with impaired muscle. Activities of daily living (*ADL*) in normal muscles may cause impaired muscle to act as though in training. Exercise that improves normal muscles may cause overwork damage in impaired muscle. (*EX* = Common exercise program level)

progressive neuromuscular disorders because the therapeutic window is narrowed. Although remaining motor units do respond to training, the amount of strengthening possible is proportional to the number of undamaged motor units. These motor units must work harder to handle a given amount of exercise stress. The same amount of exercise that causes a vigorous training effect in normal muscle can cause overwork damage in impaired muscle (Fig. 15–4).

Effect of Exercise in Progressive Neuromuscular Disorders

The effect of exercise in progressive neuromuscular disorders is more difficult to demonstrate because exercise-induced improvement may be offset by progressive weakness. Unlike nonprogressive disorders, further motor units are damaged or lost by the ongoing disease process. Nevertheless, there is evidence that muscles that are not yet end-stage can respond positively to exercise without damage.

The rate of disease progression is important in determining a muscle's response to exercise. The slower the progression, the more adequate the compensation, and the better the response of muscle to exercise. Brown (1973) has shown that in normally aging muscle, progressive but relatively slow loss of motor neurons occurs constantly, yet muscle size and strength are maintained. Estimates are that only 50% of motor units remain by the sixth decade, yet strength is preserved because of compensatory collateral sprouting of remaining motor neurons. With aging, clinical evidence of weakness and atrophy does not occur until 80% of motor neurons are lost. Moritani and deVries (1980) have shown remaining muscles still respond to strength and endurance training.

In amyotrophic lateral sclerosis, because of rapid progression, compensatory collateral sprouting cannot occur fast enough to maintain strength. Accordingly, the response to exercise is blunted. In one study, only three of ten muscles showed any response to isometric strengthening and only one muscle improved functionally. Interestingly, there was no evidence of overwork damage even with strenuous exercise.

Other important factors that determine a muscle's response to exercise are the degree (mild or severe) and the stage (early or late) of the disease. In animal models the severity of disease (extent of involvement and rate of progression) differs between various breeds. In those animals with mild or early dystrophic-like disease, muscle responds to exercise, whereas in animals with severe or late disease, muscle shows exercise damage. In certain "dystrophic" mice that have a severe, rapidly progressive neuropathic disease, even mild treadmill exercise is detrimental, producing greater weakness and shortening of the exercised animal's life span. In young dystrophic hamsters with a milder, more slowly progressive disorder, weight-lifting exercise (forced climbing, carrying weights to reach food and water) produces muscle hypertrophy and increased strength. However, adult hamsters with more advanced disease show an increased rate of cardiac and skeletal muscle degeneration after forced swimming or heavy weight-lifting. Dystrophic chickens that have mild weakness and myotonia improved righting and wing-flapping with practice, which is associated with decreased lipid infiltration in the exercised muscle. The improved performance may, in part, be attributable to decreased myotonia and the associated lipid reduction is consistent with improvement in dystrophic muscle.

Although evidence is indirect, many of the aforementioned studies suggest that the therapeutic window continues to narrow as a neuromuscular disease progresses and the range of overwork damage broadens. Johnson and Braddom (1971) found greater weakness in the most-used upper extremity in members of a family with fascioscapulohumeral (FSH) dystrophy. Usually the dominant (normally the most used) arm was weaker, but in one case a heavily used nondominant arm was more affected. Although asymmetric weakness in FSH dystrophy is usual, the relationship of the asymmetry to chronic exercise has not been thoroughly investigated. Several studies have shown greater serum creatine phosphokinase (CPK) levels after exercise in dystrophic patients than in normal patients, suggesting a possible injurious effect of exercise. In one study, the cumulative effects of prolonged exercise in dystrophic patients caused higher serum CPK levels than one to three daily episodes of brief maximal exercise. Bonsett (1963), in a postmortem examination of all the muscles of a 16-year old patient with end-stage Duchenne dystrophy, suggested that even daily activities caused overwork at that stage. Postural muscles, as well as muscles that had become postural and therefore were forced to work continuously, showed the most degeneration, presumably from chronic overwork.

In Figure 15–5, as the amount of functional muscle decreases, the absolute amount of exercise required for each effect also decreases, but the percentages of maximal tension remain the same. Less force is required to elicit each effect. For instance, in moderately severe disease, muscle reacts in a training mode with minimal activity, which may explain, in part, the increased fatiguability experienced by patients. Chronic high-intensity exercise (i.e., heavy relative to the amount of muscle available to respond to exercise) is most likely to cause overwork stress and should be avoided even with early or mild disease. In end-stage disease, even activities of daily living may act as heavy stress and contribute to muscle fiber damage (Fig. 15–5).

An exercise training program should only be prescribed when there is some reasonable chance of improving function of the muscle or at least slowing the progression of weakness. Many early exercise studies in dystrophic patients reported no significant improvements in severely involved, usually wheelchair-bound patients with little functioning muscle. When weakness is first clinically apparent in a rapid disease where compensation has not taken place, 30% to 50% of motor units are already nonfunctional. With few motor units remaining in severely impaired patients already functioning at their limit, exercise should not be expected to improve strength or endurance.

It is equally important to prescribe enough activity to maintain baseline strength to avoid additional weakness from disuse atrophy (Fig. 15–5). Because dystrophic patients may feel fatigued and tend to avoid activities, and are known to be adversely affected by prolonged bed rest, Vignos (1983) has recommended prescribing two to three hours daily of standing, walking, or swimming for ambulatory patients. As long as the patient feels rested after a night's sleep, Vignos suggests that the patient will not be seriously overexercised. Activity should be alternated with rest periods in patients with limited endurance. Any time a patient becomes immobilized for more than two to three days, an active physical therapy program should be started to reverse the disuse and deconditioning effects of bed rest.

Well-supervised and relatively brief strengthening and endurance training in early or mild disease can still improve strength and slow the rate of progression. deLatuer and Giaconi, studying the effect of submaximal quadriceps isokinetic exercise in one group of dystrophic patients, found some improvement in strength compared to the unexercised group of dystrophic patients, although the gains were not statistically significant because the number in the study group was small.

In a study of patients with early Duchenne dystrophy and other

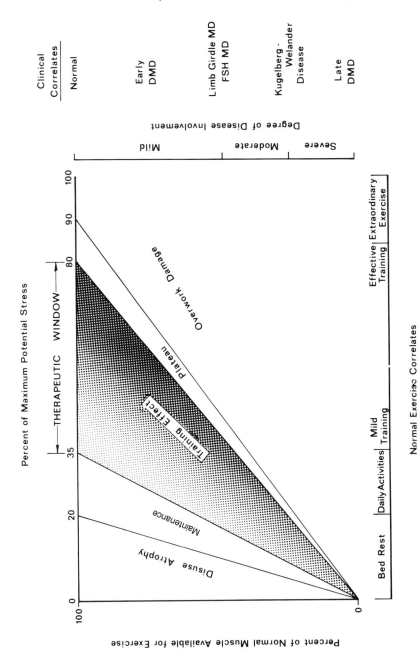

Figure 15-5   Idealized response of normal and impaired muscle to exercise. The therapeutic window of safe exercise narrows progressively. Activities (lower x axis) causing normal exercise effects in normal muscle (upper x axis) correlate to different effects in impaired muscle.

milder dystrophies receiving closely supervised maximal resistive exercise, Vignos and Watkins (1966) found that the muscles increased an average of 50% in strength in the first four months and maintained these gains for the entire year the patients exercised. Antigravity and stronger muscles had a greater response.

Summary

This chapter has focused on the effects of exercise in improving strength and endurance in denervated and myopathic muscle. Although current literature is incomplete, the following implications can be drawn:

1. Exercise is most effective when begun as early in the disease process as possible.
2. Daily activity is important to maintain baseline strength and prevent disuse atrophy.
3. Supervised exercise training can maximize strength while avoiding overwork in early and mild disease.
4. In mild to moderate diseases, the need for direct supervision becomes more important as the therapeutic window narrows.
5. When disease is advanced, muscle is already functioning maximally so that it is more profitable to emphasize other aspects of a comprehensive rehabilitation program.

Further studies are needed using modern techniques to measure and statistically define the effects of exercise within the framework of the therapeutic window outlined in this chapter.

Suggested Readings

ANDERSON AD, LEVINE SA, GELLERT H: Loss of ambulatory ability in patients with old anterior poliomyelitis. Lancet 2:1061, 1972

BONSETT CA: Pseudohypertrophic muscular dystrophy: Distribution of degenerative features as revealed by an anatomical study. Neurology 13:728, 1963

BROWN WF: Functional compensation of human motor units in health and disease. J Neurol Sci 20:199, 1973

DELATEUR BJ, GIACONI RM: Effect on maximal strength of submaximal exercise in Duchenne muscular dystrophy. Am J Phys Med 58:26, 1979

DEMOS MA, GITIN EL, KAGEN LJ: Exercise myoglobinemia and acute exertional rhabdomyolysis. Arch Intern Med 134:699, 1974

EDGERTON VR: Neuromuscular adaptation to power and endurance work. Can J Appl Sports Sci 1:49, 1976

FOWLER WM, TAYLOR M: Rehabilitation management of muscular dystrophies and related disorders. I. The role of exercise. Arch Phys Med Rehabil 63:319, 1982

FOWLER WM, TAYLOR M: Rehabilitation management of muscular dystrophies and related disorders. II. Comprehensive care. Arch Phys Med Rehabil 63:322, 1982

GARDINER PF, HIBL B, SIMPSON DR, et al: Effects of a mild weight-lifting program on the progress of glucocorticoid-induced atrophy in rat hindlimb muscles. Pfluegers Arch 385:147, 1980

GONYEA WI, SALE, D: Physiology of weight lifting exercise. Arch Phys Med Rehabil 63:235, 1982

HAGBERG, IM, CARROLL IE, BROOKE MH: Endurance exercise training in a patient with central core disease. Neurology 30:1242, 1980

HERBISON GI, JAWEED MM, DITUNNO JF JR: Exercise therapies in peripheral neuropathies. Arch Phys Med Rehabil 64:201, 1983

HERBISON GI, JAWEED MM, DITUNNO JF JR: Muscle fiber types. Arch Phys Med Rehabil 64:227, 1982

HETTINGER T: Physiology of Strength. Springfield, Ill, Charles C Thomas, 1961

HOLLOZY JO: Muscle Metabolism during exercise. Arch Phys Med Rehabil 63:231, 1982

JOHNSON EW, BRADDOM R: Overwork weakness in fascioscapulohumeral muscular dystrophy. Arch Phys Med Rehabil 52:333, 1971

KOTTKE FJ: Therapeutic exercise. In Krusen FH (ed): Handbook of Physical Medicine and Rehabilitation, 2nd ed. Philadelphia, WB Saunders, 1971

MORITANI T, DEVRIES HA: Potential for gross muscle hypertrophy in older men. J Gerontol 35:672, 1980

REITSMA W: Skeletal muscle hypertrophy after heavy exercise in rats with surgically reduced muscle function. Am J Phys Med 48:237, 1969

SALMININ A, VIHKO V: Susceptibility of mouse skeletal muscle to exercise injuries. Muscle and Nerve 6:596, 1983

SHARRARD JW: Discussion: Neuromuscular factors in rehabilitation after poliomyelitis. In Fourth International Poliomyelitis Conference, Geneva, 1957, p 568. Philadelphia, JB Lippincott, 1958

TAYLOR RG, FOWLER WM JR, DOERR L: Exercise effect on contractile properties of skeletal muscle in mouse muscular dystrophy. Arch Phys Med Rehabil 57:174, 1976

VIGNOS PJ: Physical models of rehabilitation in neuromuscular disease. Muscle and Nerve 6:323, 1983

VIGNOS PJ, WATKINS MP: The effect of exercise in muscular dystrophy. JAMA 197:121, 1966

16

Marcia B. Smith

Physical Therapy and Management of Neuromuscular Disease

This chapter outlines the therapist's role in the long-term management of patients with neuromuscular diseases. There are 220 muscular dystrophy association (MDA) clinics in the United States, many of which use a team approach for patient management. The physical therapist, a valuable member of the team, will find the role challenging and constantly changing, depending on the patient's disability.

The clinical course of many neuromuscular diseases is influenced not only by the rate of nerve and muscle degeneration but also by the care the patient receives. The earlier physical therapy is instituted, the greater the patient cooperation and subsequent benefit. The goal of the physical therapist in the management of neuromuscular disorders is to allow the patient to lead as normal a life as possible. To this end, treatment should prevent or correct losses of range of motion of the joints, allow locomotive mobility for as long as possible, and maintain strength. The therapist should also educate the family in the progression and management of the disease, provide training in activities of daily living, and offer support for a patient's emotional needs.

Evaluation

A baseline evaluation of the patient should be performed so that the efficacy of a treatment program can be assessed (see Evaluation of the Neuromuscular Patient).

1. During the initial visit with the patient and family, as much background history as possible should be obtained, including developmental milestones in children as well as preferred rest position. If

Evaluation of the Neuromuscular Patient

Date and examiner ————————————————

Left   Right

Goniometry
Shoulder

				Abduction				
				Flexion				
				Elbow				
				Extension				
				Supination				
				Wrist				
				Extension				
				Hip				
				Extension				
				Adduction				
				Knee				
				Extension				
				Ankle				
				Dorsiflexion				
				Eversion				

Left   **Manual Muscle Test**   Right
Shoulder

				Abduction				
				Flexion				
				Extension				
				Protraction				
				Elbow				
				Flexion				
				Extension				
				Wrist				
				Extension				
				Abdominals				
				Hip				
				Abduction				
				Flexion				
				Extension				
				Ankle				
				Dorsiflexion				
				Eversion				

0 = absent; 1 = trace; 2 = poor; 3 = fair; 4 = good; 5 = normal

Evaluation Form (*Continued*)

Gait Analysis

Swing: _____

_____

Stance: _____

_____

Assistive devices: _____

Time (10 meters): _____

Functional Abilities (upper time limit 120 sec)
(Check descriptions that apply)

Stair climbing (four 7″ steps): Without railing _____   Time: _____

With railing _____

Gower's _____

Foot over foot _____

Assume sit from supine: Without trunk rotation _____   Time: _____

Rotates to L / R _____

Unable _____

Stand from supine: Time: _____

Activities of Daily Living:

Lifts telephone receiver _____   Time: _____

Lifts glass of liquid _____   Time: _____

Writes _____   Time: _____

Upper extremity dressing _____   Time: _____

Respiratory
Breathing pattern: _____

Functional cough: _____

Chest expansion: _____

Scoliosis
Convexity to _____

Film ordered _____

subjective information differs from objective data, this difference may help the therapist in assessing the family's attitudes and acceptance.

2. Accurate goniometric measurements are recorded at least every 6 months, but preferably every 3 months, in patients in whom contractures develop quickly.

3. Muscle strength can be determined using standardized manual muscle tests or with a myometer. To simplify the examination, only key muscles need to be tested. For example, in myopathies with proximal weakness, key muscles include trapezius, deltoid, latissimus dorsi, serratus anterior, pectoralis, biceps, triceps, wrist extensors, abdominal musculature, iliopsoas, gluteus maximus, gluteus medius, and quadriceps ankle dorsiflexors, and evertors. In distinction, in neuropathies, distal muscles are typically affected (i.e., tibialis anterior, extensor digitorum longus, gastrocnemius, and peroneus longus in the lower extremities; lumbricals, opponens pollicis, and other intrinsic hand muscles in the upper extremities). Accurate recording of antagonistic muscle strength facilitates proper decisions concerning bracing or surgery. Myometers are expensive, time-consuming, and difficult to standardize. They are useful in quantifying weakness during therapeutic trials, but, to provide reliable objective data, they must be repeatedly used by the same therapist.

4. Ambulation can be assessed by analyzing swing and stance phases on both extremities. The necessity of assistive devices (orthosis, walker, cane, or crutch) and amount of assistance required for safety should be included. Speed of ambulation is best recorded using a fixed distance (i.e., time to walk 10 meters).

5. Assessment of functional abilities should include climbing stairs, sitting, standing, and raising arms over the head. Many functional classifications have been proposed, although all have inherent disadvantages. Most assess maximum, not daily, function. Additionally, the majority of scales pay little attention to upper extremity function, so they are less useful once the patient becomes wheelchair-bound. The functional scale, below, is designed to reflect the total range of patient function. Timing of functional activities is of additional value, however, because of long plateaus in function followed by sudden loss; even timed functional tests do not provide an absolute, graded indicator for determining efficacy of new therapies.

FUNCTIONAL CLASSIFICATION

1. Walks and climbs stairs without assistance
2. Walks and climbs stairs with aid of railing
3. Walks but unable to climb stairs
4. Walks unassisted but cannot rise from chair
5. Walks only with assistance or with braces

6. In a wheelchair; sits erect, can propel wheelchair, and independent in transfers and activities of daily living
7. In a wheelchair; sits erect, limited manual propulsion, assisted in transfers and activities of daily living
8. In a wheelchair; cannot sit independently, unlimited electric propulsion, performs minimal activities of daily living, cannot raise arms 8 inches off arm rests
9. In bed; no activities of daily living without assistance

Classification of Neuromuscular Disease

Over 40 separate diseases affect the lower motor neuron (see Chap. 12). Although many of the diseases share common signs and symptoms, the physical therapist should have a working knowledge of each disease so a specific program can be designed to maximally benefit the patient. Within our neuromuscular disease clinic at the University of Colorado, nearly 25% of the patients have a progressive muscular dystrophy. Of patients treated by the physical therapist, the largest majority (9%) have Duchenne muscular dystrophy (DMD), while fewer have limb girdle, (LG) dystrophy, facioscapulohumeral (FSH) dystrophy, and Becker's dystrophy. Of all patients, 5% have some form of spinal muscular atrophy (SMA). Peroneal muscular atrophy (Charcot-Marie-Tooth disease), a hereditary neuropathy, comprises 7% of the clinic population. A variety of rare congenital and inflammatory myopathies are also seen. Although a large percentage of patients have myasthenia gravis, painful neuropathies, myotonic syndromes, and other cramping disorders, the physical therapist has less involvement with these patients.

Most myopathies have progressive loss of strength, but each disease has a different prognosis, which influences the physical therapy program. The management of DMD (see Figs. 12–6 and 18–3), the most severe of the muscular dystrophies, serves as a model for treatment of other neuromuscular disorders. Boys with DMD are affected from birth, and although they may attain normal developmental milestones for sitting and crawling, ambulation is often delayed. Throughout the toddler period they have difficulty performing gross motor activities, including running and jumping. In early childhood they do acquire new skills, which may lead the family to incorrectly assume that the child is improving.

Becker's dystrophy has a later onset and a less rapid course than DMD (see Figs. 12–7 and 18–14). Patients with LG dystrophy may have involvement in either shoulder or pelvic girdles and usually do not become wheelchair-bound until adulthood, if at all. FSH dystrophy usually has the most benign course of the dystrophies (see Fig. 12–8). As the name implies, involvement includes oral–bulbar musculature,

proximal upper extremities (winging of scapulae), and distal musculature of the legs (dorsiflexors and evertors of the ankle).

Spinal muscular atrophies are classified according to age of onset. In
the most severe infantile form, Werdnig-Hoffman disease, the gross
motor skills of an infant of several months are rarely attained. Patients
with intermediate types of spinal muscular dystrophy (SMA) exhibit
normal developmental milestones for the first six months but generally
do not ambulate. In juvenile proximal SMA (Kugelberg-Welander), the
least severe form, patients are already ambulatory when they develop
progressive proximal weakness.

In peroneal muscular atrophy, the patient may have a stocking–glove
pattern of sensory loss, a finding not seen with myopathies or anterior
horn cell diseases. The most prominent disturbance in this neuropathy
is weakness in the lower legs and intrinsic hand muscles (see Fig. 12–4).

Clinical Problems

General principles used in the management of DMD apply to many other
neuromuscular disorders. Modifications for particular disorders are
presented when indicated.

FATIGUE

Maintenance of activity is important in any neuromuscular patient, but
overexertion may lead to increased instability with falling and unnecessary injuries (see Chap. 15). Activity should be such that recovery from
fatigue follows a night's sleep. The patient should be encouraged to take
naps or rest periods during the day to prevent fatigue.

CONTRACTURES

In every patient it is easier to prevent than to correct contractures,
which occur because of habitual postures and unopposed muscle action.
In ambulatory DMD patients, contractures initially involve the weight-
bearing joints and are related to the upright posture the boy assumes
when standing. Sutherland and co-workers (1981) report that the initial
postural change is an increase in lumbar lordosis that develops as the
child attempts to keep the line of the center of gravity behind the hip
joint (see Fig. 18–1). Inadequate strength in the abdominal–gluteus
maximus force–couple causes the pelvis to tilt anteriorly, producing a
hip flexion contracture. To compensate for this shift in the center of
gravity, the boy increases his lumbar lordosis, placing the weight of the
upper trunk posteriorly. The child also rises on his toes to help shift the
center of gravity during ambulation, creating an equinus deformity. To

make himself more stable, the child will abduct the legs using the tensor fascia lata. During stance, this abduction is often asymmetric so that the extremity on which the majority of weight is placed will have greater dorsiflexion range. The opposite leg, which is abducted for balance, often has a greater equinus contracture and more tightness in the iliotibial band and knee flexors (see Fig. 18–3).

When forefoot evertors become weakened in DMD, unopposed invertors create a varus deformity in the feet. Simultaneously, quadriceps weakness creates knee flexion contractures, which are reinforced by tightness of the iliotibial band. If the patient attempts to maintain knee extension using the action of the soleus, further equinovarus deformity develops. Ober's test is useful to detect tightness of the iliotibial band and as a position of stretch (Fig. 16–1). The Thomas test position, with one leg flexed on the trunk and the other dropped into extension, detects hip flexion tightness (Fig. 16–2). Contractures of the hamstrings are noted during straight leg–raising.

About the time a boy with DMD enters school (age 5–6), a 5-degree dorsiflexion loss may be noted along with a slight hip flexion contracture. Unless the family is instructed in proper exercises, these contractures will increase as the deforming mechanical advantage increases.

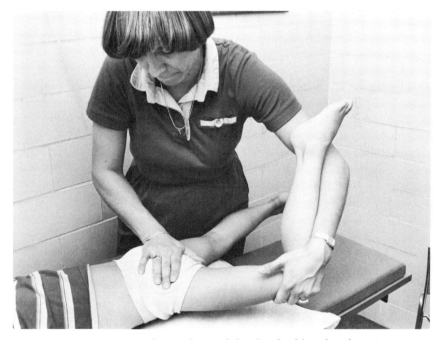

Figure 16–1 Testing and stretching of the iliotibial band is done in a prone position; the abducted hip is hyperextended, then adducted while extension is maintained. Pelvic stabilization is achieved by pressure over the buttocks.

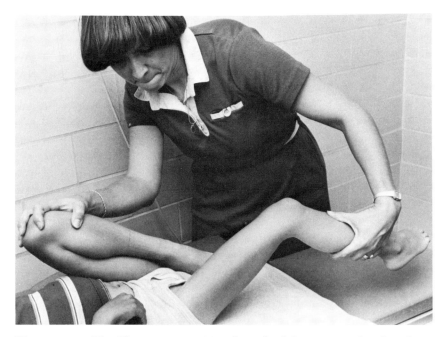

Figure 16–2   The Thomas test position flexes both legs against the chest from an extended supine position. As one leg drops into extension, the therapist's hand should be placed on the pelvis (in the presence of mild hip flexion contractures) to detect when pelvic motion occurs. Measurements are recorded at this position.

To counteract deformities at the hips, knees, and ankles, the family should be taught daily stretching exercises to retard the development of soft-tissue contractures in the gastrocnemius–soleus, hamstring muscle group, and tensor fascia lata. Repeated instruction in heel cord stretching (Fig. 16–3), straight leg–raising (Fig. 16–4), and stretching of hip flexors and abductors is generally required before the family can perform the method correctly.

Once a child with DMD is confined to a wheelchair, acceleration of lower extremity contractures will occur (see Fig. 18–12). The iliotibial band's mechanical pull into hip flexion and abduction is reinforced in the sitting posture. Simultaneously, increasing upper extremity tightness occurs in biceps, pronators, and wrist flexors (see Fig. 18–13). At this time, less emphasis is placed on stretching the legs and greater emphasis is given to maintaining arm and hand function. However, an attempt is made to keep loss of range in the legs to a minimum to ensure a comfortable sleeping position and greater ease in hygiene.

Contractures are often less severe in other myopathies and juvenile proximal SMA. When loss of motion does occur, the physical therapist should instruct the patient and family in independent stretching exer-

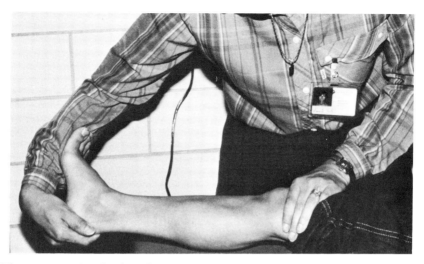

Figure 16-3 For heel cord stretching, cup the heel while applying distracting force to the calcaneus to passively stretch the heel cords. Allow the sole to rest against the forearm to increase leverage (pressure against only the forefoot causes breakdown of longitudinal arch). If resistance to stretch is encountered, place the hand on the foot and flex the knee to relieve tension on the gastrocnemius, and then straighten the knee.

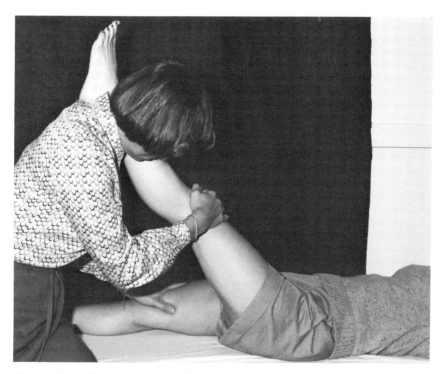

Figure 16-4 Hamstring musculature is stretched by straight leg-raising. The knee is extended while the hip is flexed. The opposite leg is stablizied to prevent pelvic movement and inaccurate measurement.

cises. Flexion contractures of the hips, knees, and ankles develop quickly in individuals with type 2 SMA because of an inability to stand or ambulate. Infants with Werdnig-Hoffman disease may exhibit slight tightness of the rotators of the shoulders, elbow flexors, and long finger flexors. Limited range may also be found in hip adduction and knee extension because of habitual froglike positioning. Patients with Charcot-Marie-Tooth disease, Becker's dystrophy, and Friedreich's ataxia may have a characteristic pes cavus deformity at the foot and ankle. Stretching exercises of all posterior compartment musculature can delay surgical intervention.

A program of slow, prolonged stretch performed twice daily is most effective in delaying the onset or progression of contractures. The program should be reviewed with the family or individual at regular intervals so improper techniques can be corrected and programs upgraded. The physical therapist should always reinforce the value of stretching, because contractures become more rigid and difficult to stretch if sessions are missed.

In addition to passive stretch to reverse the flexed posture assumed throughout the day, prone sleeping with toes dangling over the edge of the bed is encouraged. This positioning of the feet will prevent reinforcement of plantar flexion contractures at the ankles. Molded long leg night splints or casts have been advocated to maintain extension during sleep. Although some clinics have found that splints work well when instituted early in the patient's management, I have observed that parents easily become noncompliant in the application of splints because their children experience discomfort using them at night.

The use of massage or hydrotherapy for contractures is of unproven value and as such should not be a primary treatment for soft-tissue deformity.

WEAKNESS

Hypotonia occurs in all myopathies, spinal muscular atrophies, and other lower motor neuron disorders. Proximal tone and strength is usually involved to the greatest degree in all but the neuropathies. When lifting a hypotonic child, the child's scapulae and arms often slip through the examiner's grasp. In DMD patients, weakness is first noted in the trunk, anterior neck, shoulder, and pelvic girdle. The most rapidly deteriorating muscles include the gluteus maximus and medius, quadriceps, and serratus anterior. Loss of muscle strength occurs symmetrically at a rate of about one-half grade per year (see Evaluation of the Neuromuscular Patient). Some boys, especially in the early years, may show no decline in strength.

Weakness in the spinal muscular atrophies ranges from mild to profound. Although some authors have suggested that SMA types 2 and 3 do not deteriorate beyond two years after onset of symptoms, Russman and co-workers (1983) report that a predictable, continuous deterioration of shoulder and neck muscles can be expected even in patients who never achieve the ability to walk.

The treatment of weakness should be individualized. Sedentary activities (i.e., watching television) should be interrupted by some physical activity. For young patients with DMD, we have a goal of at least 3 hours of ambulation or standing a day to maintain strength. No specific exercise program is given unless requested by the family. Instead, recreational activities such as riding a bicycle or tricycle, swimming, and childhood games are stressed to provide a more natural, acceptable form of exercise (see Chap. 27). Resistive exercises can be employed to strengthen musculature of DMD patients, but this is best done during the early stages of the disease (fair or better strength).

Patients must be cautioned not to perform an exercise routine that is too tiring. Serum levels of the muscle enzyme creatine phosphokinase increase in patients following heavy exercise, suggesting that exercise is breaking down rather than building up muscle (see Chap. 15). LG and FSH dystrophics tolerate more prolonged exercise programs. Following 4 months of resistance exercise, increased strength has been noted for 8 additional months in these disorders.

Any type of exercise, including straight plane or spiral diagonal patterns along with facilitation techniques, may be employed to strengthen patients. When writing a home program of exercise, resistance may be provided by rubber dental dam or small sandbag weights. Because the range of safe and effective exercise narrows as disease progresses, direct supervision of a home program by a responsible party is needed to avoid overwork damage (see Chap. 15). Although facilitation techniques can be employed to try and activate anterior horn cells, considerable controversy exists over whether or not children with type 2 or type 3 SMA can be strengthened.

If an ambulatory neuromuscular patient becomes immobilized for a prolonged period of time, rapid loss of muscle bulk and strength will jeopardize ambulation. For each day spent convalescing in bed, a 3% loss of strength occurs. Skeletal muscle need only lose 30% to 50% of strength before residual losses become permanent. An exercise program should be begun immediately following a fracture or a childhood illness to strengthen weakened muscles. Exercise of proximal hip musculature is critical in the bedfast patient if he is to retain the ability to ambulate.

SCOLIOSIS

Scoliosis impairs sitting balance, contributes to skin breakdown when the rib hump overlaps the pelvic crest, and restricts ventilation. Patients with adult-onset neuromuscular disease seldom develop as severe a scoliosis as patients in whom the curve develops during the adolescent growth spurt. Scoliosis is also less severe in ambulatory patients because the lordotic posture assumed to maintain balance also locks the posterior facet joints, deterring a lateral curve. In infants and children with weakness (DMD, type 2 SMA), the development of kyphoscoliosis correlates strongly with wheelchair confinement. If the patient slumps in the chair, the loss of the lumbar curve and declining trunk strength promote a long thoracolumbar curve with pelvic obliquity. The convexity of the curve is generally toward the dominant hand.

The importance of a proper-fitting wheelchair cannot be over-emphasized (see Chap. 25). If a chair is too wide, a patient will lean to one side, reinforcing scoliosis. Correctly adjusted arm rests provide additional passive support. If the curve is less than 20 degrees, the deformity can be managed by attachment of scoliosis pads and lumbar roll to the wheelchair. A change to a full-length scoliosis pad (from axilla to greater trochanter), which is adjustable every 2 inches to accommodate curve changes and clothing, has proven unsuccessful. If the curve is greater than 20 degrees, a polypropylene body jacket (thoraco–lumbar–sacral orthosis—TLSO) should be used (see Fig. 18–16). Neither pads nor a TLSO totally prevents progression of scoliosis, but they both improve sitting posture and may retard advancement.

Recently, improved function in the presence of scoliosis has been attempted using custom-molded seating orthoses with or without head rests. We used a polypropylene shell contoured to the body, from the thighs to the upper thorax, in 10 patients with varying severity of scoliosis (Fig. 16–5). Only two patients were comfortable enough that they were willing to continue using the inserts. For individuals with severe scoliosis, leveling the pelvic obliquity created seating imbalance to which the patients were unable to adapt because of muscle weakness. In patients with milder scoliosis, the seating orthosis was abandoned because it didn't allow the individual enough trunk mobility. In all cases, the extra seat height of the insert necessitated extra caution when entering and exiting vans.

Others have recommended wheelchair inserts that maintain increased lumbar lordosis and tilt the patient posteriorly 15 degrees (see Fig. 18–16). When head and upper extremity control is poor, this amount of incline may prevent the child from driving his wheelchair.

The biomechanical factors causing scoliosis in DMD patients have been analyzed in detail by Gibson and Wilkins (1975). A few patients will maintain a stable spine while sitting on their ischial tuberosities if they maintain lumbar lordosis. In these individuals, the pelvis remains level and an extension contracture of the spine develops, locking posterior facets to limit lateral curvature.

A Milwaukee brace is not useful to control scoliosis in weak patients

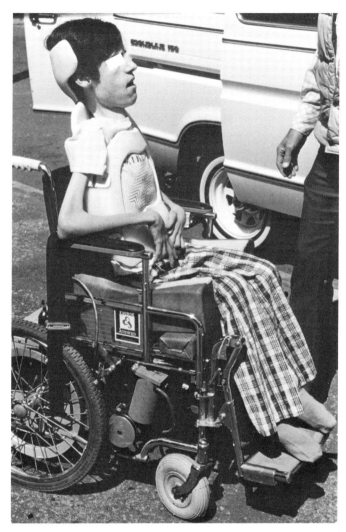

Figure 16–5 Custom-molded seating orthosis for severe DMD. Severe scoliosis and pelvic obliquity prevented this boy from sitting. The seat may be removed and placed in the family car for travel.

with neuromuscular disease because this brace requires an active system of muscle contraction to correct a curve. A physical therapist can provide valuable assistance in monitoring the progression of scoliosis in the fitting of an orthosis and wheelchair, and by instructing a patient in sitting postures that reinforce lumbar lordosis. The role of a physical therapist during surgical correction for scoliosis is discussed in Chapter 18.

FRACTURES

Fractures can easily develop in individuals confined to a wheelchair because loss of muscle mass and decreased weight-bearing lead to osteoporosis. Seemingly insignificant falls from the wheelchair or twisting of a lower extremity during transfer will result in an incapacitating leg fracture. Upper extremity fractures are more frequent in unsteady, ambulatory patients using knee–ankle–foot orthoses (KAFO) because of unprotected falls.

GAIT ABNORMALITIES

The therapist should be familiar with the biomechanical sequence that occurs in standing postures with Duchenne dystrophy (see Contractures, above, and Chap. 18). All dystrophic patients with proximal weakness walk with increased lumbar lordosis to compensate for hip extensor weakness. Two typical gait patterns are seen. One is a Trendelenburg gait (hip dip) where the pelvis drops downward on the swinging leg due to abductor weakness of the stance leg. The other is a gait that compensates for abductor weakness with a lateral shift of trunk and shoulders over the stance leg. This raises the pelvis on the unsupported side to allow toe clearance. When the compensated pattern is combined with gluteus maximus weakness, the patient leans backward and laterally to stabilize the hip.

In DMD, the concept of braced ambulation should be introduced to the child and his family at an early stage of the stretching program when the child is not falling frequently. By subjective and objective measures, a decision must eventually be reached whether to assist safe ambulation with braces or whether mobility will be provided by a wheelchair. Ambulation can continue until the quadriceps strength is graded poor plus (2+) if contractures are not present, or fair minus (3−) if they are present. DMD children generally stop ambulating within 6 months of the time they are no longer able to move from supine to standing (see Evaluation of the Neuromuscular Patient). By the age of 10 years, most DMD children fall frequently, and ambulation time and standing time total less than 15 minutes a day.

Surgical release of fixed contractures is necessary (heel cords greater than 5 degrees of plantar flexion; hip flexion greater than 15 degrees; abduction greater than 20 degrees) if a child is to ambulate with orthoses (see Chap. 18). Our approach is to introduce braces when the child is still ambulatory but unable to move from supine to standing. At this time significant tightness or range limitations are minimal, and the patient may be fitted with orthoses without surgery. The appliance most often selected for use in our clinic is the polypropylene vacuum-formed knee – ankle – foot orthosis (KAFO) with drop-locks at the knees (see Fig. 18 – 6). Occasionally, double metal uprights with spring-loaded drop-locks at the knee and double adjustable locked ankle joints on high-topped orthopaedic shoes are used for greater stability (see Fig. 18 – 7). The adjustability of the ankle joint allows for changes in range of motion that may occur and greater adjustability during growth.

After a child receives braces, a program of gait training and instruction of the family in brace care is begun. The family should be encouraged to continue vigorous stretching exercises. Because of shoulder girdle instability and very weak latissimus dorsi muscles, axillary crutches are generally not used in dystrophic patients. Instead, a rolling walker provides the assistance required for balance. The use of braces markedly slows walking but improves energy cost per meter. Occasionally, braced DMD boys continue to ambulate for up to 4 years. More typically, in our clinic, orthoses extend limited ambulation 1 to 3 years, after which the patient is no longer able to balance or swing his legs because of advanced weakness.

Polypropylene ankle – foot orthoses (AFO); (Fig.16 – 6) can relieve the toe drag or steppage gait of an individual with Charcot-Marie-Tooth disease. If a patient with a footdrop also has poor gastrocnemius – soleus control and a weakened quadriceps (fair), then a metal AFO with an

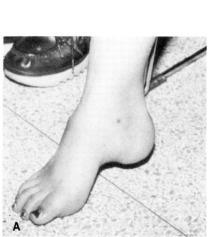
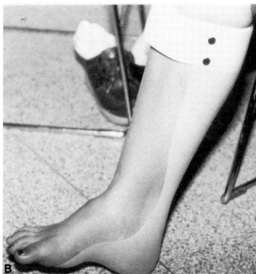

Figure 16 – 6 (A) Dropfoot, pes cavus, and mild inversion deformity associated with Charcot-Marie-Tooth disease. (B) Polypropylene ankle foot orthosis (AFO), used to position the foot and ankle during stance and prevent toe drag during swing. The patient must be cautioned not to vary his shoe heel height once fitted with this AFO.

adjustable, locked ankle will provide better control of both knee and ankle by improving tibial stability. Additionally, some patients benefit from a cane or a single Lofstrand crutch to assist with balance.

Recently, a reciprocating orthosis developed at Louisiana State University has been used to maintain ambulation in very weak neuromuscular patients. The ability to perform some shoulder depression allows for success with this brace because the biomechanical action of the brace causes the foot to swing when the leg is unloaded. The presence of contractures at the hips prohibits use of this orthosis.

SELF-CARE DEPENDENCY

Even when a patient is ambulatory, a wheelchair can be used for long distances to decrease fatigue. Teachers in school systems often request a chair either for convenience or to protect the child from falling on the playground or in hallways. If a patient is confined to a wheelchair, the therapist should teach him and the caretaker assisted and dependent transfer techniques. If a child has KAFOs and a chair, a pull-to-stand maneuver for stand–pivot transfers may be used. For the patient with-

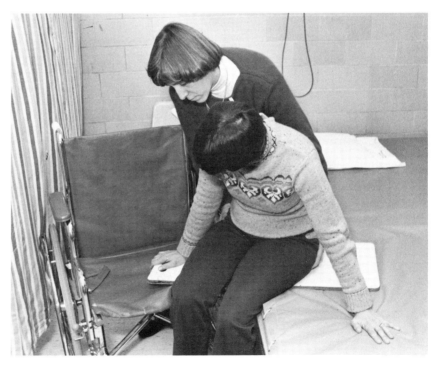

Figure 16–7 Correct position for sliding board transfer. With adequate arm strength, the patient can assist with the transfer.

out braces, an assisted stand–pivot transfer is preferable. Eventually, a dependent pivot transfer is necessary as weakness accelerates. In addition, a two-man through-the-arms lift can be used. The presence of scapular instability requires a firm but comfortable grasp.

A transfer or sliding board may be used in any neuromuscular patient for wheelchair transfers to and from the bed, car, or raised toilet seat (Fig. 16–7). If possible, the patient assists by performing a modified shoulder depression while the caretaker slides the patient's hips across the board. With increasing weakness, correct positioning for balance and having the patient move his head in a timely fashion helps the caretaker with the transfer. If a sliding board is used in a very weak patient, caretakers must be thoroughly familiar with a totally dependent sliding-board transfer.

Mechanical lifts, including a Trans-Aid and Hoyer, are available when manual transfers are unsafe for the patient or the caretaker. Correct positioning of the sling is important to ensure the safety of the patient when transferring from wheelchair to tub, toilet, car, or floor (Fig. 16–8).

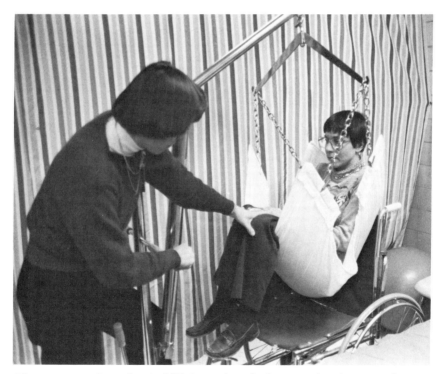

Figure 16 – 8 A mechanical lift is employed when a patient is too weak or too heavy for his caretaker. Transfers should be broken down into steps for the family, including demonstration of and practice in removing and positioning the sling while the patient is in the wheelchair.

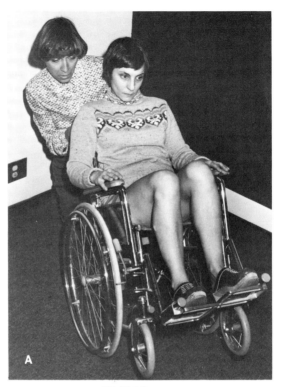

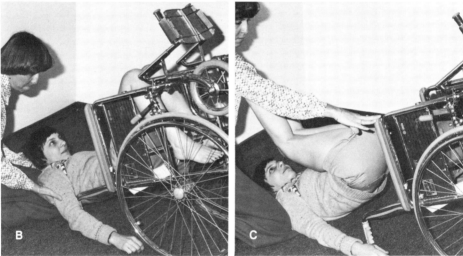

Figure 16–9 (A) "Beach" or emergency transfer allows one person to place a wheel-chair-bound person on the floor. The wheels are locked, and the arm rests are secured before the chair is tilted backward. (B) The back of the wheelchair is placed on the floor, and the patient's feet are allowed to dangle behind the footrests. The patient may place his hands on his knees to control hip flexion. (C) A caretaker grasps the patient's ankles and flexes his hips (as in changing a diaper); the buttocks will rise out of the chair seat. While holding this position, the brakes are unlocked and the chair is pushed away. Finally, the patient's legs are lowered to the floor.

If a patient wishes to be on the floor, the caretaker is instructed in a "beach," or emergency, transfer. The patient is removed from and repositioned in the chair after it has been tilted posteriorly (Fig. 16–9).

IMPAIRED RESPIRATION

A therapist should always anticipate the development of ventilatory failure in patients with neuromuscular diseases (see Chap. 14). Complications occur because of scoliosis, respiratory muscle weakness, poor cough, and tracheal aspiration. Assessment should include evaluation of functional cough as well as pulmonary function tests using a spirometer.

If a patient reports an increase in upper respiratory infections, he should be instructed in the use of a good diaphragmatic breathing pattern, postural drainage (see Fig. 19–1), percussion, and assisted coughing. In patients with severely compromised pulmonary functions, glossopharyngeal breathing patterns may automatically occur to augment restricted vital capacity. To maintain lung function, respiratory exercises using inspiratory resistors (see Fig. 14–6) or incentive spirometers (see Fig. 19–2) are helpful. Such techniques can be supervised by the family and by the therapist in the school system.

Conclusion

The physical therapist's work extends beyond the neuromuscular clinic in advising teachers and school nurses on the most advantageous method of walking or transferring a child. The neuromuscular therapist may also be asked to provide information to other therapists within the community who have limited experience in the management of neuromuscular disease.

When a neuromuscular patient undergoes a surgical procedure, the physical therapist must evaluate and encourage the patient to regain function. In spite of neuromuscular deterioration, it is the therapist, using knowledge of neuromuscular disease and kinesiology, who provides the patient with a sense of accomplishment and the best possible adjustment to his disability.

Suggested Readings

ALLSOP KG, ZITER FA: Loss of strength and functional decline in Duchenne's dystrophy. Arch Neurol 38:406–411, 1981

ANGELINI C, RINGEL SP: Italian multicenter therapeutic trials in Duchenne dystrophy. I. Protocol. Ital J Neurosci 5, 1983

BROOKE MH: A Clinician's View of Neuromuscular Disease. Baltimore, Williams & Wilkins, 1977

GIBSON DA, WILKINS KE: The management of spinal deformities in Duchenne muscular dystrophy. A new concept in spinal bracing. Clin Orthop 108:41–51, 1975

HYDE SA, SCOTT OM, GODDARD CM, et al: Prolongation of ambulation in Duchenne muscular dystrophy by appropriate orthoses. Physiotherapy 68(4):105–108, 1982

RUSSMAN BS, MELCHREIT R, DRENNAN JC: Spinal muscular atrophy: The natural course of the disease. Muscle Nerve 6:179, 1983

SCOTT OM, HYDE SA, GODDARD C, et al: Effect of exercise in Duchenne muscular dystrophy. Physiotherapy 67(6):174–176, 1981

SCOTT OM, HYDE SA, GODDARD C, et al: Prevention of deformity in Duchenne muscular dystrophy: A prospective study of passive stretching and splinting. Physiotherapy 67(6):177–180, 1981

SIEGEL IM, SILVERMAN O, SILVERMAN M: The Chicago insert: An approach to wheelchair seating for the maintenance of spinal posture in Duchenne muscular dystrophy. Orthotics Prosthetics 35(4):27–29, 1981

SPENCER GE: Orthopaedic care of progressive muscular dystrophy. J Bone Joint Surg 49-A:1201–1204, 1967

STERN LZ, RINGEL SP, ZITER FA, et al: Drug trial of superoxide dismutase in Duchenne's muscular dystrophy. Arch Neurol 39:342–346, 1982

SUTHERLAND DH, OLSHEN R, COOPER L, et al: The pathomechanics of gait in Duchenne muscular dystrophy. Dev Med Child Neurol 23:3–22, 1981

VIGNOS PJ: Physical models of rehabilitation in neuromuscular disease. Muscle Nerve 6:323–338, 1983

VIGNOS PJ: Rehabilitation in the myopathies. In Handbook of Clinical Neurology, vol 41, Part II, Chap. 13, pp 1–44. Amsterdam, Elsevier North Holland Biomedical Press, 1979

ZITER FA, ALLSOP KG, TYLER FA: Assessment of muscle strength in Duchenne muscular dystrophy. Neurology 27:981–984, 1977

Assistive Devices for Patients With Neuromuscular Diseases: The Role of Occupational Therapy

The occupational therapist (OT) has a basic and important role in identifying, prescribing, and filling assistive devices for patients with neuromuscular diseases. In order to fulfill the therapist's responsibility and to optimize the outcome for the patient, the following *principles* must be recognized and remembered:

1. Treatment is designed to augment home care and daily activities.
2. Techniques and assistive devices should be based on a realistic evaluation and understanding of the patient's needs, capabilities, and limitations, and should include an awareness of the attitudes and acceptance of the family to the patient's progressive disability. At times, family members may feel guilty if the family's daily routine does not allow for all the well-meaning suggestions or instructions given by the therapist and doctors. Unnecessarily difficult and time-consuming exercises or daily living routines will be burdensome to the family, will impede progress, and will result in increased frustration for all concerned. The success of home treatment programs rests with an understanding of the needs and activity schedule of the entire family.
3. The goal of therapy is to maintain function rather than to improve strength. Traditional goals of increasing function and strength have to be altered because, in most neuromuscular patients, function and strength progressively worsen. In the neuromuscular patient, function must be maintained as long as possible, thereby retaining the maximal quality of life, independence, and freedom.
4. A therapeutic program should consider those who live with and assist the patient. People involved in the patient's care must be served in such a way that all emerge as winning participants. For

example, it may not be in the patient's best interest to do as many activities of daily living as possible independently. A patient with stand-by assistance can reserve strength and energy for school, work, or a much-needed recreational venture. Families often find it easier for their daily routine to assist the patient in self-care activities. Then, while going to work or school, the patient has reserve energy to be more self-sufficient. Adaptive equipment for patients with advanced weakness serves the additional purpose of making the caretaker's task easier. Clearly, work simplification for a caretaker is as necessary as for a patient so that a family does not become hopelessly discouraged.

Evaluation

In our University Hospital neuromuscular clinic, the occupational therapist's evaluation tools include the following.

General Information

General information is gained from a checklist that patients fill out as they arrive. Patients are asked to identify problems encountered at school, on the job, or with daily activities resulting from weakness and fatigue (Fig. 17 – 1).

Activities of Daily Living

We have developed a practical form for evaluating activities of daily living (ADL), which uses a scale of 0 to 5 (Fig. 17 – 2). A 5 indicates that the activity is performed independently and optimally. A 0 indicates that the activity cannot be performed. The ADL checklist includes communication, eating skills, mobility, hygiene, dressing, and a miscellaneous category that includes such diverse functions as operating a radio or television, opening and closing doors, and preparing a snack.

Wheelchair Evaluation

Occupational therapists most often assess the need for a wheelchair, motorized scooter, safety/travel chair, or stroller, and for accessories including scoliosis pads, a ball-bearing feeder, head support, and neck collar. The wheelchair prescription procedure is detailed in Chapter 25.

Manual Muscle Testing

Although usually performed by a physical therapist, a briefer assessment of muscle function should be done by the occupational therapist.

NEUROMUSCULAR CLINIC   DATE: _____

To assist in your care, please <u>check</u> any of the items below that are a problem for you today.

_____	Breathing	✓	Sleeping
_____	Heart	_____	Adaptive equipment (body jacket, brace, etc.)
_____	Conflicts at work	✓	Loss of weight or appetite
✓	Pain (where *hip & bottom*)	✓	Diet
_____	Bladder	✓	Bathing
_____	Anxiety, depression or anger	_____	Financial problems
_____	Bowels	✓	Wheelchair
_____	Skin	_____	Personal adjustment to illness
✓	Speech or swallowing	_____	Difficulty relating to doctor
_____	Family quarreling	✓	Physical therapy program
✓	Teeth *Can't open mouth wide*	_____	School problems
_____	Family adjustment to illness	✓	Occupational therapy program
✓	Medication	✓	Wish to speak to doctor alone
_____	MDA Patient service		

Other (specify): *toilet too low — can't write*

_____

_____

Please return this form to the clinic nurse when you are called for your appointment.

Figure 17-1 Neuromuscular check list. This check list is used to alert physicians to concerns of patients. After discussing the points with the patient, the doctor calls the occupational therapist (OT). By using the check list and the ADL check sheet, it was determined that this patient needed an alternating air mattress to relieve pressure on the hip and buttocks that occurred while the patient was in bed. A universal cuff and pencil holder were ordered, as well as a bath transfer bench and a hand-held flexible shower attachment. A raised toilet seat with toilet safety frame was also prescribed to assist the patient and the caretaker. A wheelchair equipped with ballbearing feeders was ordered so that the patient, while seated in the chair, could use his arms to operate a computer and perform simple hygiene. (Used by permission. University of Colorado Health Sciences Center. All rights reserved.)

UNIVERSITY OF COLORADO MEDICAL CENTER
Department of Physical Medicine and Rehabilitation
Evaluation of
ACTIVITIES OF DAILY LIVING

Date
Ward
Name
Hosp. No.
Address

		Date	Date	Date	Comments	METHOD OF SCORING
C	Summon aid	5				Performs activity:
O	Speak intelligibly	5				5 — independently and
M	Read and interpret	5				in optimal manner
M	Turn pages	4				4 — Independently but in
U	Write adequately	3			*pencil holder*	less than optimal
N	Complete phone call	4				manner in relation to
						time and adaptations
E	Eat with spoon/fork	3			*built up utensils cuff*	3 — independently but
A	Drink from cup/glass	3				impractically
T	Cut with knife	2			*rocker knife*	
	Carry own dishes/tray	0				2 — with standby
						attendant only
	Roll side to side	3				1 — with human assistance
	Sit up in bed	3				0 — unable to perform
M	To W/C and back	0				
O	Operate W/C	3			*consider scooter*	SUMMARY:
B	Site-stand-sit	2			*? lift*	
I	Ambulation	2				
L	Stairs	0				
I	Toilet on/off	2			*raised toilet seat*	
T	Shower in/out	N/A				
Y	Tub in/out	1			*water powered bath lift*	
	Braces/prosthesis on/off	N/A				
	Car in/out	2				
	Bus on/off	N/A				
H	Wash hands and face	3			*need arms supported - work simplification*	
Y	Brush teeth	3			*handles needs to be built up*	
G	Comb hair	3			*arms supported - increase handle*	
I	Shave/make up	3			*support arms*	
E	Bathe	2			*bath mitt - long handled sponge*	
N	Care for nails	2			*suction brush*	
E						
D	Dress/blouse/shirt on/off	3			*modify clothing*	
R	Slacks on/off	3				
E	Manage fastenings	3			*needs button hook*	
S	Socks/stockings/shoes on/off	2			*sock aid - long handled shoe horn*	
S	Clothes in/out of storage	3			*lower clothing rod*	
M	Operate radio and TV	4			*needs handles built up*	
I	Manage eyeglasses	4				
S	Pick up object from floor	2			*needs reacher*	
C	Operate light switch	3			*extension knob*	
E	Operate doors	3			*extension levers*	
L	Wind watch	N/A			*digital*	
L	Use matches safely	N/A				
A	Use money	3			*coins difficult*	
N	Object from pocket/purse					
E	and replace	2				
O	Prepare snack					
U						
S						

Figure 17-2   ADL evaluation cues the therapist to direct questions to safety, adaptive equipment needs, and work-simplification techniques. (Used by permission. University of Colorado Health Sciences Center. All rights reserved.)

Splinting

The occupational therapist should determine if splinting of an extremity is beneficial to the patient. Splints should be light and designed to assist remaining function. Correction of deformity may impede function and is not a primary goal of splinting in the neuromuscular patient.

Conversation and Work Simplification

After conversing with a patient as to how activities of daily living are performed, work-simplification techniques should be suggested. The occupational therapist's goals should ensure patient safety while increasing function and decreasing fatigue.

As a therapist becomes more skilled and familiar with the different types of neuromuscular diseases, it becomes easier to ask the right questions and to bring out problem areas patients are hesitant or embarrassed to mention. Following the assessment procedures, patients often come to the OT clinic for more extensive trials in performing ADL tasks and to select appropriate adaptive equipment (commercial or custom-made). Splinting can often be done during or immediately following the clinic visit. If complicated patient problems are reviewed prior to the clinic visit, the therapist can anticipate and budget time accordingly.

Adaptive Aids

Adaptive aids allow the patient to perform a lost or deteriorating function in an optimal manner related to muscle capability, strength, and range of motion. Many adaptive aids are successfully used by patients with proximal weakness, particularly to maintain effective hygiene. A patient with proximal weakness of the shoulders and hips has difficulty bending over without losing balance or lifting an arm over the head without support of the other arm. Because hygiene is an area that most people consider private, questions concerning bathing, toileting, and other personal tasks must be direct and specific. The following is a short list of frequently used devices and a brief description of their functions:

Extension-handle comb/brush. Long-handled brushes are designed with numerous angles to eliminate the need for a patient to lift the arms above the head.

Long-handled sponge. The long-handled sponge increases reaching ability and decreases the need to bend over.

High bath/shower chairs (preferable with a position back rest). The chair decreases the distance required to come to a stand and provides the patient with a secure supported posture while bathing.

Lifts. Hydraulic lifts operated by a caretaker lower and raise a patient in and out of a tub, chair, bed, or car, or on and off the floor (Fig.

17–3). Light-weight, water-powered bath lifts are used only in the tub. Crank lifts (see Fig. 16–9) must be manually operated by a caretaker, but they function similarly to a hydraulic lift. Unfortunately, most lifts cannot be operated by the patient independently unless the lifts are customized with special controls.

A *transfer bench*. The transfer bench provides for easy transfer from chair to tub with little break in sitting surface. The bench works well with a flexible shower hose attachment.

Grab bars. These ensure safety by preventing falls.

A *flexible shower hose and adapter* (see Fig. 8–13). These can be attached to a shower or bathtub fixture to control water flow. If hooked to the shower head, the patient can still fill the tub with his feet in the water.

A *toilet paper holder*. This assists a person with limited reach and poor balance.

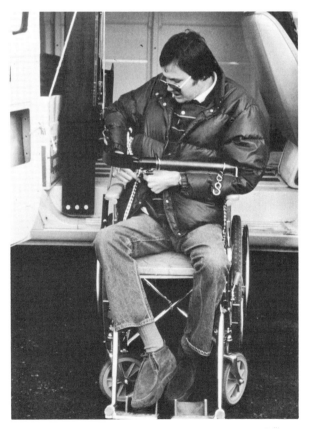

Figure 17–3   Van lift. This type of van lift can be operated by a patient with neuromuscular disease.

A raised toilet seat (Fig. 17–4). A raised toilet seat is used when a patient cannot rise from a standard chair height or must pivot transfer from a wheelchair. The elevated seat avoids back strain and allows greater independence.

Whenever possible, a patient's preference (*i.e.*, bath or shower) should be considered so that customary lifestyle can be maintained. The following examples highlight typical patient problems and solutions.

Problem No. 1: The Walk-in Shower Many patients do not use adaptive aids, either because of pride or through ignorance. As a result, they do not volunteer details of how a task is actually performed, preferring a face-saving, "I manage O.K." This response must not be accepted! With detailed questioning, dangerous practices and inadequate care frequently surface. A patient describing showering (walk-in type) often says, "My spouse helps me step up over the edge to get into the shower. I hold onto the side of the shower door or onto the shower curtain. I steady myself with the soap rack and am just fine." In this case, by hanging on throughout the shower, the patient cannot adequately clean his hair, feet, and legs, and if he is quite weak, a slip is sure to result in a fall.

Solution The patient needs grab bars installed both outside and inside the shower. It is unsafe for a person to use a shower door, shower

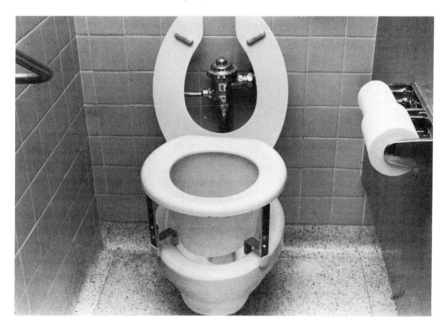

Figure 17–4 Raised toilet seat. The seat, portable for travel, helps any person with proximal weakness come to a standing position more easily.

curtain, soap dish, towel rack, or other fixture to hold his weight. If the patient needs walls to be steady while bathing, a tall shower chair with a back support is safer and still allows the patient the pleasure of leisurely showering. A long-handled sponge will enable the patient to reach his feet and back. An extension-handle brush with attachments can also help a patient to scrub and wash his hair. Some spouses shower with the patient, a practice that improves cleansing and can be a mutually rewarding time together.

Problem No. 2: The Bathtub Shower The patient has moderate proximal weakness, fatigues easily, and needs support to bathe.

Solution This patient could successfully bathe independently by using a bath transfer bench to get in and out of the tub and a seat in a secure position in the tub. A flexible shower hose is helpful to eliminate sitting with a constant flow of water in the face from a fixed shower head. (Remember, since bathtubs are lower, bathtub transfer seats must also be lower.) Grab bars on the wall are useful at the side of the tub if the patient can stand. When transferring directly from a wheelchair to the tub, grab bars may not be needed. A long-handled sponge and hair scrub brush are helpful. If there are sliding glass doors on the bathtub, this bathing technique is almost impossible, so the doors should be removed.

Problem No. 3: Bathing a Moderately Weak Patient If the patient retains sitting balance and head control, a tub bath remains possible but is difficult.

Solution Patients with head and trunk control can use a water-powered bath lift (Fig. 17–5) that has a swivel seat that extends over the bathtub edge. The lift is small, making it ideal for small bathrooms and trailers, and is easily removed so the tub remains accessible to other family members. Other previously described adaptive equipment can be used depending on the patient's particular needs. Importantly, grab bars are not easily attached in trailers because of trailer construction.

Problem No. 4 A patient has marked weakness, limited range of motion in the upper extremities, poor trunk and head control, and is totally dependent.

Solution This patient needs a caretaker to assist with sponge-bathing and requires a lift with a total body sling as well as a commode seat for tub bathing. Many lifts cannot be maneuvered into small bathrooms. However, a sling apparatus can be placed under the patient so he can be moved into the bathroom on a utility chair or in a wheelchair. The sling can then be attached to a lift and secured to the bathtub or a floor fixture, and the patient lowered into the tub. A commode sling allows easy

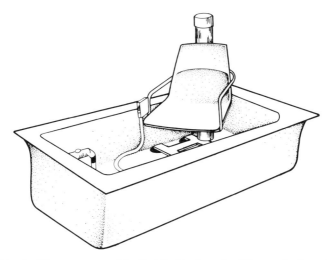

Figure 17–5 Water-powered bath lift. Designed with a swivel seat that extends over the tub edge, this lift is ideal for small bathrooms and in mobile homes. The lift is easily removed so that the tub is accessible to other family members.

access for cleansing the genital area. A full tub of water allows the patient to move more freely and to use remaining muscle power.

Problem No. 5 Because many patients experience great frustration in getting on and off a toilet without help, they may avoid visiting friends or traveling.

Solution A 6 inch to 8 inch raised portable toilet seat is most helpful for adults because it is easily removed and light-weight. If a patient needs extra assistance to get off a raised toilet seat, adjustable-height toilet aid assist frames or strategically positioned grab bars are useful. A patient should be cautioned never to use a free-standing sink or towel rack to hoist himself off the toilet because these objects pull away from the wall.

Raised toilet seats come with a variety of openings around the rim to allow the patient to wipe. If there is a problem with limited range of motion or weakness, a tong-shaped toiletpaper holder should be suggested. For those patients confined to a wheelchair who cannot get into the bathroom because of an architectural barrier, a movable commode is recommended. The commode can be used with a movable lift and commode seat sling apparatus as well.

Mobility and Independent Activity

Adaptive aids for mobility can provide increased independence for the patient and the caretaker. Some patients who are too weak to stand up from a seated position can still ambulate with the aid of crutches or a walker. A patient lying supine who cannot push to a sitting position can hook his arms through a series of loops attached to the foot of the bed and gradually pull up to a sitting position. An easy-lift power chair is useful for patients who cannot get out of a sitting position to stand (despite employing work-simplification techniques). The back of the chair reclines as it gently elevates the seat and the attached arm rests up and forward. Chairs without arm rests are dangerous for the patient with poor trunk control. These chairs cannot be used for standing by patients with marked quadriceps weakness because they lack the strength to complete the standing maneuver. A somewhat mobile catapult seat with various strengths of pushing power can be used in the home, car, or on other pieces of furniture. A drawback of the catapult seat is that it gives a rapid push and does not have arm supports, making it unsafe for patients with poor balance and stability. The weight of the seat precludes easy carrying from place to place.

In patients with advanced weakness, even moving in bed may not be possible without help, and they may become caught in the blankets. An alternating air mattress or waterbed fitted with bed hoops can add comfort and prevent total dependency. The alternating air mattress slowly shifts the patient's weight, allowing more sleep for both the caretaker and patient before turning is required. In patients with severe hip and knee contractures, a waterbed works well because the water volume can be adjusted to permit weight shifts with little effort, minimizing discomfort and optimizing independent movement. Bed or burn hoops, by elevating covers, relieve discomfort and minimize ankle contractures from plantar flexion.

Dressing

Simple solutions to dressing problems for weak patients include teaching easier dressing techniques and suggesting modifications in type and style of clothing. Commonly used adaptive aids include a zipper pull, button hook, sock aid, and long-handled shoehorn. When selecting clothing, garments with many tiny buttons and zippers in the back should be avoided. A woman should choose slacks with an elastic waistband rather than a pair with buttons and zippers. A male patient may require a zipper pull or a button hook, depending on the style of trouser. A small thumb loop inside the trouser waistband permits added leverage for fastening the pants. Velcro fasteners are easiest to open and close. In active patients, jogging suits are easily donned and are suitable for many activities and environments. Comfortable, well-fitting shoes are difficult to find because of dependent edema, contractures, pressure, and orthoses. Hiking boots that open to the toe provide ankle support and easily accommodate an orthotic. Orthotics can also be worn with loafers if there is elastic or a buckle on the top of the shoe to prevent pressure-induced pain and sores. Patients with mild to moderate weakness and irreversible shortening of the Achilles tendon require footwear with a heel (i.e., cowboy boots) for both comfort and mobility. Lightweight tennis or running shoes provide maximal comfort but no support.

Difficulty in putting on a shoe can occur from inability to bend down, from inadequate strength to pull the shoe on, or from lack of strength or dexterity to tie the shoe. Devices that assist a patient in putting on shoes include elastic shoelaces, zipper fastenings, and long-handled shoehorns. A variety of sock aids can make putting on socks easier.

Homemaking/Kitchen Aids

Many assistive devices make cooking easier. An under-the-counter jar opener allows weak patients to open jars with very little effort. For the person whose counter or tables are too high, a lap-tray apron provides an excellent small work surface. In addition, in the event that something hot is spilled, the apron protects the patient from burns.

An all-purpose utility knob fits over most knobs, is easy to hold, and, because of its long handle, increases leverage for turning on/off stoves, televisions, and radios (Fig. 17–6). Doorknob extenders can make door opening easier for the weak patient. A voluntary-opening, long-handled reacher allows patients to pick up light-weight articles. A one-handed cutting board, secured to a work surface by suction cups, has aluminum nails that spear vegetables or other difficult-to-hold products. With this board, a patient with one weak arm can function almost as well as if he had two strong arms.

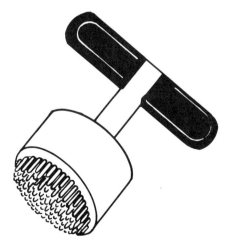

Figure 17–6 Turning knob. The tiny projections form around different shaped and sized knobs, and the long handle allows added leverage for turning on and off stoves, televisions, and so on.

Eating

Naturally, patients prefer to eat independently and inconspicuously. Correct positioning and correct table height can facilitate independence. If a person can use his arms against gravity for only a limited time before fatiguing, etiquette must take a backseat. By resting the elbows on the table, gravity is eliminated and more motion at the elbow, wrist, and hand is possible. Rather than bringing the head forward to the food, a table surface should be raised so the patient's arms rest closer to the mouth. A raised tray at the patient's place avoids having the table too high for other family members. Desk arms enable a patient in a wheelchair to get closer to the table. If a utensil is difficult to hold, the handle should be enlarged to increase its gripping surface. Alternatively, a universal cuff will hold a variety of eating utensils (Fig. 17–7).

With marked shoulder, arm, and hand weakness, a ball-bearing feeder/mobile arm support should be considered (Fig. 17–8). The feeder bracket is permanently attached to the wheelchair uprights, but other parts are removable so that nonfeeding activities can be performed without interference. A feeder arm holds the forearm in a trough, leaving the wrist and hand free for eating. By pulling the arm toward midline and leaning into the forearm trough, the patient's hand will come to the mouth with little effort. Adjustments are needed to balance the feeder arm and bracket, and a patient must be willing to practice to make the device work. Although one mobile support is sufficient for fine motor tasks and feeding, some patients prefer two supports for other activities and for range-of-motion exercises.

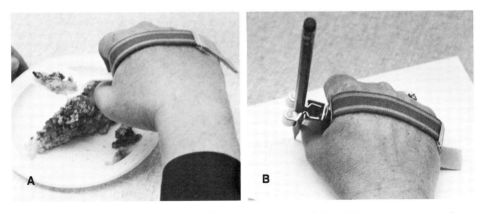

Figure 17–7 Universal cuff. When slipped on a patient's hand(s), no active grasp from the patient is required, because a slot holds different items, such as a spoon for feeding (A). A klick pencil holder with pencil in place allows writing to be accomplished using a more general wrist and arm motion (B).

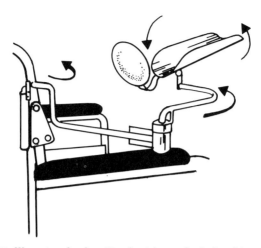

Figure 17–8 Ballbearing feeder. Used with marked shoulder, arm, and hand weakness, the bracket is the only part permanently attached to the wheelchair uprights.

Communication

There are many phone systems available to assist an individual who is unable to speak clearly or dial (pushbutton phones are easier than dial phones). A clear-plastic communication board can be used in the hospital or at home by patients who have difficulty articulating or who speak softly. The patient directs his eyes to the words or letters on the communication board while the doctor or caretaker looks on from the opposite side to obtain the message. Written communication aids are commercially available for patients who are unable to hold a pen or pencil. Frequently used pencil holders include a pencil grip, sarong pencil holder, and klick holder, which fits into a universal cuff slot. Many patients have little wrist and finger motion but can write "from the shoulder" using large, gross motions. The patients must be positioned with arms supported in order to use these adaptive devices.

It is both challenging and rewarding to fabricate a specific piece of equipment that improves a patient's performance at work (Fig. 17–9). A creative bioengineer and occupational therapist, working with the patient, can usually identify limitless possibilities for improving function for a specific need (see Chap. 8).

Splinting

Splints are used to prevent contractures and to maintain function. They must be light in weight and designed to assist residual function by

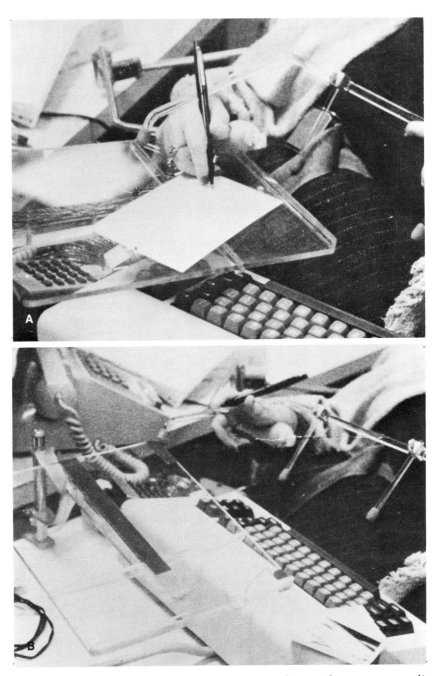

Figure 17–9 A patient with spinal muscular atrophy rests her arm on a modified ballbearing feeder. (A) The clear plastic writing surface has a strip of dycem applied to prevent the paper from slipping. The writing surface can be swung over the typewriter and calculator to be next to the telephone. Rubber tips applied to a clear plastic rod allow the patient to reach a pad and pull it forward. (B) The plastic projections with rubber tips also allow the patient to strike a typewriter keyboard or to flip a cardex file.

capitalizing on residual muscle strength. A patient's remaining ability is the key to splint design. The ankle and hands most frequently benefit from splinting. In a patient with Achilles contractures, an exercise and stretching program is the most effective treatment but can be augmented by dorsiflexion night foot splints. Unfortunately, compliance is poor because of discomfort. Wrist-extension splints improve hand function in severely weakened Duchenne muscular dystrophy (DMD) and spinal muscular atrophy (SMA) patients. Positional hand splints improve functional use, slow the rate of contracture, and decrease edema in patients with amyotrophic lateral sclerosis (ALS). Individual finger splints are used in specific cases to stabilize finger joints and to retard contractures.

Work Simplification

Work-simplification techniques are energy-saving, common-sense adjustments to activities that do not require assistive devices. The following principles should be followed:

1. Use common sense—eliminate all unnecessary work.
2. Organize tasks (*i.e.*, get everything from the refrigerator that is needed for a cooking activity in one rather than multiple trips).
3. Change the pacing of activities (*i.e.*, instead of doing all cleaning, bathing, and other chores in the morning, space activities throughout the day).
4. If possible, use both hands to work in opposite and symmetrical motion; use smooth-flowing motions in a curved path with no angles (*i.e.*, when ironing, rather than a push/pull technique, use a curved path; it is much easier to the stop the iron).
5. Lay out work areas within easy reach.
6. Slide, don't lift and carry (*i.e.*, slide pots from sink to range). Use a wheeled utility cart where work surfaces are broken.
7. Have fixed work stations. Have a special place to do each job so that supplies and equipment are kept ready for immediate use.
8. Use the fewest tools possible. Select equipment that may be used for more than one job.
9. Avoid holding. Use utensils that are fixed by suction cups or clamps so that both hands are free to work (*i.e.*, use a regular mixer instead of a portable hand mixer).
10. Let gravity work. Rather than carrying laundry, toss it down stairs. Rather than lifting items from a cutting board, place a pan below the board and scrape items off the board into the pan.
11. Store small tools so you can grasp them and start work immediately without excessive bending and reaching motions.

12. Locate controls and switches within easy reach; change the location of switches if necessary or insert switches in electric cords for easier use. Use adaptive devices to increase leverage.
13. Sit to work whenever possible (*i.e.*, sit to iron). Work at a sink to prepare vegetables or at a counter to mix foods. Adjust the chair height to the work surface for maximum comfort.
14. Modify work surface height. Jobs requiring hand activity (slicing, typing) require a higher work surface than tasks needing pressure (kneading bread, ironing).

It is helpful to raise the height of sitting, sleeping, and work surfaces for patients with hip weakness (*i.e.*, put the bed or couch on blocks). Combing hair, applying make up, or shaving is easiest when seated at a raised work surface. Similar modifications should be tried for a familiar and enjoyable hobby. Try to find creative solutions because it is important to a patient to function independently.

A proper chair should have a seat large enough to give full support; a low back support so that shoulder and elbow movement is not inhibited and the trunk is held well balanced over the hips; and a footrest at the proper height to avoid excessive pressure behind the knees or on the buttocks.

There are many additional money-saving and energy-efficient work-simplification methods that can be used. It is important to listen to your patients because they often have many worthwhile suggestions that can be passed on to other handicapped people.

Functional Loss

One of the most difficult problems for the occupational therapist is the patient who no longer can ambulate. The use of a wheelchair is a sensitive issue for the patient and family because the wheelchair is society's symbol for the handicapped and tangible evidence that the patient is deteriorating and perhaps even closer to death. Whenever possible, the OT should advise the patient and family in advance of the need for a chair so there is time to adjust to this change.

There are many types of wheelchairs, scooters, and strollers. The terminology, types, and adaptations are detailed in Chapter 25. For maximal efficiency, a wheelchair should be the proper size and have accessories that increase function and quality of life for the patient. If a chair is too wide, a patient will lean to one side, accentuating scoliosis. In addition, a wide chair requires more energy to push because the patient alternates from side to side rather than pushing simultaneously with both arms.

If a chair is too deep, circulation at the back of the knees can be compromised and the patient will find it difficult to propel the chair because of a kyphotic sitting position, head forward and scapulae retracted. Footrests should be the swing-away style for ease in transferring. If footrests are too high, patients experience unnecessary buttock pressure, and hip and knee flexion contractures worsen. If footrests are too low, the patient's feet hang in plantar flexion, promoting Achilles contractures. Solid seat and back inserts with foam padding promote good posture and keep the chair upholstery from stretching, particularly if a patient is obese. An electric wheelchair, although it does not encourage use of muscles, is important for the severely handicapped patient to allow participation in activities outside of the home.

For patients with Duchenne dystrophy, we normally provide scoliosis pads when an electric wheelchair is ordered because these children frequently develop progressive spinal collapse and lean to the side of the controls (Fig. 17–10; see Chaps. 16 and 18). Slender patients with marked lordosis sit erect and do not require scoliosis pads, but, because these children lean forward in the chair, a custom harness with a wide band or material across the chest is necessary for support and to facilitate breathing. A homemade or custom-made harness is usually more comfortable than conventional H-strap harnessing or a chest strap and seat belt.

A head support is important for patients with neck weakness and can be custom-fitted if the patient needs to fully recline or have his head supported throughout the day. Without support, the head can fall back with extreme force, so the support should fill in all space between the patient's head and the back of a recliner.

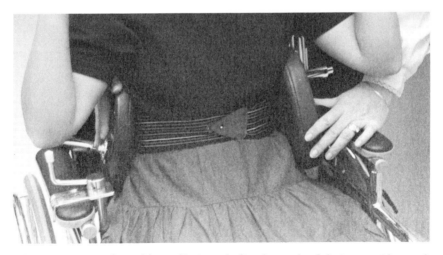

Figure 17–10 Adjustable scoliosis pads fitted on wheelchairs provide trunk support and retard development of scoliosis.

Soft or firm neck collars also provide some head support. A wire-frame cervical collar is cool and allows clothing to fit more normally; we therefore recommend it if a patient's head bobs when starting or stopping a wheelchair or while a passenger in a car (see Fig. 25–13).

Summary

The OT has an important role in teaching the patient and all those in his environment how to make daily living tasks easiest for everyone concerned. In turn, families, school teachers, and employers may have good suggestions that can benefit an individual and that the OT can share with colleagues and other patients. Treatment and adaptive equipment should be realistically formulated based on an understanding of a particular patient's needs, capabilities, and limitations. The OT's goals for the patient are to maintain function for the longest possible time, retain maximal quality of life, and set priorities within the patient's capabilities for activities of daily living. The therapeutic relationship provides a chance for creativity for both the therapist and patient to develop ways to ensure maximal independence with optimal freedom and quality of life.

Suggested Readings

BROOKE MH, FENICHEL GM, GRIGGS RC, et al: Clinical investigation in Duchenne dystrophy: 2. Determination of the "power" of therapeutic trials based on the natural history. Muscle and Nerve 6:91, 1983

GIBRETH IM, THOMAS OM, ELEANOR C: Management in the Home, rev ed. Binghamton, Vail-Ballou Press, 1964

HALE G (ed): The Source Book for the Disabled. London, Imprint Books, 1979

MAY EE, WAGGONER NR, BOETTKE EM: Homemaking for the Handicapped. New York, Dodd, Mead & Co, 1966

WILLARD HS, SPACHMAN CS: Occupational Therapy. Philadelphia, JB Lippincott, 1963

18

Irwin M. Siegel

Orthopaedic Management of Muscle Disease

Alteration in the dynamics of postural maintenance in muscular dystrophy, particularly Duchenne muscular dystrophy (DMD), occurs as a result of functional imbalance between muscle groups or because of the pattern of muscular involvement used to compensate for weakness. This ultimately results in hip and knee flexion contracture, ankle equinocarovarus, and spinal distortions in the sagittal plane (lordosis) in the patient who is still ambulatory and in the coronal plane (scoliosis) in the patient who is confined to a wheelchair.

In DMD, the hip flexors, tensor fascia lata, and the triceps surae develop ambulation-limiting contractures. As long as the patient can maintain the line of gravity behind his hips, in front of his knees, and within his base of support, the upright posture can be maintained (Fig. 18–1). As the processes of the disease advance, however, stance and gait become typified by hip flexion and abduction, progressive lumbar lordosis, and ankle and foot equinocavovarus (Fig. 18–2). Generalized weakness makes it increasingly difficult to attain alignment stability with the trunk balanced over unstable lower extremities. Proprioceptive abilities are also affected, and sufficient strength to execute those postural adjustments necessary to compensate for selective weakening and contractures is often lacking (Fig. 18–3; see Chap. 16).

Surgical Treatment

The aim of surgery is to release ambulation-limiting contractures sufficiently to maintain adequate standing and walking equilibrium. Appropriate orthoses offering satisfactory support without undue weight are fitted afterward.

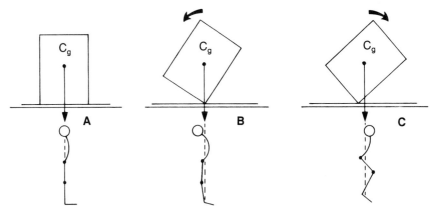

Figure 18–1 (A) Line of gravity maintained behind hips, in front of knees, and within base of support. (B) Lumbar lordosis, equinus, and knee extension permit upright posture. (C) Line of gravity is no longer as it was in A or B. Standing is no longer possible. (Cg = center of gravity) (Siegel IM: Diagnosis, management, and orthopaedic treatment of muscular dystrophy. In The American Academy of Orthopaedic Surgeons: Instructional Course Lectures, Vol XXX. St Louis, CV Mosby, 1981)

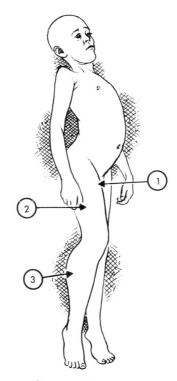

Figure 18–2 Ambulating–limiting contractures occur in (1) hip flexors; (2) tensor fasciae latae; and (3) triceps surae. (Siegel IM: The Clinical Management of Muscle Disease. London, William Heinemann Medical Books, 1977)

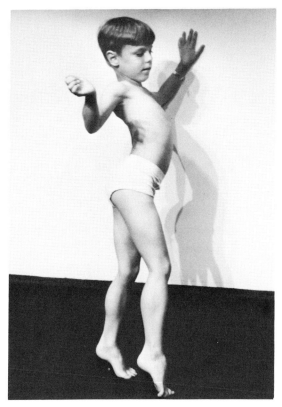

Figure 18 – 3   Posture in Duchenne muscular dystrophy. (Siegel IM: Diagnosis, management, and orthopaedic treatment of muscular dystrophy. In The American Academy of Orthopaedic Surgeons: Instructional Course Lectures, Vol XXX. St Louis, CV Mosby, 1981)

Operative intervention in the lower extremities is usually indicated between the ages of 9 to 12 years. Patients generally lose the ability to rise easily from a seated position and to ascend stairs and walk (in this sequence) at yearly intervals. When the sum of knee and hip extension lag reaches or exceeds 90 degrees in the face of ankle equinus of 15 degrees or more, the patient can no longer maintain the upright posture and ambulation ends (Fig. 18 – 4).

Surgical management must permit early postoperative mobilization. Even brief restraint can lead to rapid decrease of strength (approximately 3% loss per day) in the dystrophic patient. During surgery, anesthesia must be closely monitored, paying particular attention to providing adequate ventilation, avoiding gastric dilatation, prohibiting potassium overload, and preventing malignant hyperthermia.

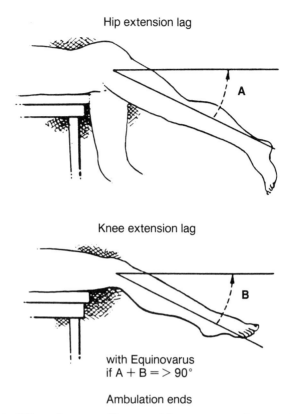

Hip extension lag

Knee extension lag

with Equinovarus
if A + B = > 90°

Ambulation ends

Figure 18–4   When the sum of knee and hip extension lag reach 90 degrees, ambulation ends. (Siegel IM: The Clinical Management of Muscle Disease. London, William Heinemann Medical Books, 1977)

Surgery and Bracing of the Lower Extremity

Maintenance of the upright posture and ambulation can often be extended 2 to 4 years beyond the time it would ordinarily cease by contracture release and appropriate bracing of the lower extremity. Percutaneous release of heel cords, iliotibial bands, bipolar tensor fasciae (if distal release alone proves inadequate), and superficial hip flexors (when degree of hip flexion contracture prevents torsopelvic balance in spite of tensor fascia release) is performed (Fig. 18–5). This is followed by long leg plasters, allowing the patient to stand on the day of surgery and to walk the next day.

Casts are worn for 3 weeks and then knee–ankle–foot orthoses (KAFOs) are fitted (Fig. 18–6). As the patient grows, braces require lengthening. Care must be taken to bring the thigh cuff to approximately 2 cm below the ischial tuberosity to permit ischial seating (Fig. 18–7).

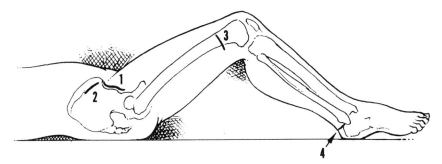

Figure 18-5 Sites for percutaneous tenotomy. (1) Hip flexors; (2) and (3) bipolar tensor fascia; (4) heel cord. (Siegel IM: The Clinical Management of Muscle Disease. London, William Heinemann Medical Books, 1977)

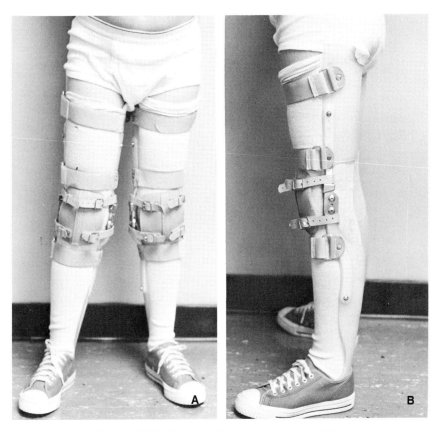

Figure 18-6 Plastic KAFO (knee-ankle-foot orthoses). (A) frontal view and (B) lateral view. (Siegel IM: Diagnosis, management, and orthopaedic treatment of muscular dystrophy. In The American Academy of Orthopaedic Surgeons: Instructional Course Lectures, Vol XXX. St Louis, CV Mosby, 1981)

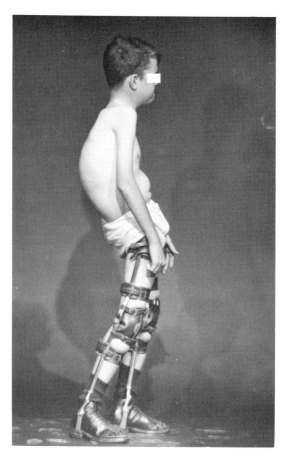

Figure 18-7 Kyphosis secondary to short braces. Patient is attempting to project line from center of gravity posterior to hips, anterior to knees, and within base of support. (Siegel IM: The Clinical Management of Muscle Disease. London, William Heinemann Medical Books, 1977)

Orthoses are vacuum-formed plastic and incorporate a molded foot-plate, obviating the need for an attached orthotic shoe. Ankle mobility can be regulated by varying the width of the posterior strut connecting the calf piece to the footplate. These appliances are less bulky than a standard brace, and are more comfortable and can be worn under an ordinary stocking without requiring special clothing adaptations. Tubular braces, which are more resistant to superimposed torsion stress than are the open models, use even lighter copolymer in their fabrication (Fig. 18-8).

Lengthening of the heel cord as an isolated procedure will not succeed unless the quadriceps is graded fair or better. When performed, a below-knee orthosis (AFO), modified for floor reaction, is prescribed postoperatively (see Chap. 16).

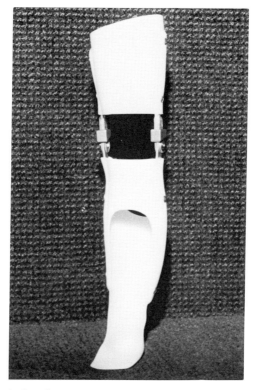

Figure 18–8 Tubular plastic KAFO. (Siegel IM, Silverman O: Double cylinder plastic orthosis in the treatment of Duchenne muscular dystrophy. Phys Ther 61:1290–1291, 1981. Used with the permission of the American Physical Therapy Association)

Posterior tibial transfer or release can be of prophylactic value in the younger patient. Transfer is through the interosseous membrane to the dorsum of the foot. The procedure obviates the deforming force of this motor. It loses one grade in transfer. Often the transferred muscle is active on command but not in phase. Nonetheless, even functioning as an active tenodesis, a progressive inversion deformation of the foot can frequently be avoided.

Postoperative Care

Postoperative care includes the following:

CircOlectric bed
Nasal oxygen
Intermittent positive-pressure breathing
Standing bed position on afternoon of surgery

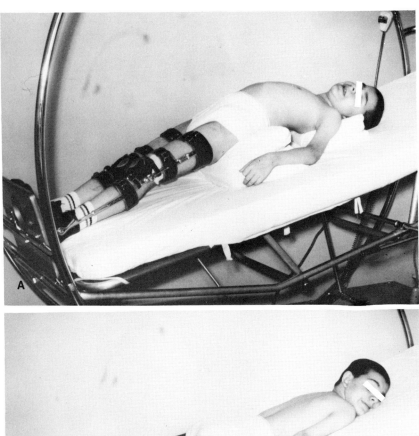

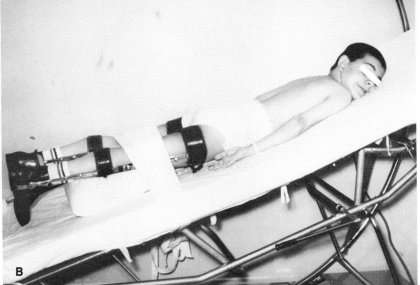

Figure 18–9 Postoperative positioning on circular electric bed with (A) hips elevated when the patient is supine, and (B) knees elevated when the patient is prone.(Siegel IM: Orthopedic correction of musculoskeletal deformity in muscular dystrophy. Adv Neurol, vol 17, 1977)

1. Day of surgery — passive hip stretching
2. First postoperative day — ambulation
3. Hospitalization one week — hip stretching and ambulation
4. Home physical therapy continues program
5. Braces fitted three weeks postoperatively

Figure 18-10 Physical therapy sequence.

The use of nasal oxygen and intermittent postitive-pressure breathing facilitates postoperative respiratory toilet. A revolving bed permits the patient to stand with his feet resting on the footboard attachment the afternoon of surgery. The hips are stretched into extension and abduction by elevating the sacrum when the patient lies supine and by elevating the knees when he lies prone (Fig. 18-9). Physical therapy (standing in bed and passive hip exercise) is initiated the afternoon of surgery. The patient is ambulated on the first postoperative day (Fig. 18-10). Initially the use of a light aluminum walker may be necessary until he adjusts to his rediscovered balance. During walking, torso shift over the supporting limb is still necessary, but lumbar lordosis lessens when the patient sits, hence the ischial weight-bearing feature of the orthosis.

The child is hospitalized for a week or less, after which a program of physical therapy, including walking and hip stretching, is continued at home. Braces may be worn as night splints if tolerated. With surgery and bracing, one can break the vicious cycle of weakness–imbalance–contracture–deformity, thus delaying progression of disability. Patients continuing to walk in braces maintain better alignment of weight-bearing joints and suffer less sedentary osteoporosis and disuse muscular atrophy. After surgery, a patient can usually handle his toilet needs with minimal help. The operation facilitates chair transfer when the braces are locked at the knees and the legs used as a long lever to tilt the child to the standing postition. Finally, the additional period of independent ambulation may represent up to 20% of the life span of these patients. Thus, it is of benefit to both the patients and their caretakers because maintenance of the upright posture has extended the ability of the patients to attend to the tasks of daily living for a significant period of their lives.

Foot Deformity

Footdrop (equinus) in facioscapulohumeral (FSH) dystrophy and dystrophia myotonica (MyD) can usually be managed with an AFO. Where the quadriceps is weak, a floor reaction feature can be incorporated in the brace. Patients suffering from the hereditary motor and sensory neuropathies (e.g., Charcot-Marie-Tooth disease) may tolerate plastic orthoses poorly, because the footplate blocks the kinesthetic input they require for balance. Because of distal sensory and proprioceptive loss, such patients may consistently shift their weight at the ankles or knees, attempting to "sense" the supporting surface at more proximally placed joints where proprioception is still intact. Equinus in this class of disease is best managed with a light spring-loaded dorsiflexion assist orthosis. Posterior tibial transfer or tarsal osteotomy (when bony deformity is severe) or arthrodesis may be indicated.

In DMD, isolated forefoot equinus secondary to plantar fascia tightness is best treated by plantar release. Hindfoot equinus is managed with Achilles tenotomy, posterior tibial transfer, and adequate bracing as indicated.

Equinocavovarus ultimately occurs in DMD because of progressive selective weakening and asymmetric contracture of foot musculature (Fig. 18–11). Although this condition may temporarily respond to passive stretch and heel control (UCB) shoe inserts, more aggressive treatment is ultimately necessary.

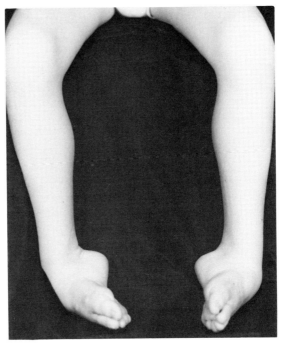

Figure 18–11   Equinocavovarus deformity in Duchenne muscular dystrophy. (Siegel IM: The Clinical Management of Muscle Disease. London, William Heinemann Medical Books, 1977)

Before bony deformity has occurred, correction can be obtained by soft tissue release (heel cord, posterior tibial, plantar fascia) and bracing, again remembering that heel cord lengthening removes the stabilizing equinus force that hyperextends and locks the knee during stance, so that, unless quadriceps is graded as having fair strength or better, the knee must be braced.

Later, with bony deformity, soft tissue releases are augmented by percutaneous tarsal medullostomy of the talar head and anterior portion of the calcaneus. Correction is obtained by manipulation of the foot with collapse of the enucleated bones. A short leg plaster, in which ambulation is permitted immediately, is worn for three weeks, followed by an appropriate orthosis.

Miscellaneous Foot Procedures

Metatarsus adductus is an isolated deformity sometimes seen in childhood polymyositis. It can be treated with percutaneous proximal osteotomy of the metatarsals followed by immediate ambulation in a cast with application of an AFO three weeks later.

Isolated forefoot inversion is also occasionally seen in polymyositis and is usually managed by dorsolateral transfer of the tibialis anticus tendon or by split tibialis anticus transfer. These procedures remove a deforming inversion force and create an active dorsiflexor working in neutral or eversion.

Cavus, such as that found in Charcot-Marie-Tooth disease and Friedreich's ataxia, is best managed by a lateral closing wedge proximal displacement calcaneal osteotomy. This is augmented by dorsal proximal closing wedge osteotomies of the metatarsals (usually only the first and second) as indicated. This procedure is preferred over the standard triple arthrodesis, which can result in a heavy and sometimes awkward gait. Foot height may be decreased after such an operation to the point where oxford shoes are difficult to fit because the malleoli impinge on the counter of the shoe.

Clawtoes, present in the hereditary motor and sensory neuropathies and allied conditions, are best treated with waist resection of the proximal toe phalanges.

Knee Problems

Chondromalacia patella is sometimes seen in patients who are unable to extend their knees because of flexion contracture. Pain is usually not severe enough to warrant treatment beyond symptomatic care. Genu recurvatum occurs in cases in which lower extremity weakness is severe and contracture is minimal. If quadriceps strength is adequate, knee position and stance can be controlled by an AFO that locks ankle motion in neutral or slight dorsiflexion, thus preventing back-knee.

A judicious choice among the relatively simple surgical procedures outlined above, followed by immediate postoperative mobilization, can often prolong walking. The earlier surgery is done, the better the result. Except for prophylactically performed operations (e.g., early transfer of posterior tibial muscle), the indications for surgery are contractures sufficient to threaten the patient's ability to maintain the upright posture.

Upper Extremities

Weakness of the hand is not a problem in DMD until late in the disease, and then is usually best treated with adaptive equipment. In DMD, distal myopathy, or certain neuropathies, thumb opposition is often weakened enough to require a plastic post orthosis to strengthen opposition pinch. Surgery to compensate for median or ulnar motor loss may be necessary in treating the hand weakness seen in advanced hypertrophic Charcot-Marie-Tooth disease.

Elbow and wrist flexion contractures found in wheelchair-confined DMD patients are best treated with passive stretch. Some elbow flexion contracture (less than 60 degrees) may be functional in these cases. Dorsiflexion splinting is also of use in managing wrist flexion problems.

Shoulder weakness in DMD or limb girdle dystrophy is best handled in the wheelchair with a forearm orthosis balanced to allow the arms to

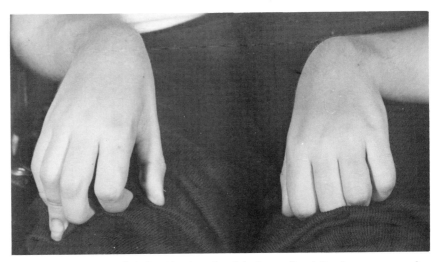

Figure 18–12 Hand deformity in wheelchair-confined Duchenne muscular dystrophy requires dorsiflexion wrist-splinting and balanced forearm orthoses.

move across rather than against the field of gravity (Fig. 18–12). In FSH dystrophy, where deltoid strength is preserved, tasks such as eating and overhead dressing can be significantly enhanced by scapulothoracic fusion. After scapular fixation, patients no longer require a thrown movement to elevate the arm. The scapula should not be fixed with its vertebral border more than 20 degrees from the vertical, and it is necessary to allow at least one upper extremity the freedom to attend to toileting tasks.

Scoliosis

Neuromuscular scoliosis comprises 15% to 20% of all spinal deformity treated by the orthopaedic surgeon. It occurs in many types of neuromuscular diseases, including chronic infantile and juvenile spinal mus-

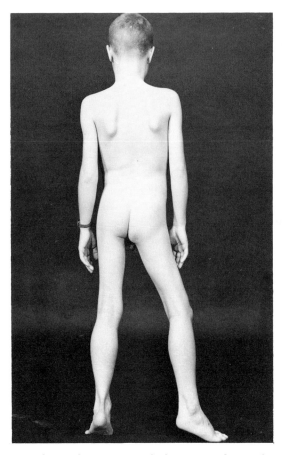

Figure 18–13 Early scoliosis in ambulatory Becker's dystrophy. Note equinus, pelvic tilt, and winged scapulae.

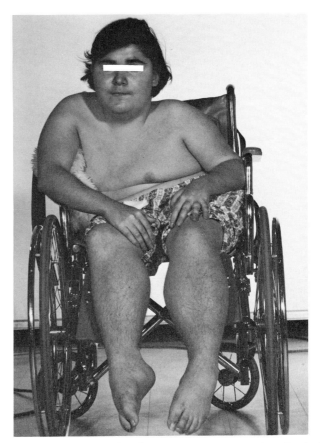

Figure 18–14 Obesity with fixed equinocavovarus and scoliosis in wheel-chair-confined Duchenne muscular dystrophy.

cular atrophy; the various spinal cerebellar ataxias; the myopathies, such as DMD, childhood FSH dystrophy, Becker's dystrophy, and the childhood form of MyD; and in other neuromuscular conditions of as yet uncertain etiology, such as nemaline rod disease, central core disease, Prader-Willi syndrome, and oculocraniosomatic neuromuscular disease with "ragged-red" fibers.

Neuromuscular scoliosis differs from its idiopathic cousin in that deformity and disease are often progressive in neuromuscular curves, their patterns develop earlier and are more likely to progress beyond skeletal maturity, and the disease includes a deformity involving not only the spine, but also the pelvis, hips, and legs. Bone stock is usually quantitatively and qualitatively poor, there is less tolerance for orthotic devices, and, with spinal fusion, the rate of pseudarthrosis is increased.

Paralytic scoliosis in muscular dystrophy occurs with advancing dis-

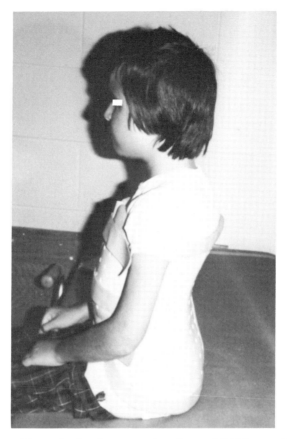

Figure 18-15 Thoracic–lumbar–sacral orthoses (TLSO), providing lumbar lordosis to lock lumbar and lumbo–sacral facet joints.

ability. Although a functional spinal curve is occasionally seen in limb girdle dystrophy, severe scoliosis is an uncommon finding. Progressive scoliosis, however, is often seen in childhood MyD and in the childhood type of FSH dystrophy, as well as in the Becker form of muscular dystrophy (Fig. 18–13). In these conditions, asymmetry of spinal muscle weakness can cause scoliosis while the patient is yet ambulatory. In DMD, paraspinal weakness is symmetric and scoliosis rarely occurs in the patient still up and walking. Once wheelchair-bound, almost all patients with DMD develop scoliosis (Fig. 18–14). Although approximately one-third of paralytic curves in this disease are minimally unstable, scoliosis (commonly thoraco–lumbar–kyphotic with unstable axial rotation) may progress rapidly, especially during the adolescent growth spurt.

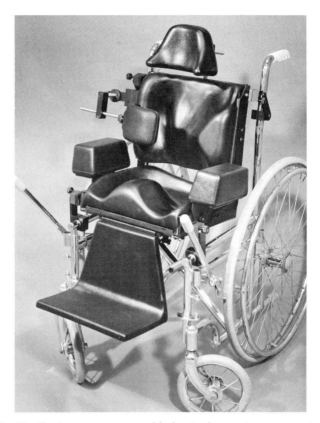

Figure 18-16   Custom vacuum-molded spinal containment seating system. (Siegel IM, Silverman M: Fully contoured seating for the wheelchair-bound patient with neuromuscular disease. Phys Ther 63: 1625–1626, 1983. Used with the permission of the American Physical Therapy Association)

Treatment of scoliosis includes the use of thoracic orthoses providing three-point fixation. For a brace to be successful, it must exaggerate lumbar lordosis and lock the lumbar and lumbosacral facet joints, thus inhibiting lateral bend (Fig. 18–15). The Milwaukee brace is a dynamic appliance requiring enough residual muscle strength for exercise in the brace and has not proved useful in the treatment of neuromuscular scoliosis. Use of the thoracic suspension orthosis has benefited patients with severe respiratory problems and has been effective in curves too advanced to lend themselves to more conventional orthotic treatment.

Specialized wheelchair seating may also achieve spinal containment. Systems are designed to mold the spine into lordosis and provide lateral stability (Fig. 18–16). It is essential that the spine be extended in such an apparatus and this usually requires at least 15 degrees of posterior tilt in the adapted wheelchair.

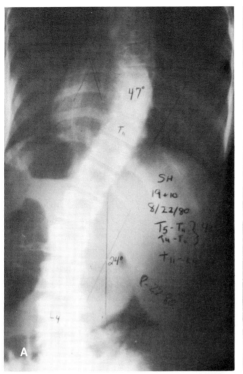

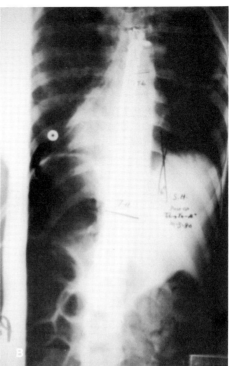

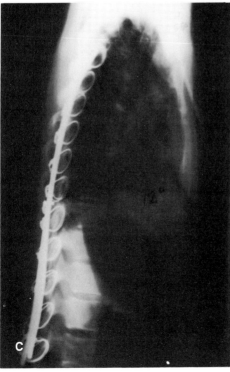

Figure 18-17 Luque segmental spinal stabilization. (A) Preoperative scoliosis; (B) AP view, postfusion; and (C) lateral view, postfusion.

A proper orthosis or seating system can delay but not prevent scoliosis. If the curve is 35 to 40 degrees and unstable, and the vital capacity is within 35% to 40% of predicted normal, the patient is usually a good candidate for spinal fusion. This includes most wheelchair-confined DMD and yet-ambulatory childhood DMD patients, Becker's dystrophy patients, and childhood FSH dystrophy patients, as well as wheelchair-confined patients with spinal muscular atrophy, Friedrich's ataxia, or Charcot-Marie-Tooth disease. In the wheelchair-bound patient, the spine must be fused to the pelvis to provide stability and prevent pelvic tilt.

Surgical techniques include Harrington compression–distraction instrumentation, anterior fusion, use of the Dwyer cable technique (seldom indicated), and the L-rod segmental stabilization of Luque. This latter is the preferred technique, because adequate spinal stabilization may be obtained with (and sometimes without) accompanying bony fusion, allowing early postoperative mobilization without the necessity for casting or bracing (Fig. 18–17).

Intraoperative supervision requires close monitoring of arterial blood gases, cardiac output, and urine output, as well as spinal cord function. Blood transfusions (usually numerous) are indicated. Hemodilution, hypotensive anesthesia, and autogenous blood transfusion or red blood cell-saving techniques have been used.

Postoperative care entails daily range-of-motion exercises to prevent contractures, resistance exercises to maintain muscle strength, and, later, appropriate training in body mechanics and transfer techniques. Intensive respiratory rehabilitation is necessary to compensate for loss of vital capacity secondary to poor pulmonary reserve and loss of chest compliance secondary to splinting because of pain.

Stabilization of the spine, whether through orthotic or surgical means, improves body image, enhances cardiorespiratory function, obviates discomfort, frees the upper extremities from a supportive role for more functional use, and facilitates transfer. Obtaining spinal stability with the head in the midline through the correction of pelvic obliquity allows the patient both improved cosmesis and function.

Summary

Orthopaedic treatment in muscle disease must be aimed at realistic functional goals (transfer, standing, walking) and must enable immediate postoperative mobilization because dystrophic patients suffer rapid loss of strength when even briefly confined. Techniques are available for the surgical release of lower extremity contracture, the correction of foot, ankle, knee, and hip deformity, shoulder stabilization, improvement of elbow and wrist function, and correction of hand and finger deformity. Bracing should be suitably staged and orthoses constructed to provide maximal support with minimal weight. Spinal deformity must be prevented, where feasible, through the use of spinal orthoses and special seating assistance. Spinal fusion is available when indicated.

Management conducted in an atmosphere of intelligent concern can minimize the frustrating aspects of these conditions while maximizing the benefits obtained through available care, thus significantly enhancing the patient's quality of life, and perhaps even his life expectancy.

Suggested Readings

BOWKER JH, HALPIN PJ: Factors determining success in reambulation of the child with progressive muscular dystrophy. Orthop Clin North Am 9:431–436, 1978

BUNCH W: Scapulo-thoracic fusion. Minn Med 56:391–394, 1973

COBHAM IG, DAVIS HS: Anesthesia for muscular dystrophy patients. Anesth Analg 43:22–29, 1964

DRENNAN JC: Orthopaedic Management of neuromuscular Disorders. Philadelphia, JB Lippincott, 1983

EYRING EJ, JOHNSON EW, BURNETT C: Surgery in muscular dystrophy. JAMA 222:1056–1057, 1972

GIBSON DA, KORESKA J, ROBERTSON D, et al: The management of spinal deformity in Duchenne's muscular dystrophy. Orthop Clin North Am 9:437–450, 1978

HENSINGER RN, MACEWEN GD: Spinal deformity associated with heritable neurological conditions: Spinal muscular astrophy, Friedreich's ataxia, familial dysautonomia, and Charcot-Marie-Tooth disease. J Bone Joint Surg 58A:13–23, 1976

HSU JD: Management of foot deformity in Duchenne's pseudohypertrophic muscular dystrophy. Orthop Clin North Am 7:979–984, 1976

JOHNSON EW, KENNEDY JH: Comprehensive management of Duchenne muscular dystrophy. Arch Phys Med Rehabil 52:110–114, 1971

ROBIN GC, BRIEF LP: Scoliosis in childhood muscular dystrophy. J Bone Joint Surg 53A:466–476, 1971

SIEGEL IM: Diagnosis, management, and orthopaedic treatment of muscular dystrophy. In Murray D (ed): The American Academy of Orthopedic Surgeons Instructional Course Lectures, vol XXX. St Louis, CV Mosby, 1981

SIEGEL IM: The Clinical Management of Muscular Disease. London, William Heineman, 1977

SIEGEL IM: The management of muscular dystrophy: A clinical review. Muscle and Nerve 1:453–458, 1978

SPENCER GE, VIGNOS PJ JR: Bracing for ambulation in childhood progressive muscular dystrophy. J Bone Joint Surg 44:234–242, 1962

YATES G: Molded plastics in bracing. Clin Orthop 102:46–57, 1974

Emmajean Amrhein
Gretchen Branowitzer

19

Nursing Management of Neuromuscular Disorders

Nursing care of the patient with neuromuscular disease requires both a thorough knowledge of medical – surgical nursing and neurophysiology. Patient management and rehabilitation are best accomplished by a nurse using a multidisciplinary health-care team approach. The overall goal of the multidisciplinary team should be to provide maximum quality of care while assisting the patient in obtaining his optimal level of wellness.

This chapter divides the nursing management of neuromuscular patients according to common symptoms, including weakness of arms and legs and difficulty in speaking, swallowing, and breathing. Consideration is also given to patient stress and discharge planning. Although some details of pathophysiology are included, the reader is referred to other chapters for a more comprehensive analysis.

Successful neuromuscular nursing care requires the cooperation of a physician; physical, occupational, and respiratory therapists; speech pathologist; nutritionist; and social worker. This chapter emphasizes how the nurse can best interact with each of these health-care specialists.

Weakness

Weakness, the most common symptom of patients with neuromuscular diseases, can cause a myriad of problems, depending on the muscle groups involved, the patient's lifestyle, and the rate of progression of the disease. A patient with slowly progressive weakness may develop a limp, footdrop, or waddling gait, or may have difficulty in getting into or out of a bed or a chair. Loss of fine motor movements can impair writing, feeding, and dressing. Facial weakness can make it difficult for the patient to whistle or drink through a straw. If a patient has a more rapidly progressive neuromuscular disease, the nurse must be prepared to assist the patient totally should he become paralyzed and unable to breathe or swallow voluntarily.

Careful attention should be given in both questioning and observing a newly admitted patient. During the initial interview, the nurse can ask leading questions to determine if the patient understands his illness. If not, a family member may volunteer information about the location and extent of the patient's weakness. Questions should address the patient's safety (i.e., frequency of falls) and whether symptoms fluctuate throughout the day.

After the nurse charts her assessment and initiates a nursing plan, she should discuss her independent observations with the patient's primary physician. Because the nurse often has more contact with the patient than do other members of the health-care team, she may more readily identify difficulties in independent performance of activities of daily living (ADL).

Exercise is important to maintain strength but, if overdone, can also produce muscle fatigue (see Chap. 15). A patient with a neuromuscular disease may be stronger in the morning, but needs a mid-day rest period to conserve strength. Thus, the patient's care plan should include an early shower or bath before breakfast, with a rest period before physical therapy. Additional rest periods may be necessary to conserve energy.

Stretching exercises should be done either by the patient or with the assistance of the nurse several times throughout the day to help prevent extremity contractures, which worsen if muscles are not used. A physical therapist can develop an exercise plan for evening or night hours when routine therapy sessions may be unavailable.

Because weakness causes difficulty in ambulation, assistive devices may be necessary to prevent falls. Until a patient feels comfortable and safe with an assistive device, a nurse or a family member should accompany the patient when he is ambulating.

As a neuromuscular disease progresses, muscle weakness may become so severe that a patient may be unable to sit in a chair without support. A high-backed reclining chair is useful to prevent such a patient from sliding off the chair. A loose safety belt on a seated patient will also prevent further complications from a fall. It is important that the patient be informed why such measures are taken so that there is no misunderstanding about "being restrained."

If a patient is virtually immobile, the nurse involved in his care must be extremely sensitive to the patient's feelings and loss of independence. Unless medically contraindicated, the patient should be encouraged to sit in a chair for several periods during the day. Although several people may be needed to lift the patient into a chair, it is useful to let the patient make helpful decisions concerning the transfer to promote his self-esteem.

Dysarthria

If muscles of the lips, tongue, and larynx are weak, speech will be impaired. A speech language pathologist can teach a patient techniques to communicate more easily (see Chap. 9). Although speech therapy does not reverse weakness, a patient can learn to increase the efficiency of oral muscles.

Inability to enunciate clearly is extremely frustrating for the neuromuscular patient who remains intellectually intact. Therefore, it is particularly important that a nurse acknowledge if the patient can be understood verbally or nonverbally. To relieve patient anxiety, some type of communication must be established and maintained.

If a patient is mute and cannot move his arms and legs, a creative method must be established for the patient to request help while in the hospital. A sensitive nurse call-light that the patient can use is often enough (i.e., a string attached to a bell and operated by the patient using his teeth). Alternatively, if a patient can tap a finger, a code can be developed that all can understand. Whatever communication system is established in the hospital, the same system should also be encouraged at home to provide a patient with the ability to interact. If the disease progresses, adaptations for communication may also have to be changed.

Dysphagia

Weakness of the tongue, palate, pharynx, and larynx produces dysphagia, or difficulty in swallowing. Complications of dysphagia include dehydration, aspiration, and inability to control saliva.

A patient who still has some gag reflex left can be taught various swallowing techniques by a speech pathologist (see Chap. 9) to control saliva. A change to a mechanically soft diet can make eating easier and prevent weight loss (see Chap. 23).

Patients with dysphagia can suddenly aspirate so that a nurse feeding such a patient must be prepared to do a Heimlich maneuver (hug of life; see Chap. 14) or to suction the patient if he aspirates. Some patients, because of an ineffective cough reflex, aspirate without overtly choking. If a patient develops recurrent pneumonia or coughs while eating, a barium swallow should be done to rule out unrecognized aspiration. In a patient with a tracheostomy who resumes eating, aspiration can be detected by observing food (*i.e.*, colored liquids) while suctioning the trachea.

Drooling because of the inability to swallow saliva is embarrassing and frustrating to the patient. A patient can be taught to suction his mouth using a small aspirator, or he can receive atropine, which reduces secretions but produces undesirable side-effects. Surgical section of salivary nerves or parotid irradiation may be necessary if symptoms persist.

When a patient no longer has a gag reflex and the risk of aspiration is significant, or if the patient is unable to maintain proper nutrition, feeding through a nasogastric, gastrostomy, or cervical esophagostomy tube becomes necessary. A variety of small nasogastric feeding tubes (No. 8 French) can be inserted for long periods of time (2 – 3 weeks) with little irritation. One disadvantage of these tubes is that they clog easily. To dislodge the contents from the tube, small amounts of warm water, sodium bicarbonate, or alcohol can be infused. If unsuccessful, a new tube must be inserted.

For long-term nutritional supplementation, a gastrostomy or cervical esophagostomy is preferable. The advantages of a cervical esophagostromy are that it can be inserted under local anesthesia and removed between feedings, and skin erosion does not usually develop. Gastrostomy tubes are more difficult to insert under local anesthesia, are permanent, and can result in skin breakdown from gastric acid. Regardless of the location of a tube, a nurse should instruct the patient and his home support in the proper care of the tube and stoma area:

1. Check placement of tube before each feeding (the tube should be marked).
2. Keep tube secure with twill tape if necessary.
3. Wash skin around tube with soap and water, dry at least once daily.
4. Apply zinc oxide to area.
5. Apply dry dressing over site.

Multiple feeding formulas are available, the majority of which contain 1 calorie per milliliter (see Chap. 23). For most patients 1 cal/ml is sufficient. If additional calories are necessary, a few formulas containing 1.5 calories/ml are available. To avoid diarrhea, feedings must be started slowly. The rate of infusion and the concentration of formula are increased separately.

Day 1 — 200 ml ½-strength feeding followed by 50 ml to 100 ml of water 4 times a day

Day 2 — 200 ml ¾-strength feeding followed by 50 ml to 100 ml of water 4 times a day

Day 3 — 200 ml full-strength feeding followed by 50 ml to 100 ml of water 4 times a day

Day 4 — increase the amount given at each feeding as necessary to achieve desired caloric supplementation

If diarrhea develops, the rate and strength of the tube feeding should be decreased and medications that slow bowel motility (Kaopectate or Paragoric) can be prescribed.

Commercial tube-feeding formulas are practical but expensive. Alternatively, a dietitian can teach the patient how to prepare a regular vitamin-supplemented diet, using a blender.

Feedings can be administered by using a funnel, asepto syringe, or feeding bags with regulators that ensure a fixed-delivery rate. The bag is secured above the level of the feeding tube to provide delivery.

Before discharge, the patient and his home support must demonstrate the ability to care for the tube, stoma, and infusions, and should be instructed to look for common complications such as tube displacement, aspiration, and infection.

It is helpful for a family to continue to include a patient in the social functions associated with regular meals no matter how much modification is required. At all times the patient must be given an opportunity to verbalize concerns and frustrations about his lifestyle changes.

Impaired Ventilation

A nurse must be familiar with the ventilatory changes that occur with neuromuscular diseases in order to anticipate and avoid potential complications (see Chap. 14). An assessment of the patient and his respiratory status on admission should include observation of respiratory and pulse rates, effectiveness of cough, ability to clear secretions, changes in speech pattern, dyspnea, restlessness, confusion, and cyanosis. Pulmonary function tests that record vital capacity (VC), tidal volume (TV), maximum voluntary ventilation (MVV), and inspiratory and expiratory pressure are often of additional value. A bedside spirometer available for repeated examinations is useful to document changes during hospitalization.

A respiratory care plan developed from criteria obtained during admission should include the following:

1. *Positioning.* The patient is encouraged to maintain correct posture when standing or sitting to reduce visceral pressure on the diaphragm and to increase expansion of the chest. If a patient slumps in a chair, restricting ventilation, a safety belt should be tied loosely around his body. While a patient is resting or sleeping, the head of the bed can be elevated approximately 15 to 30 degrees to assist in ventilation by allowing gravity to reduce visceral pressure on the diaphragm.

2. *Cough, deep breathe.* The patient is encouraged to cough and deep breathe at least once every 4 hours. An incentive spirometer can be used to encourage a patient to reach a goal while deep breathing (Fig. 19-1).

3. *Postural drainage, percussion, and vibration.* Because many neuromuscular disease patients have an insufficient cough to clear secretions spontaneously, postural drainage of secretions should be taught to the patient and his home support system. A patient should not be left unattended when in various positions because he may be too weak to clear his own oral airway as secretions pool in his throat (Fig. 19-2). A suction apparatus should be available in case this occurs. Proper percussion and vibration effectively remove secretions and stimulate coughing. The entire procedure can be repeated every 4 hours in the hospital, although twice a day is usually adequate at home.

4. *Suctioning.* Proper suctioning can be used to clear the lungs and oropharynx of any secretions. A patient can usually be taught how to suction himself orally to prevent drooling. The patient's family or home attendent usually is able to suction orally or through a tracheostomy, but rarely is able to suction endotracheally.

With chronic neuromuscular diseases, respiratory complications are frequently life-threatening. Therefore, a patient, his family, and the

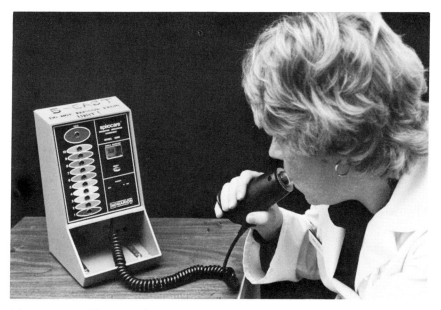

Figure 19-1   The use of an inspiratory incentive spirometer (Spirocare) promotes deep breathing and strengthens the respiratory muscles.

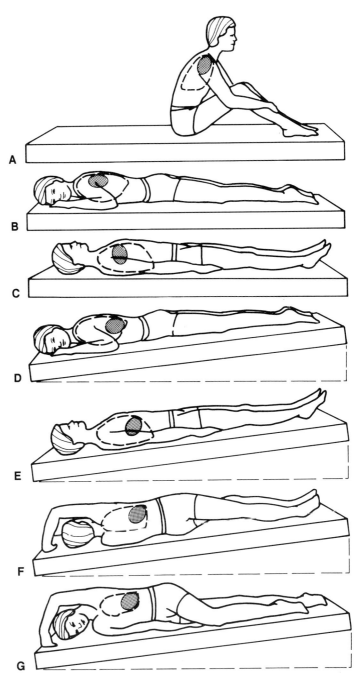

Figure 19–2 The seven most commonly used positions for postural drainage and clapping. (*A*) Apical segments for draining right and left upper lobes. (*B*) Superior segments for draining right and left lower lobes. (*C*) Anterior segments for draining right and left upper lobes. (*D*) Basal segments for draining right and left posterior lower lobes. (*E*) Basal segments for draining right and left anterior lower lobes. (*F*) Lateral segments for draining right middle and lower lobe. (*G*) Lateral segments for draining left lower lobe.

physician must openly discuss to what extent life-support measures will be used (see Chap. 14). Although these discussions are very difficult and painful for all involved, they are better discussed before a life-threatening complication occurs. Whatever decision is made, the nurse is obligated to act as the patient's advocate. Certain nursing measures are always provided, including adequate suctioning to ensure patient comfort and to prevent airway obstruction.

With acute reversible neuromuscular diseases, such as Guillain-Barré syndrome and myasthenia gravis, temporary intubation and mechanical ventilation may be necessary until respiratory muscle strength returns. Such intubated and mechanically ventilated patients are understandably depressed and usually fear that they are going to die. A nurse can be extremely comforting at this time by reassuring the patient that he will improve with time. While on the ventilator, communication between the nurse and patient should be established immediately to relieve some of the fears and anxiety that develop (see Chap. 9).

Instruction in respiratory care in preparation for discharge is frequently the responsibility of the nurse. Early detection of respiratory complications, particularly infection (fever, decreased energy, change in color and amount and character of sputum) must be emphasized. After a nurse demonstrates effective coughing, use of incentive spirometry, postural drainage, percussion of the chest, and oral suctioning, the patient and his home support system should show familiarity and comfort with these procedures as well.

Stress Reaction

Although a biological organism is believed to require a certain amount of stress for its well-being, when the balance in stress is interrupted, pathologic change can occur (see Chap. 21). One patient may react to the stress of illness with excessive feelings of anger and fright, while another, threatened by dependency, may deny symptoms and incapacity. Therefore, it is not only important to treat a person's illness, but it is also important to assist him in identifying stresses and coping mechanisms.

A patient with myasthenia gravis can have an exacerbation of weakness from many causes, including emotional stress. Dysarthric speech and weakened facial expressions can cause communication difficulties and embarrassment. During periods of facial weakness, a patient with myasthenia gravis may even be unable to convey his thoughts with a smile. Some patients refuse to go out in public because of embarrassment over their disability. A vital function of the nurse is the ability to recognize a patient's behavioral patterns and stresses. Since a patient and nurse have a time span of 8 hours per day to react and to build communication, trust will readily develop. Such familiarity can enable

UNIVERSITY HOSPITAL
DEPARTMENT OF NURSING SERVICE

STANDARDS OF CARE

AMYOTROPHIC LATERAL SCLEROSIS

Pt = Patient

SO = Significant Other

* = Refer to Progress Notes for Details

Date initiated ______

Patient Outcome Criteria		Instructed Pt	Instructed SO	Assess Learning				Understands Pt	Understands SO
I. Pt/SO has some basic knowledge of amyotrophic lateral sclerosis (ALS):									
A. Verbalizes that he/she has ALS	A	8/15	8/15	8/16				8/17	8/17
B. Progressive neuromuscular disease with no cure at this time	B	8/15	8/15	8/16				8/17	8/17
C. Verbalizes knowledge of possible symptoms: Dysphagia, dyspnea, weakness, discomfort, constipation, communication, depression	1	8/15	8/15	8/16				8/17	8/17
II. Pt/SO has understanding of management of ALS:									
A. Verbalizes symptoms of dysphagia and demonstrates care to prevent aspiration:	A	8/20	8/20	8/21	8/22			8/23	8/23
1. Specific diet ______ ______	1	8/22	8/22	having difficulty adjusting rate				8/27	8/27
2. Take time eating	2	na	na						
3. Six small meals/day	3	na	na						
B. Pt/SO demonstrates care of cervical esophagostomy tube:									
1. Tube placement	1	8/22	8/22	8/23	8/24	8/25	8/26	8/27	8/27
2. Preparation and administration of food	2	8/23	8/23	8/24	8/24			8/27	8/27
3. Care for insertion site:									
a. Wash skin with warm water and soap	a	8/23	8/22	8/23	8/24	8/25	8/26	8/27	8/27
b. Apply zinc oxide around site	b	8/22	8/22	8/23	8/24	8/25	8/26	8/27	8/27
c. Apply dry dressing	c	8/22	8/22	8/23				8/27	8/27
C. Pt/SO verbalizes symptoms of dyspnea:									
1. Build-up of secretions	1	8/15	8/15					8/17	8/17
2. Atrophy of tongue	2	8/15	8/15					8/17	8/17
3. Anxiety reactions	3	8/15	8/15					8/17	8/17
4. Flexion of hypertension of neck	4	8/15	8/15					8/17	8/17

Figure 19–3 Criteria used by University Hospital nursing personnel for teaching the patient with ALS. (Used with permission of University of Colorado Hospital. All rights reserved.)

a patient to more fully describe his anxieties and should provide a nurse ample opportunity to suggest ways of coping with problems.

Contemporary medical approaches advocate diagnosis and treatment of a family as a unit. Proper identification and teaching of a patient's support systems early in his illness can bring positive results in a nursing treatment plan. As a patient progresses and more time is required of the primary caregiver, other members of the family must be encouraged to provide assistance without feeling resentful or guilty.

D. Pt/SO demonstrates ways to prevent increased weakness and discomfort:											
1. Physical therapy	1	8/23	8/23							8/27	8/27
2. Rest	2	8/23	8/23							8/27	8/27
3. Use of water bed, various mattresses	3	8/23	8/23							8/27	8/27
E. Pt/SO verbalizes ways to prevent constipation:											
1. Record all bowel movements:	1	8/24	8/24							8/27	8/27
2. 2500–3000 cc fluid a day	2	8/24	8/24							8/27	8/2
3. Diet high in fiber	3	8/24	8/24							8/27	8/2
F. Pt/SO demonstrates ability to communicate:											
1. Inform others length of time it may take to express self	1	8/25	8/25	appears depressed about this						8/27	8/27
2. Communicate with letter board, cue cards, magic	2	8/25	8/25							8/27	8/27
3. Use of talking book system	3	8/25	8/25							8/27	8/27
G. Verbalizes knowledge of medications (name, dose, peak, duration, administration, and side-effects): Name of Medication											
1. _____	1	8/25	8/25							8/27	8/27
2. _____	2	8/25	8/25							8/27	8/27
3. _____	3										
4. _____	4										
5. _____	5										
III. Pt/SO verbalizes understanding of need for follow-up and how to obtain:											
A. Regular appointments: knows when to make	A	8/26	8/26							8/27	8/27
B. Interim care: knows when and how to call clinic for interim problems	B	8/26	8/26							8/27	8/27
C. Acute: knows when to use emergency room instead of clinic	C	8/26	8/26							8/27	8/27
D. Knows of community resources	D	8/22	8/22							8/27	8/27

Name	Int	Name	Int	Name	Int
Jane Doe	JD				
Salley James	SJ				

Figure 19–3 (Continued)

Discharge Planning

Discharge planning and patient instruction actually begin at the time of the patient's admission to the hospital. After a nurse identifies a patient's primary caregiver and support systems, all of these individuals should be included in decision-making and instructions. The nurse can often facilitate the discharge arrangements of the physician or other members of the health-care team. An off-shift nurse may assume the

UNIVERSITY HOSPITAL	Hosp #
PATIENT DISCHARGE FORM	Pt. Name

UNIVERSITY HOSPITAL

PATIENT DISCHARGE FORM

Admit Date _____

Discharge Date _____

Physician _____

Phone # _____ Service _____

TEACHING SHEET GIVEN _____

DIAGNOSIS/PROCEDURE

Amyotrophic Lateral Sclerosis/Cervical Esophostomy

ACTIVITY   Continue exercises provided by the physical therapist at least 3 times each day.

RECOMMENDED DIET   1800 cal tube feeding – 2 cans Ensure four times a day. Follow each feeding with at least 100 cc of water. Check placement of tube before each feeding.

AFFECTED CARE   Wash the area around the tube at least once a day with soap and water. Cover with a dry dressing.

SEEK MEDICAL ATTENTION IF   1. Increased difficulty in breathing. 2. Increased difficulty in ambulating. 3. Any problems with the esophostomy tube.

SPECIAL INSTRUCTIONS   1. If diarrhea occurs, decrease rate and concentration as necessary. 2. Remember that respiratory infection such as a cold can be harmful. 3. Rest periods during the day are important for you.

MEDICATION	DOSE	TIMES TO TAKE	PURPOSE OF DRUG	OTHER INFORMATION
Multivits.	5 cc	once a day Take in the morning with first feeding	Supplementation	
Kaopectate	1 tbsp	Take after each loose stool	To prevent diarrhea	Do not take more than 8 tbsp per 24 hours

RETURN APPOINTMENT DATE __8/23/83__   NURSE SIGNATURE __Jane Doe, RN__

I UNDERSTAND ABOVE INSTRUCTIONS

Pt./S.O. SIGNATURE _____

Trial aMR2100 040 [3/83]   PATIENT COPY

Figure 19-4   Patient discharge form, showing information necessary for patient use at home. (Used with permission of University of Colorado Hospital. All rights reserved.)

responsibility of patient instruction because the primary caregiver may only have time to visit during the evening or may need to arrange time according to a work schedule to attend patient-care conferences.

Ideally, a patient conference should include all members of the health team (physician, nurse, physical therapist, occupational therapist, speech pathologist, social worker, and visiting nurse coordinator). Prior to discharge, the team must thoroughly assess and review what a patient needs at home and what resources are available in the community in order to provide the highest optimal level of wellness (Fig. 19–3).

A visiting nurse can arrange for an assessment of the home environment and safety before discharge. A social worker and the muscular dystrophy association patient-service coordinator can often arrange for equipment and support systems for the patient (Fig. 19–4; see Chap. 26).

It is important to establish alternative support systems to allow a patient's family a break from health care, because everyone needs a few hours away to regroup and gain understanding. A nurse should encourage family members to take this time without feeling guilty, since the disease process can be trying for even the most stable family unit.

Outpatient appointments and follow-up care are arranged prior to a patient's discharge. Between appointments a patient should be made aware of how to obtain necessary emergency treatment should it become necessary.

Summary

Nursing of the neuromuscular patients offers a tremendous challenge for potential growth and development in today's specialized health-care environment. Although its development is still in the early stages, this nursing specialty offers the interested and committed nurse a new challenge. A nurse can interact with numerous health-care specialists, participating and contributing to the care of patients with neuromuscular diseases.

Suggested Readings

BLOUNT M, BRATTON C, LUTTRELL N: Management of the patient with amyotrophic lateral sclerosis. Nurs Clin North Am 14:157–170, 1979

DUBOVSKY S: The psychophysiology of health, illness, and stress. In Simons R, Pardes H (eds): Understanding Human Behavior in Health and Illness, 13, pp 86–95. Baltimore, Williams & Wilkins, 1981

EARNEST M: Neurological Emergencies. New York, Churchill Livingstone, 1983

HARTLEY FD: A nurses's view: Amyotrophic lateral sclerosis. J Neurosurg Nurs 13:89–95, 1981

HICKEY J: The Clinical Practice of Neurological and Neurosurgical Nursing, pp 448–463. Philadelphia, JB Lippincott, 1981

LAVIGNE JM: Respiratory care of the patient with neuromuscular disease. Nurs Clin North Am 14:133–143, 1979

OLSEN B: Motor neuron disease: Amyotrophic lateral sclerosis. J Neurosurg Nurs 13:83–87, 1981

RINGEL SP: Clinical presentations in neuromuscular disease: In Vinken PJ, Bruyn, G (eds): Handbook of Clinical Neurology, pp 295–348. New York, North Holland Publishing, 1979

SNEDDEN J: Myasthenia gravis: A study of social, medical and emotional problems in 26 patients. Lancet 1:526–528, 1980

SNYDER M: A Guide to Neurological and Neurosurgical Nursing. New York, John Wiley & Sons, 1983

Lyle O. Johnson

20

Educational Imperatives for Children With Muscular Dystrophy

Alan is a 6-year-old boy who has progressive muscular dystrophy. Special education laws require that the focus of intervention not be on Alan's handicap of muscular dystrophy, but rather on his individual educational needs that result from his physical condition and disability. His handicap alone does not identify his unique educational needs. Every child with muscular dystrophy is not affected in the same way or to the same extent. Alan may require only the special services of itinerant help and may be able to spend most of his day in the general education program with his nonhandicapped peers. On the other hand, he may require a modified educational program with a shortened day schedule and an aide to help him with feeding and lavatory activities. He may be in a special classroom with other children with needs like his own, with little or no integration with his nonhandicapped fellow pupils, but it is unlikely that he will be totally segregated.

The law requires that the special education provided for Alan involve only instruction that is specially designed and directed to meet his unique needs, such as those that result from the adverse effect of his handicap on his ability to function in the general education program.

The following is a discussion of the laws that give handicapped students such as Alan their legal mandated rights.

Overview of the Laws

PL 94–142

On November 29, 1975, President Gerald Ford signed into law Public Law 94–142, the Education of All Handicapped Children Act of 1975. (The regulations implementing Part B of the Education of the Handicapped Act [20 United States Constitution (U.S.C.) 141101420], as amended by PL 94–142, were transferred to title 34 [Education] of the Code of Federal Regulations [CFR] [45 FR 77368, November 21, 1980] and redesignated as 34 CFR, Part 300. However, the individual section numbers have not changed. For example, under the discussion of individualized educational programs [IEPs], previously 45 CFR 121a.340–121a349, have been designated as 34 CFR, Part 300; 340–300.349. The citations in this chapter use the original reference numbers for PL 94–142 regulations as issued on August 23, 1977, and coded in the Code of Federal Regulations [CFR] as 45 CFE, Part 121a.) This Act guarantees all children the right to a free appropriate public education. This means that any child between the ages of 3 years and 21 years who has special learning needs is entitled to services designed to meet those needs. These services must be provided by the public school at the expense of the school district in which the child resides. Until this federal legislation was mandated, a free public education was not available to many handicapped children and youths.

PL 94–142 is unique in several aspects. Actual instruction at the classroom level is more explicitly addressed than in any other federal statute. The statute is the mandate for the development of an IEP for each handicapped child. This Act is coded as both education and as civil rights legislation. Specific definitions of critical terms have given the Act the clarity needed for understanding:

1. *Handicapped children.* As used in the law, the term "handicapped children" refers to those children who are mentally retarded; hard of hearing; deaf; speech-impaired; visually handicapped; seriously emotionally disturbed; orthopaedically impaired; otherwise health-impaired, including those with diabetes, leukemia, tuberculosis, heart conditions, and so forth; deaf–blind; multi-handicapped; or who have specific learning disabilities. It involves children who, because of those impairments, need special education and related services ([121a.5(a)] Code of Federal Regulations [CFR] 121).

The definition of handicapped children sets two criteria for determining whether a child is eligible for special education. First, the child must have been evaluated and found to have one or more of the handicaps listed in the definition. The second criterion is that the child must need special education and related services because of the handicap. A pupil may have one or more of the handicapping conditions but not necessarily need special educational services. It is important to emphasize that a child who does not require special education services is not considered handicapped for purposes of the law.

2. *Special Education* (CFR, 121–24 [a] [1]). As used in this part of the law, the term *special education* means specially designed instruc-

tion, at no cost to the parent, to meet the unique needs of a handicapped child, including classroom instruction, instruction in physical education, home instruction, and instruction in hospitals and institutions. From this definition of special education, coupled with the concept of least-restrictive environment embedded within the Act, the goals of general education predominate for all children. Special education becomes appropriate only when a handicap impairs a child from functioning in a general school program. Even then, special education is appropriate only to the extent that it is necessary to bridge the gap between the child's ability to function in the general school program and the deficits in doing so because of the handicap. For most handicapped children, special instruction will not be the totality of their education. Handicapped children will participate in the general education program to the maximum extent possible.

3. *Related Services.* A child who is handicapped and needs help as a result of the impairment is eligible for special education and "related services." The term "related services" as used in the law is defined (CFR, 121a.13) as:

The term 'related services' means transportation and such developmental, corrective, and other supportive services as are required to assist a handicapped child to benefit from special education, and includes speech pathology and audiology, psychological services, physical and occupational therapy, recreation, early identification and assessment of disabilities in children, counseling services, and medical services for diagnostic or evaluation purposes. The term also includes school health services, social work services in schools, and parent counseling and training.

Related services can be termed additional services necessary for the child to benefit from special education. The definition of "related services" is based on the need of special education services first, then related services may follow.

Six Major Educational Components of PL 94–142

Within the parameters of the Act are six educational components that are most open to controversy and challenge. These are (1) the right to a free appropriate public education, (2) priority for services, (3) identifying children in need, (4) safeguards for parents in decision-making, (5) a written IEP for each child, and (6) the least-restrictive environment.

Priority for Services The Act requires that the highest priority for services must be given, first, to handicapped children who are not receiving an education, and, second, to the most severely handicapped who are receiving an inadequate education.

Identifying Children in Need   The local educational agency is responsible for ensuring that all handicapped children within its jurisdiction are identified, located, and evaluated, including those is all public and private agencies and institutions in its area. Congress believed that early identification was crucial to preventing a child's handicap from becoming worse or leading to further learning problems. In meeting this requirement most school districts have "Child Find" programs that employ various approaches to discover children with handicaps. Screening, evaluation, diagnosis, and referral are elements of the Child Find activities.

Safeguards for Parents in Decision-Making   State and local education agencies must guarantee parents and children strong safeguards to protect their due process rights in all steps of the special education decision-making process. Notice and consent are often mentioned together as procedural safeguards, but consent need not be obtained for every step for which notice must be given. Consent is specifically required for only four things: (1) the initial evaluation of the child; (2) the initial placement of the child; (3) evaluation before a "subsequent significant change in placement"; and (4) before release of records to persons not already authorized to see them. Steps for due process are listed under Due Process Procedures, below.

DUE PROCESS PROCEDURES: PARENT AND/OR LEGAL GUARDIAN RIGHTS UNDER RULES OF THE EDUCATION OF THE HANDICAPPED ACT, PL 94–142

1. To examine your child's records
2. To confidentiality of information relating to records and proceedings
3. If you disagree with the assessment made, you may secure an independent evaluation at no cost to you.
4. To grant written consent prior to preplacement evaluation or initial placement of your child into a program
5. To have your child protected in evaluation procedures
6. To have your child be provided a surrogate parent
7. To have your child provided an appropriate educational program in the least restrictive environment
8. If you disagree with assessment and/or placement results, you may have an impartial due process hearing on the issues of disagreement.
9. To be given written notice within a reasonable time of action relating to identification, evaluation, or educational placement of your child and other matters
10. To revoke this consent at any time

The difference between consent and notice is that notice is now required to be given before any step is taken in regard to the child.

According to 45 CFG 121a.504 (a) (1)–(2) written notice is required "a reasonable time before the public agency proposes to initiate or change (or refuses to initiate or change) the identification, evaluation or placement of the child or the provision of a free appropriate public education to the child." This means that at each step the agency must tell the parents whether it plans to go ahead with any special education process for the child.

A Written IEP for Each Child The intent of a written IEP is to (1) guarantee the availability of special education programming to handicapped children and (2) ensure fairness and appropriateness in decision-making about the provision of special education to handicapped children. The IEP results in a document that reflects the child's strengths and indicates what special education and related services to the child will receive.

The Least-Restrictive Environment The law mandates that handicapped children should be educated to the maximum extent possible with their nonhandicapped peers. Pupils must be placed in special education or separate classes only when it is impossible to work out a satisfactory placement in a regular class with supplementary aids and services. State and local education agencies must ensure that a range of alternative placements is available to accommodate handicapped children in the least-restrictive environment or setting possible.

SECTION 504 OF THE REHABILITATION ACT OF 1973

Section 504 is the basic civil rights provision for ending discrimination against America's handicapped citizens. The section was enacted through the Rehabilitation Act Amendments of 1973, PL 93–112. The Act prohibits discrimination against any qualified handicapped person in any program or activity receiving financial assistance:

> No otherwise qualified handicapped individual in the United States . . . shall, solely by reason of his handicap, be excluded from the participation in, be denied benefits for, or be subjected to discrimination, under any program or activity receiving federal 29 U.S.C. 794 financial assistance. (Sec. 504, 1973)

The rules and regulations of Section 504 are similar to those for PL 94–142 in their comprehensiveness and detail. They explain how the federal government will interpret and enforce its responsibilities under the Rehabilitation Act to ensure that handicapped children are protected from discrimination in federally funded programs.

Access. No qualified handicapped person may be excluded from or be denied the benefits of a public preschool, elementary, secondary, or adult education program because the facilities are inaccessible to or unusable by the impaired.

Facilities. Section 504 stresses barrier-free facilities and program accessibility. Programs in existing facilities must be operated so that, when viewed as a whole, they are readily accessible and usable. Therefore, a school need not make each and every part of the existing facilities accessible if it can relocate or reschedule enough classes and activities so as to offer all required courses and a reasonable selection of electives and other activities in already accessible areas. A school district's newly constructed facilities must be designed and built so that they are accessible to and usable by handicapped persons.

Transportation. Transportation must be provided for the handicapped child as a "related service" if a child needs transportation in order to benefit from special education. If, to carry out its obligations under the law, a school system places a handicapped child in a program it does not operate, it must ensure that adequate transportation is provided to and from the activity. The system may charge the parents an amount no greater than would be incurred if the child were placed in a program operated by the school.

Education Programs and Services

Historically, treatment of the physically disabled, including persons with muscular dystrophy, evolved from a medical model. Most children with orthopaedic or health impairments received medical treatment in hospitals or state institutions. Education received little consideration. As health problems gained maximum attention, the long-term needs of the "whole person" received little attention. Gradually, however, special classes developed and with them evolved home and hospital instruction for bed-ridden patients. As the importance and relevance of special education were realized, children with more severe physical problems—cerebral palsy, muscular dystrophy, spina bifida—were added to the educational group. Interdisciplinary teams began to work with the physically disabled in an effort to provide medical and educational services in recognition of the importance of each.

When viewing the child with muscular dystrophy vis-à-vis the educational system, the child must be kept as active as his physical condition will permit. Disuse of muscles may lead to more rapid deterioration. Since the child is not affected intellectually and there are no specific learning problems associated with this disorder, he should be retained in the regular classroom as long as he is physically able to adjust to the program. When he becomes so weak that he cannot participate in a regular class, he may be assigned to a special education class for the physically handicapped or for the home-bound tutoring program.

Educational programming for children with muscular dystrophy involves an interdisciplinary team approach to a number of problem areas. The team is comprised of professionals from a variety of disciplines including, but not limited to, physical and occupational therapy, social work, nursing, psychology, speech therapy, rehabilitation counseling, and recreation (see also other chapters and related subjects). In a hospital setting, these disciplines plus the medical team provide a full range of direct services, but in the school setting many disciplines provide only consultation services.

The team should work with the child toward fulfillment of four basic developmental goals:

1. Physical independence, including mastery of daily living skills
2. Self-awareness and social maturation
3. Academic growth
4. Career education, including constructive leisure activities

These goals create certain needs for curriculum planning: the needs for adaptive equipment, procedures for adequate assessment, and realistic goal planning incorporating the above four developmental goals.

ADAPTIVE EQUIPMENT AND MATERIALS

The crux of programming and modification for the physically disabled lies in adapting tasks to allow the student to develop maximum independence. This often requires the creation of adaptive devices that facilitate or aid in the completion of tasks. Often, a student can be independent with minimal adaptation of usual techniques or provision of an adaptive device. For example, for those who have impaired arm and hand control, a headwand (pointer stick fastened to a headband) may be used to type out letters on either a typewriter or a computer keyboard.

Daily living skills also may require adaptive methods and devices. A special non-tippable cup may help to prevent spilling by a youngster with muscular dystrophy who has poor motor control. Another child may need a spoon with a special large handle that permits grasping for easy feeding.

ASSESSMENT

Criterion-referenced assessments are suggested for physically disabled students. In this method the child's progress is compared only to his own earlier performance, rather than to a standardized test framework. Many tests leave the physically disabled child at a cultural or experiential disadvantage because the physical problem hampered his development. The situation is analogous to a child from a cultural minority group tested using the majority language.

GOAL PLANNING

Proper assessment should reveal data that are useful in developing both short-term and long-term goals for the child with a neuromuscular disease. The following four developmental factors, previously cited, should be considered.

Physical Independence

Physical and occupational therapists are valuable resources in developing programs for maximum independence. Physical independence includes a number of skill areas related to physical function, including activities of daily living (see Chaps. 8, 16, and 17). Task analysis may be a crucial evaluative tool in determining which skills have developmental potential. Task analysis is based on pinpointing task subskills or components the disabled person cannot do and devising adaptive means for independent completion.

Self-Awareness and Social Maturation

Blanket generalizations about the disabled, although convenient, are erroneous by virtue of oversimplification. Some people assume that the greater the physical disability, the greater the psychological consequences, or that certain disabling conditions produce specific psychological results. These popular beliefs are not supported by available data. The impact experienced by each individual is related to the significance of the disability for that person, the pattern of events that have contributed to personal values, self-perception in relation to the rest of the world, and personal stress reactions. Furthermore, the sense of loss experienced by individuals with an acquired disability differs from the experience of those born with a physical handicap.

Psychological problems experienced by the physically disabled, listed below, are not only self-imposed but can also result from societal barriers that hinder emotional development.

1. Unresolved dependency feelings that may create an excessive need for affection attention
2. Excessive submissiveness that actually may be covering a deep-seated hostility toward physical dependence on others
3. Extreme egocentricity and inability to deal with loneliness
4. Fantasy as compensation for feelings of inferiority or inadequacy
5. Resignation to, rather than recognition of, limits
6. Superficial conscious recognition of a handicap, but a subconscious rejection of self

Because concepts of ability and disability are integrated into self-image, a child's self-concept certainly may be affected by muscular dystrophy. Body image, life experiences, social relationships, emotions, and intellectual performance also affect the sense of self. As we interact with others and compare ourselves with our peers, our self-concept develops. Parents, teachers, and other significant individuals in a child's life must therefore nurture the development of a positive self-concept (see Chap. 22).

In the classroom, children with muscular dystrophy need to explore their attitudes toward themselves and to express their true feelings. Teachers and therapists can readily provide opportunities for introspection and interaction related to topics on family life, human sexuality, and death. Disabled students need to learn that experience of a wide range of feelings is normal; to accept constructive criticism in order to better meet frustration and disappointment without experiencing ego loss; and to evaluate each experience and use this information for future planning.

Personal development and independence should be fostered throughout the school experience, along with traditional academic training. Education of life and death issues should be a part of one's personal development. Generally, students with neuromuscular disease are exposed to death more than their nondisabled peers are, yet they have little or no preparation for this stress. Basic information about death and its part in the natural cycle of life provides students with factual knowledge to aid understanding. This supportive atmosphere is best intertwined with parental involvement so as to promote a totally positive, yet realistic, climate for the child.

Parents of children with muscular dystrophy often have trouble coping with their child's condition and experience difficulty in giving needed support. Regardless of whether a child's disability is genetic, traumatic, or of unknown cause, parents often feel responsible and guilty. Such guilt leads to over-protection and fosters dependency. Parents should be reminded that their child will benefit from learning adaptive methods independently, even if it takes extra time, rather than having parents intervene in task completion (see Chap. 17).

Academic Growth

Because of the varied educational needs of children with muscular dystrophy, curricula must integrate adaptive techniques with the numerous educational materials used in standard curricula, with learning disabilities, and with mentally retarded, sensory handicapped, or gifted children. Educational programming can be realistic if new or adapted material is used creatively to meet the needs of each child.

Infant stimulation and early childhood education programs emphasize gross and fine motor developmental skills, activities of daily living, and social interaction. Physical and occupational therapists can contribute a great deal to the program development of young children because the therapists are more familiar with developmental milestones.

Apart from emphasis on development of physical skills, coordination and readiness for academic work should also be developed, incorporating the beginnings of activities referenced to specific criteria. Environmental exploration and movement experiences should be encouraged. Success in simple self-help skills, such as dressing, builds motivation for learning.

In elementary education, academic skills receive increasing attention. Although basic skills in reading, arithmetic, language arts, and social studies are important, some students will need to continue readiness activities. Educational programming requires integration of special needs with the regular core curriculum.

Adolescents need to develop academic skills for information finding, and precision in such mathematical skills as basic computation. Language arts should emphasize personal writing and correspondence, because these skills are basic to independent survival. Today, most students with neuromuscular disease who are in school exceed basic survival skills and complete a general academic high school program.

Students with appropriate academic ability and perseverance should be encouraged to plan high school academic programs that prepare them for community college, university, or other professional training. Extensive adaptive methods and equipment to facilitate functional independence should promote successful completion of postsecondary education.

Life Experience Education

The goal of education is to prepare an individual for successful experiences in employment, recreation, social relationships, self-help skills, and constructive leisure activities. The following goals, suggested by Howard and Bigge, apply:

1. Ability to obtain meaningful employment (whether it be homebound, sheltered workshop, or competitive)
2. Capacity for independent living appropriate to individual's physical and mental capabilities
3. Capacity for community involvement (including a variety of daily living skills)
4. Skills for participation in meaningful leisure time activities (a well-defined free-time management system); the basic objectives are recreational experiences for enjoyment and meeting and retaining friends.
5. Development of reliable means of transportation
6. Mastery of self-care skills

7. Ability to maintain residence away from parent, convalescent hospital, or state institution
8. Development of healthy self-concept

Career education involves all those skills needed by a student after completing school. For vocational education, factors to consider include strength and stamina, mobility, independent toileting, communication skills, and the potential for future development. Students with limitations in these areas need not be unemployable if the most appropriate vocational training is provided.

For some, the choice may be between vocational training and other constructive use of time. Although a puritan work ethic is so ingrained in our society that any challenge to it may bother the family or professionals, there are alternatives that interpret the quality of life in different ways. Unproductive days in front of a television set seem inappropriate and non-rewarding, but constructive leisure-time education could teach the severely disabled student to use time wisely. Productive use of time is a key to the quality of life.

Recreation activities lead to the development of interests and hobbies that can be continued after the school years. Program planning should consider assessment of a child's strength, mobility, and balance. Group activities should be planned that meet the unique interest needs of, and allow for active participation by, each child regardless of disability. For individual activities, adaptive techniques and equipment may be needed (i.e., the child with limited hand use may benefit from numbered checkerboard squares to tell his or her partner the next move).

Community programs and public agencies have greatly expanded recreational programs for physically disabled children and adults. In addition, community college programs for the disabled learner are a valuable resource for constructive use of time following completion of public school.

Parents' Role in the Educational Process

Parents know their child best. To carry out their role effectively, parents must see themselves as equal partners with professionals in planning and programming for the child and should be aware, confident, and assertive to make sure that the program plan is appropriate and effective. Parents as partners foster independence and growth in their handicapped child and promote healthy attitudes among those who relate to the child.

Many parents feel alone because they have the responsibility of finding programs and services that provide continuity and meet their child's needs. The parents' role requires involvement, courage, assertiveness, commitment, determination, ingenuity, and humor. To some, it may be an overwhelming responsibility; to others, it is a challenge committing them to a worthy cause.

Legislation now recognizes the role of parents in the special education decision-making process (see Due Process Procedures, above) and provides effective means for ensuring that a child receives a free appropriate public education. However, rules and regulations do not automatically relieve parents of frustration. It helps for schools to include parents in decision-making, but it still takes a determined parent to make sure the process is working.

Most school districts have special education advisory committees with representatives who serve as advisors to directors of special education, school superintendants, and boards of education. These committees support, advocate, and monitor programs and services. Participation of parents in these committees, as well as in other related groups and programs, can be a potent force for change for the handicapped. Parent and professional workshops and inservice groups provide the opportunity to share issues and concerns in the educational process. State departments of education and advocacy groups support interested participants through a better use of the legislative process. Students and parents of today have demonstrated their ability to influence policies at all levels — local, state, and national.

Summary

The 1970s and early 1980s represent a period of significant progress on behalf of exceptional children. Parental and professional advocacy groups emerged as educational and legislative forces, and rights of the handicapped child became a major public issue. Landmark federal legislation included PL 94 – 142 and Section 504 of the Rehabilitation Act of 1973. The most significant feature was a mandate for free appropriate public education for all handicapped children. No child can be excluded from school because of physical barriers or because he requires special transportation. Due to the implementation of the concept of the least restrictive environment, a regular classroom, rather than a self-contained special class, is the preferred setting for most exceptional children.

Parents play an important role in the educational process of their handicapped child. Working with professionals as partners, parents can help develop and carry out educational goals and objectives.

Today, the education of the handicapped child is more a part of than apart from general education. School administrators and regular classroom teachers share in the responsibility of educating these children. The impact of the 1970s and early 1980s will be far-reaching. In some respects, it has just begun.

Suggested Readings

BIGGE JL, O'DONNELL PA (eds): Teaching Individuals with Physical and Multiple Disabilities. Columbus, Charles Merrill, 1977

HOWARD R, BIGGE JL: Life experience programming. In Bigge JL, O'Donnell PA (eds): Teaching Individuals with Physical and Multiple Disabilities. Columbus, Charles Merrill, 1977

LEVINE LS: The Impact of Disability. Address presented to the Oklahoma Rehabilitation Association Convention, Oklahoma City, October, 1959

MARTIN R: Educating Handicapped Children: The Legal Mandate. Champaign, IL, Research Press 1980

MEYEN EL: Exceptional Children and Youth — An Introduction. Denver, Love Publishing, 1978

NEFF WS, WEISS SA: Psychological aspects of disability. In Wolberg BB (ed): Handbook of Clinical Psychology. New York, McGraw-Hill, 1965

SHERRILL C: Adapted Physical Education and Recreation: A Multidisciplinary Approach. Dubuque, IA, WC Brown, 1976

SHRYBMAN JA: Due Process in Special Education. Rockwell, MD, Aspen Systems, 1982

SIRVIS B, CARPIGNANO J, BIGGE JL: Psychosocial aspects of physical disability. In Bigge JL, O'Donnell PO (eds): Teaching Individuals with Physical and Multiple Disabilities. Columbus, OH, Charles Merrill, 1977

21

Mark G. Pendleton

Psychosocial Interventions in the Rehabilitation of Adults With Neuromuscular Disorders

This chapter describes the emotional and behavioral issues frequently encountered in working with adults who have neuromuscular disorders, as well as how potential problems can be identified. Because many of these issues are encountered in patients with any disabling illness (e.g., asthma, diabetes, heart disease), successful psychosocial interventions in all chronic disease populations are relevant to patients with neuromuscular disorders. Additional consideration must be given to the particular disability produced by neuromuscular disorders as a group, and even to differences among individual nerve and muscle diseases.

Additionally, this chapter illustrates several ways in which mental health clinicians (e.g., psychologists, psychiatrists, social workers) can participate in the rehabilitation of adults with neuromuscular disorders. Different models, modes, and types of psychosocial interventions are described. Alternative treatment plans for individual patients are presented, depending on the resources that the treatment program has available.

In the past, health care was largely based on a mind–body dualism that is now questioned. The current norm is a model that (1) recognizes the complex factors that contribute to human health and illness; (2) includes subjective emotional states, beliefs, and personality styles as important among these factors; and (3) redefines the patient's role in more active, self-responsible terms. Professionals, patients, and families are all increasingly aware of the particular importance of psychosocial interventions in treatment of physical illness. Goals of health care are not only to address physical problems, but also to aid patients and their families in coping with emotional and social consequences of the disease, to minimize the need for treatment through improving patients' health-promoting behaviors, and to decrease the severity of chronic symptoms.

Treatment Issues

ACUTE SYMPTOMS

Acute neuromuscular symptoms, whether weakness or cardiorespiratory and infectious complications that result from weakness, require adjustments by the patient and his family. Additionally, an adult onset of a neuromuscular condition poses special problems as a formerly normally functioning individual becomes increasingly limited physically. Family roles and relationships must be adjusted, and marital and family conflict is common. Friendships can be strained as the patient becomes less able to participate in former social activities, and depression frequently occurs because of the physical and social losses. The patient and family need to understand each symptom, its implications for daily activities, any treatment available, and how to cope with the resulting emotional stress. Denial and intrusion frequently occur; both of these can affect the patient's adjustment negatively (these reactions are important enough that they are discussed separately below). Other expected reactions include a fear that the acute problem will happen again (which is often realistic), a fear of becoming helpless or dying (also realistic in many cases), anger at whoever or whatever may be blamed for the illness (including the "messenger" who tells them of the illness), guilt about this hostility, and sadness or depression whenever loss is involved (e.g., loss of independence, loss of trust in body functions, loss of self-esteem). Furthermore, patients are often hospitalized during acute phases of the illness, and the hospital environment can be quite stressful (see discussion below).

The patient is likely to be unusually responsive to psychosocial interventions during such periods of acute illness, but there is a risk that set, detrimental coping patterns can become established. Therefore, interventions that promote realistic adaptations and maintain the patient's self-esteem should be established quickly and effectively.

One helpful immediate intervention is training in techniques for coping with stress, using relaxation, and using cognitive coping strategies. Such training is best undertaken early, preferably at a time when the patient is still doing well physically. The skills are then available later, when the patient is confronted with the stress of additional symptoms, medical interventions, and realistic fears.

An imperative for rehabilitation staff members is to thoroughly understand coping responses of patients, as well as their own reactions to patients and illness. The staff should be prepared to provide information honestly to the patient (answering questions, clarifying misconceptions, identifying sources of support), yet tempering candor sufficiently to protect the patient. Staff members also must be willing to consistently repeat information so as not to give conflicting stories and to ensure that the patient understands his treatment plan.

Denial

Denial usually occurs early in a patient's response to an acute symptom and, as time passes, interchanges back and forth with intrusive states. Denial is characterized by an emotional "daze" and a failure to attend to or recognize many aspects of the medical condition. Horowitz (1982) has listed a number of indicators of denial: a blank stare, failure to react appropriately to external stimuli, difficulty concentrating, a lack of awareness of bodily sensations, sleep disturbance (sleeping too much or too little), withdrawal or frantic overactivity, and somatic complaints such as fatigue or headaches.

Among neuromuscular patients, myotonic dystrophy patients have been described as presenting an unusual degree of denial of their illness, even as weakness progresses and serious complications appear. Affected parents of myotonic dystrophy patients may not only deny their symptoms but their child's symptoms as well. "Confronting" the patient with "reality" is rarely an effective strategy for helping the patient, but rather may result in the patient's becoming angry which damages a therapeutic relationship. Instead, a safe, caring relationship should be established in which the patient is gradually assisted in reexperiencing the stressful event, reorganizing his thinking about it, and exploring the emotional and cognitive associations to it. Antidepressant medication may be helpful if such states persist.

Intrusion

Intrusion tends to develop later than denial, and is characterized by startle reactions and excessive alertness to potential signs that the symptom may be worsening. Horowitz' indicators of intrusive states include hypervigilance, autonomic and cortical arousal, hypnagogic phenomena (illusions, pseudohallucinations, hallucinations), sleep and dream disturbances (difficulty falling asleep, frequent nocturnal awakenings, nightmares), repetitive thoughts, preoccupation with the illness, disorganized thinking, and somatic complaints such as shaking and nausea. Relaxation training as well as brief use of mild antianxiety medications can be helpful. Symptoms of the illness can be rendered less stressful through educational efforts and cognitive coping strategies (described below).

The Hospital Environment

Although hospitalization can provide additional medical care that is not possible on an outpatient basis, patients often do not respond to hospitalization by feeling relaxed and reassured. Many aspects of hospitalization are stressful because the hospital (1) is a sign of the gravity of the patient's condition; (2) uproots a patient from familiar surroundings; (3) disrupts the patient's normal daily routine; and (4) gives a patient time to think about unpleasant aspects of the illness. Anxiety is also heightened by witnessing other patients in distress or by reading informed consent sheets that list a myriad of potential complications. In addition to interventions already covered, other helpful suggestions to alleviate patients' anxieties include involving patients in treatment decisions, encouraging them to be active in the hospital (*i.e.*, make their own beds), and consistently providing them with information as to what to expect.

NEUROPSYCHOLOGICAL DEFICITS

Some neuromuscular patients show impairment of higher mental abilities, especially those with Duchenne and myotonic dystrophies. These deficits do not necessarily affect all cognitive skills to a similar degree. For example, a comprehensive neuropsychological test battery found that myotonic dystrophy patients did particularly poorly on tests of conceptual ability, perseveration, and spatial relations, but scored only slightly lower than normal on measures of delayed recall of newly learned information (Woodward, 1982).

Neuropsychological deficits have significant implications for patients' everyday functioning and treatment. Myotonic dystrophy patients, for example, have difficulty understanding abstract information and formulating good problem-solving strategies in unfamiliar situations, and will perseverate with the same strategy in the face of negative feedback. Educational efforts and communication should be concrete, and coping and self-treatment strategies should be explicit, covering as many potential problem areas as possible.

TREATMENT COMPLIANCE

As with many other chronic medical conditions, a significant percentage of patients with neuromuscular disorders do not completely comply with a treatment program. Frequently, noncompliance is taken as a sign that there is something "wrong" with the patient. The staff may then try to cajole, beg, force, or even scare the patient into complying. Such efforts vastly oversimplify the factors that affect compliance, work only transiently at best, and have an unfortunate tendency to "backfire" (*i.e.*, the patient reacts by becoming even more noncompliant, the treatment cannot succeed, and the patient and staff regress into mutual, angry blaming).

Factors that affect compliance or noncompliance to treatment are reviewed by Davidson (1982), who also describes the following procedures to increase compliance, especially if used in combination: (1) treatment recommendations by a familiar individual who is liked and respected by the patient; (2) educational strategies with short-term treatment; (3) increased personal responsibility by the patient for his treatment; and (4) increased feelings of self-efficacy by the patient through self-monitoring, self-instructional training, and behavioral contracting with the treatment staff and the family. Increased monitoring by a rehabilitation staff, especially in combination with mild punishment for noncompliance, can also be very effective, but the improved compliance is generally lost if such monitoring is discontinued.

CHRONIC ILLNESS

The development of detrimental coping patterns can be a significant risk during periods of health crisis. These patterns can become enduring aspects of a patient's functioning, particularly with chronic, progressive neuromuscular illnesses. Chronicity does *not* mean that a successful adjustment has been made or that an unsuccessful adjustment is permanent. Intervention with chronic maladaptation is more difficult than with acute problems, but not impossible. Psychosocial interventions should only be considered effective when the physical illness and the patient's emotional reactions to it no longer interfere unnecessarily in the patient's everyday life.

Duchenne dystrophy is illustrative of the effect of chronic disability on children surviving to adulthood. Many characteristics of Duchenne dystrophy make successful adjustment difficult:

1. Because of the early onset of the disease, the physical dependence that develops, and parental guilt, these patients are often overprotected and have not developed skills for coping with disability and illness.
2. The degree of dependence increases with age as the illness progresses, making it particularly difficult for a patient to separate or form *adult* adjustments.
3. Parents and siblings can be very ambivalent toward the patient, communicating hostility, pity, and sadness intermixed with caring and love.
4. Because Duchenne dystrophy patients have long been "different" and often unable to participate in activities with peers, they may have few friends and inadequate social skills.

5. Physical deformities further isolate patients as "different" or repulsive, making it more difficult for them to make friends and develop support networks in the community.
6. Acute physical symptoms (some life-threatening) come and go.
7. Death is "imminent" (almost all Duchenne dystrophy patients are dead by age 25).
8. Many patients are painfully aware that they have never had sex and that they are unlikely to ever do so.
9. Cognitive deficits are often present that significantly affect everyday functioning.

These factors probably account for descriptions of Duchenne patients as "withdrawn, socially inept, depressed, emotionally immature, manipulative, and mentally dull." Fortunately, many still form adult adjustments that are satisfying to them and others.

A patient needs a comfortable and secure relationship with a therapist to deal effectively with such chronic difficulties. Once this relationship is established, the therapist works to assist the patient in understanding his responses, developing new perspectives and behaviors for coping with the illness, and differentiating realistic fears from fantasized fears. Change is likely to be a gradual, on-again, off-again process. Group sessions can be especially helpful because other patients with the same illness can share perspectives and serve as models for successful coping. Additionally, family meetings are essential if long-standing patterns of family relationships and communication must be changed.

Models for the Delivery of Psychosocial Interventions

STANDARD OPERATING PROCEDURE (SOP) VERSUS REFERRAL AS NEEDED (PRN)

Determining how a psychotherapist's activities should be integrated into a treatment program is a major decision. On one hand, the psychotherapist can be involved in each patient's evaluation and treatment from the beginning of the patient's participation in the treatment program. Such involvement can be routine, expected, and a required part of every patient's treatment (SOP), with the nature and frequency of contacts between the patient and psychologist determined by the patient's individual needs. One advantage of SOP is that the psychotherapist, by contributing to team treatment decisions, minimizes the chances that any patient's emotional needs will be underserved. Another advantage is that SOP lessens the possibility that a patient will be upset about or stigmatized by seeing a mental health worker. Despite increased social awareness and acceptance of mental health treatment, many people still view seeing a "shrink" as a sign that someone will think that they are "crazy." However, a patient seeing the psychotherapist because "everybody does" rather than because "something is wrong" helps minimize such reactions. A major disadvantage of SOP is that the necessary financial resources are often not available for such comprehensive psychotherapy.

Alternatively, individuals can be referred for psychotherapy as needed (PRN). The major advantage to the PRN approach is that it "triages" referrals and prevents depletion of limited resources. In addition to possible stigmatization, another disadvantage is that it is very difficult to establish good referral criteria. Reliance on patient complaints or requests for psychotherapeutic treatment runs the significant risk of only treating "squeaky wheels," and of withholding treatment from individuals who under-report and would benefit from emotional support. In our experience, neuromuscular patients tend to under-report their need for emotional support. Furthermore, a mental health worker can make contributions even when a patient is not clearly experiencing emotional difficulties. Screening criteria are sometimes supplemented by objective screening tests, but the development and demonstration of validity of such tests are difficult.

Regardless of whether the SOP or PRN model, or a combination, is used, psychological services are typically delivered in one of three ways: (1) directly to the patient independent of the team, (2) indirectly through consultation to the treatment staff, or (3) as part of a collaborative treatment team.

Direct, Independent Treatment

This model is typically used when a treatment program does not have a staff psychotherapist and has to refer patients to other agencies or private clinicians. The psychotherapist has "face-to-face" contacts with the patient and his family and carries out interventions somewhat independent of the overall rehabilitation program. Consultation and information sharing are desirable, but because the therapist is separate from team rehabilitation decisions, he must assume individual responsibility for effectiveness of attempted interventions. *Example:* The clinic staff refers a neuromuscular disease patient believed to be depressed to a psychotherapist who evaluates and treats the patient's depression.

Professional-to-Professional Consultation

Instead of direct intervention with the patient, a mental health worker can suggest possible intervention strategies to other members of the treatment staff for followthrough. Suggestions may be based on direct contact between psychotherapist and patient or, more typically, on information provided by staff. Consultation often may be based on psychological testing results. *Example:* A physical therapist reports that a patient is not complying with "homework" assignments, and the mental health clinician discusses ways in which treatment compliance can be improved.

Collaborative Treatment Team

The mental health clinician participates as part of a team that meets regularly to discuss patients and implement treatment. The psychotherapist is most responsible for evaluating the role of psychosocial factors in a patient's behavior and for suggesting appropriate psychosocial interventions. Direct treatment can be provided by the psychotherapist, or other staff members can merely seek advice about how to intervene. *Example:* During a weekly staff conference, the psychologist notes that a family's relationships are disrupted by the patient's newly diagnosed limb girdle dystrophy. A treatment plan can be devised in which the psychologist will conduct family meetings and include the family in an educational group, while other team members will make special efforts to involve the family in treatment.

MODES OF INTERVENTION

Individual treatment, group sessions, and family meetings are all valuable psychotherapeutic interventions.

Individual Treatment

Although the effectiveness of one-to-one, patient-to-therapist interactions has at times been disputed, most studies indicate that individual treatment is effective in reducing emotional distress, in helping patients make behavioral changes, and in establishing and maintaining health-promoting behavior. Both short-term and long-term psychosocial interventions can be effective.

In short-term or time-limited interventions, the patient and therapist meet only for a few sessions (usually less than 10) devoted to one or two clearly identified problem areas. Because they are oriented toward problem-solving, with the therapist taking an active role in suggesting new behaviors to the patient, such interventions are particularly useful with reactions to acute symptoms.

With long-term intervention, the patient and therapist establish a relationship that continues for as long as it is useful to the patient. This mode is usually insight-oriented or supportive, with the therapist taking a role designed to assist the patient in understanding his emotions and behavior, to increase the patient's self-esteem, and to change the patient's characteristic styles of coping. Long-term, individual therapy is most useful with bright, psychologically minded patients and with patients who do not have a well-developed support network of family and friends.

Group Sessions

It is incorrect to view group sessions as merely an expansion of individual treatment with additional patients. Groups are particularly effective in providing emotional support, decreasing a patient's sense of social isolation, increasing social skills, and exploring interpersonal issues. Groups designed for special purposes may be especially useful to neuromuscular patients. In educational groups, for example, patients and family members can be taught about neuromuscular signs and symptoms, treatment, and health-promoting behavior, such as relaxation training or stress management. In self-help groups, patients meet to discuss issues of mutual interest (emotional, medical, and even political) and to provide support to one another. Apart from emotional benefits, group sessions are cost-effective because several patients benefit from the therapist's time.

Family Meetings

Family meetings are frequently beneficial to review how a patient's disability significantly affects family relationships and roles. Some family meetings focus on educational information; others are intended to help family members to explore their relationships and communications with one another, to improve communication, to adjust restrictive roles, and to promote mutual support.

Marital counseling is often a part of family counseling, with the goals of decreasing conflict and improving communication. Conflict often results from the stress of raising a child with a neuromuscular disease or if one partner becomes similarly disabled.

TYPES OF INTERVENTIONS

Divergent theoretical orientations are represented among mental health workers. None of the above-described modes of intervention is specific to one theoretical orientation; rather, there are many different orientations, each using different techniques.

Psychodynamic Therapy

Psychodynamic therapy focuses on the interrelationships of conscious and unconscious impulses, beliefs, and emotional reactions. Emphasis is given to a patient's description of experiences, with the therapist aiding the patient in more fully understanding these experiences (gaining insight). The patient is assisted in using this insight to improve personal and social adjustments.

Behavioral Therapy

Many behavioral techniques have been developed from learning theory. The focus of behavioral therapy is on specific behaviors (motor acts, physiological responses, thinking) as learned responses, which can be changed through new and different learning experiences. Commonly used techniques include behavior modification (the use of reinforcement and punishment to discourage undesirable behavior and to encourage desirable behavior in its place), systematic desensitization (the use of relaxation to improve a patient's self-control of unpleasant emotions), and cognitive behavioral therapy (teaching the patient to change his thinking in ways that improve adjustment).

Educational Intervention

Education is an important component of comprehensive psychosocial interventions for patients with physical illnesses. Patients need adequate information to assume responsibility for and make decisions about their own health care. Information should be provided in a manner that is understandable and not psychologically damaging, so that a patient has clear understanding of necessary adjustments and can anticipate and prepare for subsequent developments. Education can be provided through group or family meetings, pamphlets, video tapes, and manuals, or through the use of mass media such as television, newspapers, and magazines. Mass media efforts can also be aimed at the general public in order to improve social opportunities available to patients.

Cognitive Rehabilitation

Many procedures are being developed to improve a patient's basic cognitive abilities in areas such as attention and concentration, learning and memory, perception, spatial analysis and manipulation, and conceptual skills. The initial reports regarding these procedures, particularly when computers are utilized, are very encouraging with patients who have sustained brain trauma, but the procedures have not yet been tested in neuromuscular patients with cognitive deficits. The effectiveness of this type of rehabilitation for neuromuscular patients should be evaluated in the near future.

Other Interventions

Some interventions are designed to help a patient directly intervene in his physical functioning. Biofeedback (the use of machines that measure aspects of a patient's physiological responses and provide the patient with this information so that he may learn to control the response) is frequently used to treat problems worsened by stress. Similar interventions center around improved diet and exercise regimens.

The Treatment Plan

Resources permitting, each neuromuscular patient should have an individualized treatment plan that explicitly considers both physical and psychosocial issues. A psychologist can contribute assessment information based on clinical interviews and formal psychological testing (e.g., personality inventories, assessments of coping skills, neuropsychological evaluations). Additionally, a rehabilitation specialist, along with the patient and family, contributes behavior observations (formal ratings, checklists, and anecdotal descriptions). A formulation of the patient's needs and desires for treatment is then completed, and the procedures for intervening are specified.

Any formulation and treatment plan should involve the patient and family as active partners. Specific components of a treatment plan may be assigned to particular staff members, but each staff member should know what every other staff member is doing. One staff member should be identified as coordinator for a treatment plan.

Evaluation of the effectiveness of treatment should be ongoing, using the same tools as the original assessment so that necessary adjustments can be made in the treatment plan.

If resources are not available to permit a comprehensive psychosocial intervention, a reasonable "fallback" strategy is to develop standardized group interventions, with only selected (on the basis of effective and fair referral criteria) patients and families being involved in more specifically planned interventions. A mental health worker's services would be offered both through independent treatment and professional-to-professional consultation whenever possible.

Suggested Readings

DAVIDSON PO: Issues in patient compliance. In Millon T, Green C, Meagher R (eds): Handbook of Clinical Health Psychology. New York, Plenum Press, 1982

HOROWITZ MJ: Psychological processes induced by illness, injury, and loss. In Millon T, Green C, Meagher R (eds): Handbook of Clinical Health Psychology. New York, Plenum Press, 1982

MEICHENBAUM D: Cognitive Behavior Modification. New York, Plenum Press 1977

WOODWARD JB, HEATON RK, SIMON DB, RINGEL SP: Neuropsychological findings in myotonic dystrophy. Journal of Clinical Neuropsychology 4: 335–342, 1982

Psychosocial Interventions in the Rehabilitation of Children With Neuromuscular Disorders

This chapter describes emotional and behavioral issues encountered in treating children and adolescents with neuromuscular disorders and illustrates ways in which mental health clinicians can promote successful psychosocial adjustment. To avoid duplication, the reader is periodically referred to information in Chapter 21. Adaptations of procedures described for adults, when more suitable for children and adolescents, are emphasized.

Pediatricians and other health-care professionals involved in treating children have been at the forefront of the movement to include psychosocial interventions as standard components of health care. All children who have serious medical conditions present a complex variety of developmental, behavioral, educational, and psychological issues. A large majority of children with progressive neuromuscular disorders will occasionally develop difficulties stemming from psychological problems. Effective psychosocial interventions can assist such children in attaining more adaptive social, mental, and physical development.

Pediatric psychology specifically addresses the psychosocial issues of children with complex medical problems. Pediatric psychologists emphasize (1) knowledge of the normal developmental process; (2) knowledge of the illness or illnesses being treated; (3) knowledge of the psychological and behavioral effects of illness in children; (4) ability to function as diagnostician, consultant, and therapist; (5) knowledge of specific, validated interventions for the problems presented by ill children and their families; and (6) ability to effectively communicate this knowledge to children, parents, and other health-care providers.

Treatment Issues

Several common psychosocial issues are relevant to the treatment of any child with a neuromuscular disease. Important differences also occur depending on the particular neuromuscular disorder. Accordingly, treatment of three chronic muscular dystrophies is highlighted, with emphasis given to treatment issues unique to each disorder.

Duchenne muscular dystrophy (DMD) poses an extremely difficult set of adjustments for affected children and their families. Although the disease can be detected at birth, symptoms are not apparent until the age of 4 or 5 years. Parents often find the delayed onset of this inherited disease difficult to understand and accept, and they may even deny that the diagnosis is accurate. Further, early spurts in motor development may result in periods where symptoms diminish, creating false hopes of a cure or that the child's condition was misdiagnosed.

Importantly, many parents have feelings of guilt because of the inherited nature of the disorder. To make "amends," parents may overprotect their child by allowing him to be overly dependent emotionally and physically, by not setting appropriate behavioral limits for him, and by not effectively disciplining him when limits are exceeded. Overprotectiveness can increase as the disease progresses and the child becomes more physically dependent and socially and educationally delayed. This pattern can result in behavior control problems (temper tantrums, not minding directions, poor treatment compliance), obesity (the parents fail to adequately control the child's diet), which further threatens the child's health, and emotional and social immaturity (withdrawal from peer contact can prevent the development of everyday skills necessary for a successful adult adjustment). As the child's condition worsens, the fear of death only magnifies the parents' tendency to overprotect.

Overprotectiveness is often intermixed with hostility directed at the child. At times, parents and siblings may resent the child's need for extra attention and effort. However, if such anger is too frequently directed at the child in either direct or indirect ways, family relationships deteriorate. The child may then begin relating to his family in a similar angry way because the child is frustrated by his dependency anyway.

In DMD, motor weakness and clumsiness usually become noticeable at a time when many new social skills are developing. In play with peers, the child's weakness interferes with the highly physical play that is particularly important among boys. The affected child may be referred to pejoratively as a "sissy" or a "whimp," placed in a subservient role in the peer hierarchy, and even purposefully excluded from activities. The boy's self-esteem suffers, his social skills lag behind, and he becomes increasingly withdrawn from peers and dependent on the family. Further damage to the child's self-esteem and social relationships is likely to occur as the disease progresses: cognitive deficits can cause the child to perform poorly at school (and can add the label "dumb"), motor deficits result in the child's eventually having to use a wheelchair (and can add the label "crippled"), contractures can distort the child's body (and add the label "freak"), and eventually the social repercussions can make the child sufficiently delayed socially so that he does not fit in with his peers (and add the label "weird" or "nerd"). If a child is ever to be expected to deal with these problems, education of peers and other individuals who interact with the child is important. Properly informed peers, neighbors, and teachers can often help affected children develop socially. The child's self-esteem is also helped by the avoidance of the pejorative labels just described.

Myotonic dystrophy (MYD) occasionally presents in the neonatal period with hypotonia, difficulty with sucking and feeding, and delayed intellectual milestones. These early difficulties may affect the parent–child neonatal bond negatively and may affect the emotional and social development of the child. Walking is often delayed in children with MYD, but once achieved, the ability is not usually lost again as it is in DMD. The combination of motor weakness, characteristic facial appearance, and cognitive deficits puts these children at a disadvantage socially and educationally. These children often develop poor social relationships and may not be able to count on the family as a source of emotional support, particularly if a parent is similarly affected. MYD children are at particular risk for retreating into fantasy and social withdrawal as a means of coping.

The heterogeneity of limb girdle dystrophy (LGD) makes discussion of a typical or common pattern difficult. Weakness that begins during adolescence or childhood represents a *loss* of previous ability and can result in depression. Progression of weakness is generally slow, affording more time for the patient to adjust to the changes in physical functioning. However, on occasion the slow onset is mislabeled as "laziness" or some other pejorative term damaging to self-esteem. For the few patients in whom progression is rapid, the patient and family must quickly make many adjustments to physical disablity and dependence, not unlike those required in DMD.

INITIAL DIAGNOSIS

Parents, much more than the affected children, often react to the initial diagnosis of their child's neuromuscular disorder with disbelief, denial, and intrusive states (see Chap. 21), and with anger, grief, guilt, and uncertainty about what to do. The diagnosis should be made in a way that promotes adjustment by the parents. The psychotherapist needs to be involved from the beginning in order to increase the likelihood that parents will adjust in ways that promote the health of their child. Golden and Davis (1974) suggest the following helpful procedures in diagnosing serious illness in a child:

1. Present the information to the parents together and with the child present, allowing the parents to include other relatives or friends if they would like.
2. Hold the child while giving the news.
3. Demonstrate actual clinical findings with the child.
4. Make similarities clear between the affected child and healthy children.
5. Encourage questions.
6. Schedule a second appointment for the near future to review this information, answer new questions, and make specific treatment recommendations.

A mental health worker can assist the parents in understanding and adjusting to the child's illness and their own emotional reactions. This approach establishes an early bond between the parents and the psychotherapist and makes further interventions easier if problems arise later in the course of the child's illness.

BEHAVIOR MANAGEMENT

Parents are especially likely to be interested in receiving assistance when their child poses behavioral problems. Some typical behavioral problems include temper tantrums, aggressiveness with siblings or peers, poor minding, and encopresis or enuresis. One effective strategy is to train parents in general behavior management strategies and programs already validated as being effective intervention techniques for specific problems. Parents can also read about these procedures ("bibliotherapy") and then consult with the psychotherapist about how to apply these techniques to their child.

Often, behavioral problems begin or worsen as the result of environmental changes that have placed the child under more stress. For example, some children develop enuresis or encopresis after being placed in a wheelchair or at other significant points in the progression of their disease. An effective intervention would teach parents a behavior management program and would involve the child in therapy interventions (individual or group). Alternatively, temper tantrums and poor minding may develop as family conflict increases. In this case, a behavioral management program could be combined with family therapy.

TREATMENT COMPLIANCE

Failures to comply with necessary treatment procedures can occur because of parental difficulties (see the discussion of treatment compliance in Chap. 21) or because of problems the child is experiencing. Useful procedures that enhance compliance by children include (1) education of parents and the child about the rationale for the treatment; (2) point or token systems as behavior management programs; (3) contracts between the parents and child; and (4) involvement of the child in individual and group therapy sessions to improve his adjustment to the neuromuscular disorder.

HOSPITALIZATION

Because a hospital environment is very stressful for children, prehospitalization preparation appears to be particularly helpful. Such preparation includes home visits by hospital staff members, teaching children anxiety-reduction and cognitive coping strategies, and showing films of other similar children coping effectively.

Adolescents, particularly, need assistance in maintaining a sense of identity and responsibility in the hospital. Interventions that allow the teenager privacy and a sense of personal territory (e.g., screens, placing beds near windows and in corners, allowing the teenager to arrange his area and to bring possessions from home) and that promote peer-group relations (social areas, telephones, favorable visiting hours for other adolescents) are important.

TERMINAL ILLNESS AND DEATH

The topic of terminal illness and death is difficult for the child, family, and treatment staff, yet a child and his family must have assistance in adjusting to this realistic fear. Family and individual interventions both appear to be particularly helpful. A special issue of the *Journal of Pediatric Psychology* (Koocher, 1977) has been devoted to specific counseling approaches for terminal illness and death, and is strongly recommended for treatment staff to read.

Models for the Delivery of Psychosocial Interventions

As with adults, a choice exists between including a mental health worker in a patient's treatment as standard operating procedure (SOP) or including the psychotherapist only when the child's difficulties indicate a referral is needed (PRN). Some factors that apply more to children than to adults make SOP even more preferable when treating children. Because children's coping styles are much less "set" than those of adults, children are both more vulnerable and more responsive to guidance. Early guidance is thus important to prevent chronic illness from resulting in chronic emotional and behavioral problems. Also, children are less able to express difficulties in a direct, verbal manner, and parents often do not detect problems early. For these reasons, pediatric psychologists prefer to take an active role in a child's treatment from the time of his initial presentation for treatment.

Three models for delivering psychosocial interventions that were discussed in Chapter 21 — independent treatment, professional-to-professional consultation, and the collaborative team — are also applicable to treatment of children. An additional role the pediatric psychologist assumes is that of consultant to the parents. In many instances, parents are capable of intervening successfully to assist their child, although parents need assistance in understanding their child's reactions. Parental intervention saves time for the therapist, preserves the parents' responsibility for their child, can stabilize family relationships, and may even enhance compliance with other components of the child's treatment.

MODES OF INTERVENTION

Individual Treatment

Individual sessions are not frequently used with children because they are less efficient than other methods. However, individual sessions can be effective for enhancing a child's self-esteem and for teaching children how to use cognitive self-instructional procedures for coping with stressful situations. Individual sessions may also help adolescents become appropriately independent of their families and smooth their adjustments to adult life.

Group Sessions

Group sessions are often overlooked in treating children, but can serve many useful purposes with children who have neuromuscular disorders. Many children with neuromuscular disease realistically feel "different" and are socially left behind by peers. In a group of similarly impaired children, a child can learn to develop improved social skills and to relate more effectively with unaffected peers and siblings.

Groups combining children and parents also provide emotional support, information sharing, and modeling of coping skills.

Family Meetings

An ill or disabled child poses a difficult task for a family to adjust to in ways that enhance the child's social and emotional development. Family meetings can foster positive adjustments and can help the family to avoid common pitfalls such as overprotectiveness, which leads to social and emotional immaturity, and expressions of hostility from over-stressed parents or siblings resentful of the special attention the ill child receives. Given the intensity of family relationships and the serious problems that can result, a mental health worker can often help a family to understand what is happening and can suggest mechanisms for change.

Parental Interventions

Raising a child who has a neuromuscular disorder causes a great deal of stress. Almost all parents benefit from some assistance in coping (see Chap. 21 for descriptions of adult coping mechanisms). Parents may feel guilty about the inherited nature of their child's illness. Rather than overprotecting the child, parents need to find more effective ways to reduce guilt.

A successful adjustment by the parents is the most important factor in determining how successful a child's adjustment to a neuromuscular disorder will be. Since children are quite sensitive and responsive to their parents' feelings, use their parents as models, and spend the majority of time under their parents' influence, improving the parents' adjustment has obvious benefits for the child.

TYPES OF INTERVENTION

Educational and cognitive rehabilitation interventions are described in Chapter 21. Two other useful interventions merit further description.

Play Therapy

Children communicate thoughts and feelings indirectly rather than by responding to direct questions or talking one-to-one. Often a child is silent or responds with an "I don't know" when asked "How do you feel about that?" Indirect communications are seen in the behavior of children — in the games they play, the pictures they draw, the stories they tell, and perhaps during explanations of other children's behavior. Play therapy is so-named because it makes use of indirect communications both as the source of information from the child and as a means for a therapist to suggest new ways of coping to the child. For example, a child may tell a story about a child who is home alone and afraid of robbers (indicating fear and also helplessness about losing things). Then the therapist may respond with a story about a child who is home alone and afraid of robbers, who makes sure the doors are locked and knows the telephone emergency number, and who spends the rest of the evening watching a good television show (fear, but with successful coping). Play therapy also enhances a child's self-esteem — if someone as important as a doctor is willing to play a game with him, the child feels that he is special in a positive way.

Behavior Modification

This method of intervention, based on the learning principle termed *operant conditioning*, can be quite effective for behavior management. As one or two specific behaviors are identified that are to be discouraged, one or two specific behaviors are identified that are to be concurrently encouraged. The consequences for each behavior are then specified: mild rewards for the desirable behavior, and mild punishment for the undesirable behavior. The program must be carried out consistently, with careful attention to record-keeping. Typically, children respond within two weeks as long as the program is managed consistently. The use of mild rewards and punishments seems to improve the likelihood that the behavioral changes will be maintained after the program is stopped.

The Treatment Plan

The treatment plan for a child follows the same three stages outlined in Chapter 21 for the adult. Assessment is done through interviews (child, parents, and family), psychological testing, screening inventories developed for use with children who have neuromuscular disorders, observations of actual behavior, and neuropsychological evaluations of cognitive abilities. A treatment plan is formulated based on this assessment, and the child and parents are included in this decision-making process. With the parents playing a central role, the plan is implemented and the effectiveness is regularly evaluated to adjust to unforeseen problems, the progression of the illness, and normal child development.

Suggested Readings

GOLDEN D, DAVIS J: Counseling parents after the birth of an infant with Down's syndrome. Child Today 3, 1974

KOOCHER GP (ed): Special issue on death and the child. Journal of Pediatric Psychology 2, 1977

MOOS RH: Coping with acute health crises. In Millon T, Green C, Meagher R (eds): Handbook of Clinical Health Psychology. New York, Plenum Press, 1982

WRIGHT L, WALKER CE: Treating the encopretic child. Clin Pediatr 16: 1042–1045, 1977

Neil L. Rosenberg

Nutrition for Patients
With Neuromuscular Disorders

Patients with progressive neuromuscular disorders may have difficulty meeting their nutritional requirements. Many nutritional concerns are common to all diseases causing progressive weakness, but others are unique to a particular disorder. Textbooks on nutrition usually refer to studies of healthy people, so that literature on nutritional assessment and management of patients with neuromuscular diseases is limited.

This chapter explores the role of nutrition in the care of patients with neuromuscular disorders. Although general principles of nutrition are included, those aspects of both malnutrition and overnutrition that are important in the proper management of progressive neuromuscular diseases are emphasized. Specific dietary manipulation and supplementation are discussed in detail.

Malnutrition (Starvation)

Several studies have evaluated the effects of starvation and malnutrition on the neuromuscular system of animals and humans. Muscle energy utilization varies almost a hundred-fold from rest to maximum metabolic activity, whereas nerve cells continually have a high metabolic rate. As a result, early neuromuscular changes following malnutrition affect peripheral nerves more than skeletal muscle. The effects of malnutrition on peripheral nerves may be related to specific deficiencies of vitamins such as B_1, B_6, or B_{12}, as well as protein–calorie malnutrition. Because skeletal muscle is the largest and most important protein reservoir of the body and is the major site for various steps in the metabolism of amino acids, severe malnutrition eventually impairs muscle function as well.

Fortunately, malnutrition secondary to starvation is infrequent in the Western world. To maintain proper nutrition, a person needs to have properly functioning mastication and swallowing, esophageal motility, gastric emptying, intestinal motility and absorption, and hormonal regulation during meals (i.e., insulin release). Several of these functions can be impaired in neuromuscular diseases. One disorder commonly associated with starvation is motor neuron disease (amyotrophic lateral sclerosis — ALS). The major cause of malnutrition is dysphagia, although defects in the other digestive steps may also be occurring. Several other neuromuscular disorders are associated with varying degrees of dysphagia (see Neuromuscular Disorders Associated with Dysphagia, below) and may even be transient and reverse with therapy (e.g., myasthenia gravis). Bulbar dysfunction in motor neuron disease occurs because of lower motor neuron and upper motor neuron degeneration. Once dysphagia develops, rapid loss in weight can occur over several weeks, alarming both the patient and clinician. During this period of bulbar dysfunction, patients with ALS are likely to choke or develop aspiration pneumonia and respiratory insufficiency. At least part of their deterioration develops secondarily from the effects of starvation on the neuromuscular control of respiration and on the immune system.

NEUROMUSCULAR DISORDERS ASSOCIATED WITH DYSPHAGIA

1. Anterior horn cell
   Motor neuron disease (amyotrophic lateral sclerosis)
   Juvenile bulbar disease (Fazio-Landau)
   Poliomyelitis
   Spinomuscular atrophies
2. Peripheral nerve
   Guillain-Barré syndrome
   Diphtheria
   Chronic progressive demyelinating polyneuropathy
   Tick paralysis
3. Neuromuscular junction
   Myasthenia gravis
   Botulism
   Organophosphate poisoning
4. Muscle
   Myotonic dystrophy
   Oculopharyngeal dystrophy
   Inflammatory myopathies

EFFECTS OF STARVATION ON RESPIRATION

Several factors predispose to fatigue of respiratory muscles. Because inspiratory muscles require energy to contract (expiration is passive), energy depletion of inspiratory muscles can result in respiratory failure in neuromuscular disorders. Malnutrition and catabolic states, by depleting energy stores, further weaken diseased inspiratory muscles and may play an important role in the pathophysiology of respiratory failure.

Apart from any primary disease process that impairs respiratory muscles, further impairment produced by nutritional deficiency should not be overlooked because the latter may be reversible. This point is illustrated by a patient with motor neuron disease followed in our clinic who sustained a 50-lb weight loss over three months and required assisted ventilation because of respiratory failure. After careful nutritional assessment and tube feedings, the patient gained 10 lb and was weaned free of the respirator. She enjoyed a reasonable quality of life until her death three and one-half months later.

EFFECTS OF STARVATION ON THE IMMUNE SYSTEM

Worldwide, malnutrition is the most frequent cause of immunodeficiency. Although more common in underdeveloped countries, similar problems can occur in patients who are elderly or who have a variety of systemic diseases. Patients with malignancies, malabsorption syndromes, or inflammatory bowel disease, or in the immediate postsurgical period, have all demonstrated a variety of nutritional deficiencies. Simultaneous defects in the immune response may include cell-mediated responses, phagocytic activity, the complement system, secretory antibodies, and antibody affinity. Such secondary immunodeficiency states lead to a higher incidence of infection, which only further prevents recovery in the malnourished patient.

The effect of malnutrition on immune function in neuromuscular disorders has not been studied. However, because patients with neuromuscular disorders often develop intercurrent infections, usually pulmonary, immune dysfunction secondary to malnutrition may be contributing to their decline. Certainly, improvement in nutritional status, whether attributable to increasing strength or immunocompetence, can significantly and favorably alter the clinical course in selected patients.

NUTRITIONAL THERAPY OF STARVATION

If a patient with a neuromuscular disorder is unable to maintain his weight and hydration, or if he is aspirating, some type of tube feeding should be instituted. Tube feedings require liquid diets that can be administered by several routes (Table 23 – 1). Feeding tubes currently in use are narrow-diameter (No. 8 French), flexible tubes that have essentially replaced the large-diameter and relatively rigid tubes used in the past. In order to decrease the risk of gastroesophageal reflux and aspira-

Table 23–1 Methods for Nutritional Support

Type of Tube	Indications	Problems
Nasogastric	Transient disorders; alert patient	Risk of tracheal aspiration Esophagitis Gastric erosion Discomfort Excessive salivation, gagging
Cervical esophagostomy	Progressive disorder; alert patient	Risk of tracheal aspiration
Gastrostomy	Progressive disorder; alert patient	Slight risk of tracheal aspiration Decreased mobility of diaphragm from pain in patients with existing respiratory insufficiency
Jejunostomy	Patient with decreased level of consciousness	Risk of peritonitis if tube inadvertently removed Complex feeding regimens High incidence of diarrhea from feedings

tion, the tip of the tube should be placed into the duodenum. The holes in the tube tip can be made larger to prevent clogging of the tube with either viscous diet supplements or pureed feedings. There are a variety of liquid supplements that are canned in a ready-to-use form and can be used as the sole source of nourishment. Pureed feedings, prepared at home in a blender, can be used as an alternative to more costly commercial preparations. When properly counseled by a dietitian, such home-prepared diets contain adequate amounts of nutrients and have the added psychological benefit of being "home-cooked." Although the patient can obtain most (if not all) nourishment from tube feedings, it may be of additional psychological benefit for the patient to be able to taste foods. In this case, the patient or concerned family members can place minute quantities of food in the patient's mouth in order for him to be able to maintain taste sense.

Tube feedings should always be administered with the patient in an upright position to minimize the risk of gastroesophageal reflux and tracheal aspiration. The solution can be infused slowly with a large syringe attached to the tube, but it is usually better tolerated when given more slowly through a volumetric infusion pump or dripped in by gravity from elevated bags. Small volumes of dilute feedings should be tried initially (one-half full strength). The volume and concentration can be

Table 23 – 2   Checklist of Problems Associated with Tube Feedings

Problem	Treatment
Continued weight loss	Check total calories. Add peripheral alimentation if necessary. Avoid weight gain over 0.7 kg/day.
Diarrhea and cramping	Decrease infusion rate. Dilute feeding mixture. Consider carbohydrate, fat, and protein sources in formula (e.g., milk allergy). Add antidiarrheal drug. Check sanitation/storage procedures.
Aspiration	Check size of tube. Elevate head. Discontinue feeding.
Esophageal erosion	Remove feeding tube. Change to gastrostomy or jejunosotomy feeding system.
Clogged tube	Flush with water. Replace tube and make holes in tip larger.
Hyperglycemia/glucosuria	Decrease infusion rate. Administer insulin.
Edema	Change to formula with reduced sodium content.
Congestive heart failure	Reduce infusion rate to less than 2000 ml/day. Reduce sodium content. Administer digoxin and diuretics.
Hypernaturemia/hypercalcemia	Adjust electrolyte content.
Essential fatty-acid deficiency	Check solution for essential fatty-acid content. Supplement orally or parenterally with Intralipid.

increased gradually as the patient tolerates the feedings. Complications that can arise during the course of tube feedings are listed in Table 23-2 and are elaborated in Chapter 10.

Obesity

Obesity is defined as an excessive ratio of fat to lean body mass and can be evaluated on the basis of weight-for-height and skin-fold thickness. Obesity can be a major problem for neuromuscular disease patients because excess weight further impairs the ability to maintain independent ambulation and compromises respiration.

The physician's goal should be to increase the patient's ratio of strength to body weight either by increasing strength or by decreasing weight. Since exercise in neuromuscular diseases is not easily accomplished and may be detrimental (see Chap. 15), an equally useful method of increasing the ratio of strength to body weight is by decreasing body weight. In such patients, relatively small gains in weight can have a major impact on physical performance such as climbing stairs or walking. An even more serious consequence of obesity in neuromuscular diseases is respiratory failure. The added force of a distended abdomen predisposes to fatigue by increasing the work of displacing the diaphragm. Loss of weight under these circumstances may not only significantly prolong the length but also the quality of life.

Reduction of caloric intake must be stressed to all patients because losing weight is more difficult for the physically handicapped, who cannot exercise easily. The dangers of excessive weight gain should be pointed out early and the patient's weight monitored at each visit. Any weight gain should be approached by evaluating the patient's diet and subsequently restricting food intake. There are many faddish methods of weight loss by dietary manipulation, some of which are as drastic as starvation. The safest and most common-sense approach is to decrease caloric intake but to maintain normal proportions of protein, carbohydrate, and fat in the diet.

Nutritional Manipulation in Specific Disorders

See Chapter 12 for clinical details of each illness.

NEUROMUSCULAR DISORDERS ARISING FROM VITAMIN DEFICIENCIES

Vitamin B_{12} Deficiency

Vitamin B_{12} deficiency can arise from a variety of causes and is commonly associated with a peripheral neuropathy. Less than 1% of vitamin B_{12} reaches the blood by passive diffusion, so that gastric intrinsic factor is necessary for its absorption. With vitamin B_{12} deficiency secondary to lack of intrinsic factor (pernicious anemia), 1000 μg of vitamin B_{12} should be given intramuscularly each month in order to achieve the levels necessary to reverse the disease process.

Vitamin B_6 (Pyridoxine) Deficiency

Deficiency of vitamin B_6 is associated with a sensory motor polyneuropathy. Although uncommon, it occurs with celiac disease and in patients receiving isoniazid for tuberculosis who have not received vitamin B$_6$ supplementation. To prevent the appearance of the neuropathy, 30 mg per day of pyridoxine is sufficient.

Thiamine Deficiency

A variety of neurologic disorders occur in chronic alcoholics who also consume a substandard diet. Although many of these problems are related to thiamine deficiency, there is growing evidence of direct alcohol toxicity. The most common manifestation of thiamine deficiency in alcoholics is a sensorimotor polyneuropathy. All alcoholics should receive thiamine supplementation.

Vitamin C Deficiency

Peripheral neuropathy is rare with vitamin C deficiency (scurvy). When it has occurred, large amounts of vitamin C have reversed symptoms.

Vitamin E Deficiency

A rare neuromuscular disorder has recently been reported that is caused by vitamin E deficiency in children with liver disease who cannot absorb fat-soluble vitamins. Weakness from nerve and muscle injury reverses with parenteral vitamin E supplementation.

DISORDERS OF GLYCOGEN METABOLISM

In several glycogen storage diseases of muscle, of which phosphorylase deficiency is most common (McArdle's disease), painful muscle cramps and even rhabdomyolysis develop following exertion. In several studies, the work capacity of patients with muscle phosphorylase deficiency was increased by intravenous glucose infusions or by the hyperglycemic effect of glucagon. This effect has not been seen in the other disorders of glycogen metabolism. Dietary manipulation by frequent oral ingestion of sugars has also been attempted to bypass the metabolic block and provide glycolytic fuels to the muscle. Unfortunately, this method is not usually effective and can cause excessive weight gain. Attempts to raise serum free-fatty acids and ketone bodies by diet or drugs might also theoretically be helpful, since patients develop a "second wind" phenomenon where they seem to improve after an initial period of pain and cramps. The mechanism of improvement has been attributed to a shift in muscle metabolism from *anaerobic* (glucose) to *aerobic* (free-fatty acids) pathways.

DISORDERS OF LIPID METABOLISM

Although glycogen metabolism is well defined for muscle, muscle lipid metabolism and the clinical disorders associated with enzymatic deficiencies have only recently been described. As a result, studies of dietary manipulation for these disorders are only preliminary.

Carnitine Deficiency

Carnitine deficiency can manifest either as a systemic disorder with episodic hepatic insufficiency, nausea, vomiting, confusion, or coma, in addition to a progressive neuromuscular disorder, or it may appear only as a muscle disorder with generalized weakness (usually starting in childhood) with slow progression but occasionally with superimposed periods of rapidly increasing weakness. Some patients with either form have responded clinically after supplementation with high doses of carnitine even though muscle carnitine levels were not altered with this therapy. Other patients with a lipid myopathy secondary to carnitine deficiency responded favorably to treatment with riboflavin or corticosteriods, but not to carnitine replacement.

Carnitine Palmityltransferase Deficiency

Clinically, carnitine palmityltransferase (CPT) deficiency is characterized by recurrent bouts of muscle aching or cramps and myoglobinuria that are often precipitated by prolonged exercise or fasting. Reduction of

Table 23–3 Gastrointestinal Problems in Myotonic Dystrophy

Problem	Area Involved	Mechanism	Treatment
Tracheal aspiration	Pharynx	Delayed relaxation	Soft diet Improve swallowing technique
Dysphagia	Pharynx	Delayed relaxation	Soft diet Improve swallowing technique
	Esophagus	Reduced motility Dilatation	Soft or liquid diet .
Bloating after meals	Stomach	Dilatation	Smaller and more frequent meals
Diarrhea	Small bowel	Malabsorption	Treat cause of malabsorption Low-fat diet
Abdominal pain, nausea, vomiting	Gallbladder	Delayed emptying, gallstones	Low-fat diet
Lower abdominal cramping	Colon	"Irritable bowel syndrome"	Bulking agents
Fecal incontinence	Anal sphincter	Myotonia of sphincter	Bowel program instruction

attacks of muscle pain and myoglobinuria has been obtained by frequent feeding with a high-carbohydrate, low-fat diet.

PERIODIC PARALYSIS

The periodic paralyses are a group of disorders characterized by episodes of weakness or frank paralysis that are often precipitated by large meals, particularly those containing a large carbohydrate load. Restriction of carbohydrates, careful regulation of potassium intake, and smaller, more frequent meals may help decrease the frequency of attacks.

MYOTONIC DYSTROPHY

Patients with this systemic disorder may have numerous gastrointestinal disturbances in addition to muscle weakness, cataracts, cardiac arrhythmias, and intellectual impairment. Table 23-3 lists typical gastrointestinal symptoms, as well as their etiology, pathogenesis, and treatment.

Nutritional Assessment of the Neuromuscular Patient

Clinical assessment of a patient's nutritional status is obtained by history and physical examination, anthropometric measurements, and specific laboratory tests. The history should stress the presence or absence of any recent weight changes, chronic conditions that may interfere with good nutritional status, any physical handicaps that may result in inadequate food intake, and any predisposing conditions contributing to poor nutrition, such as alcoholism, chemotherapy, or drug use. Analysis of a dietary history through a daily calorie count may reveal evidence of vitamin, mineral, protein, or calorie deficiencies.

Physical examination should stress appearance of hair, eyes, skin, and teeth. Changes in skin or hair color and texture, loss of muscle mass or subcutaneous fat, or morphologic changes of the tongue (such as atrophic glossitis seen in certain deficiency states) and gums may be of diagnostic significance.

Anthropometric measurements provide further quantitative measurements that are indications of nutritional status. Height and weight should be measured and compared with ideal body weight. Recent changes in weight can also be evaluated by the following formulas:

$$\% \text{ of usual body weight} = \frac{\text{current weight}}{\text{usual weight}} \times 100$$

$$\% \text{ of weight change} = \frac{\text{usual weight} - \text{current weight}}{\text{usual weight}} \times 100$$

A decrease of greater than 10% of usual weight over a 6-month period should be considered a significant weight loss. Measurement of triceps skin fold is an indirect estimate of body fat or calorie stores and correlates well with other measures of body fat when done correctly. Measurement of mid upper arm circumference is an indicator of both calorie and protein stores.

Laboratory tests commonly used to assess nutritional status include total lymphocyte count, serum albumin, serum transferrin, total iron-binding capacity, and serum vitamin levels, especially vitamins A and C.

After careful nutritional assessment, a nutritional care plan with clearly defined problems and goals is needed. Energy needs are defined by calculating basal energy expenditures (BEE) and then adding energy requirements as needed with varying amounts of stress:

$$\text{Men: BEE} = 66 + (13.7 \times w) = (5 \times h) - (6.8 \times a)$$

$$\text{Women: BEE} = 655 + (9.6 \times w) = (1.7 \times h) - (4.7 \times a)$$

where w = actual weight in kilograms; h = height in centimeters; and a = age in years.

25–30 calories/kg needed normally to maintain weight
35 calories/kg needed to gain weight
40–50 calories/kg needed for mild exertion
50–80 calories/kg needed for severe exertion

The recommended daily requirements for protein can be met with 0.8 g protein/kg of ideal body weight. Ordinary nutritional demands require 1.0 g to 1.5 g/kg. Protein needs are increased to 2.0 g to 3.0 g/kg when under stress. The type of diet and whether dietary supplements are needed (oral or through tube feedings) should be determined. Follow-up to assess results and to decide if further changes are necessary is a vital part of any dietary program.

Suggested Readings

APPENZELLER O, ATKINSON R: Nutrition for physical performance. In Appenzeller O, Atkinson R (eds): Sports Medicine, pp 53–93. Baltimore, Urban & Schwarzenberg, 1981

ASKANAZI J, WEISSMAN C, ROSENBAUM SH, et al: Nutrition and the respiratory system. Crit Care Med 10:163–172, 1982

BROWN MJ: Treatable neuropathies. In Griggs RC, Moxley RT III (eds): Advances in Neurology, vol 17, pp 235–247. New York, Raven Press, 1977

CARROLL JE, BROOKE MH, SHUMATE JB, et al: Carnitine intake and excretion in neuromuscular diseases. Am J Clin Nutr 34:2693–2698, 1981

CARROLL JE, SHUMATE JB, BROOKE MH, et al: Riboflavin-responsive lipid myopathy and carnitine deficiency. Neurology (NY) 31:1557–1559, 1981

CHANDRA RK: Immunology of Nutritional Disorders, pp 1–110. Chicago, Year Book Medical Publishers, 1980.

DASTUR DK, MANGHANI D, OSUNTOKUN BO, et al: Neuromuscular and related changes in malnutrition: A review. J Neurol Sci 55:207–230, 1982

DIMAURO S, EASTWOOD AB: Disorders of glycogen and lipid metabolism. In Griggs RC, Moxley RT III (eds): Advances in Neurology, vol 17, pp 123–142. New York, Raven Press, 1977

DIMAURO S, TREVISAN C, HAYS A: Disorders of lipid metabolism in muscle. Muscle Nerve 3:369–388, 1980

GORMICAN A: Tube feeding: Overview. Dietetic Currents (Ross Laboratories) 2:1–16, 1975

KAMINSKI MV: Tube Feeding: Tips and Techniques. Norwich, NY, Eaton Laboratory Publication, 1973

MOXLEY RT III, KEMPF C: Nutritional management. In Mulder DW (ed): The Diagnosis and Treatment of Amyotrophic Lateral Sclerosis, pp 269–289. Boston, Houghton Mifflin Professional Publishers, Medical Division, 1980

ROUSSOS C, MACKLEM PT: The respiratory muscles. N Engl J Med 307:786–797, 1982

VANITALLIE TB, YANG MU: Current concepts in nutrition: Diet and weight loss. N Engl J Med 297:1158–1161, 1977

WEISSMAN C, ASKANAZI J, ROSENBAUM S, et al: Amino acids and respiration. Ann Intern Med 98:41–44, 1983

Part IV

ADDITIONAL MANAGEMENT CONCERNS

Therapist – Patient Relationship in Chronic Care of the Disabled Patient

According to one view of the interaction with a patient, the physician or therapist, having accurately diagnosed the patient's physical, psychological, and social state, provides appropriate technical interventions and psychosocial support in a one-way interaction in which the caregiver does something for or to the patient while remaining relatively neutral himself. This concept is somewhat analogous to the old "blank screen" view of psychotherapy, in which it was assumed that since the psychotherapist did not have feelings of his own and did not reveal anything about himself, the patient's feelings about the therapist reflected only the patient's fantasies and projections.

More recent evidence suggests that the concept of a totally neutral provider of care is a goal that is not only impossible, but also one that would not be desirable even if it could be achieved. Experienced clinicians have learned — often painfully — that therapists, nurses, physicians, and other caregivers are people before they are professionals and that they cannot truly hide their emotions from their patients to whom they are very important and who observe their reactions closely. In addition, the loneliness and isolation experienced by many chronically ill patients — especially if they are depressed — are exacerbated by excessive emotional distance from those who care for them, while much of the improvement in behavioral and emotional problems that commonly accompany chronic illness and disability is encouraged by the clinician's serving as a role model for open and direct communication and more adaptive behavior. Since reactions to the patient may also be an important source of information about the patient's feelings, an awareness of the clinician's mood often provides important data about the patient. This chapter concerns ways in which the caretaker's emotions and behaviors may be used to understand the patient and demonstrates means of avoiding counterproductive interactions with patients that frequently arise in chronic care.

Reactions to Chronic Illness

Specific reactions to chronic illness depend on the personality of the patient and whether he has grown up with the illness or was previously healthy (see Chaps. 11, 12, and 22). However, all chronically ill patients must contend with certain issues regardless of the nature of their illness.

THE SICK ROLE

In Western society, the sick person assumes a social role that defines his relationship with other people: the patient gives up normal responsibilities and is cared for by others, in return for which he is expected to cooperate fully with treatment and attempt to improve. Patients who feel comfortable being cared for by others tolerate the sick role well, especially when it is of limited duration, and many people are able to take a break from their usual activities if they are sufficiently ill and if they know that they will resume these activities soon.

The sick role becomes more problematic to patients who are afraid of dependency or who crave it excessively. Patients who yearn to give up all of their responsibilities and have someone else take care of them may seek the sick role through excessive complaints that put them in a dependent position. However, those who are afraid of the sick role tend to deny illness and avoid diagnosis and treatment, becoming extremely anxious if they find that they will always be ill and will need to remain in the sick role indefinitely. Because, in certifying that a patient is ill, the physician and allied health personnel are the agents of society who both confer the sick role and help the patient to leave the sick role by becoming well as quickly as possible, they may experience difficulty carrying out their social roles when they work with patients who refuse to leave the sick role or who cannot bear to remain in the sick role when there is no guarantee that the illness will ever end.

REGRESSION

Acutely ill patients who are reminded of the dependency of childhood may adopt a way of thinking that is more appropriate to a child than to an adult; this is characterized by clinging, demanding behavior with a low frustration tolerance that may appear stubborn, depressed, or even psychotic to the observer who does not realize that psychologically the patient is a child in an adult's body. Chronically ill patients who do not assume as much responsibility as possible for their own care may remain regressed and be chronically unable to solve their own problems, as would a small child. Even patients who are not regressed tend to view their caretakers as parental or authority figures, an attitude that may be expressed as inappropriately submissive or rebellious behavior.

ANGER

Chronically ill patients are frequently angry at fate for making them sick, at themselves for being impaired, at physicians for not curing them, and at everyone else for being healthy. While the first two feelings may elicit sympathy, health-care personnel, family members, and friends often become angry, feel guilty, or act defensively in response to the latter two types of anger. When the patient or his family is angry with the physician, fear of retaliation by the doctor may result in the expression of this anger toward allied health personnel.

DENIAL

A person who ignores fears that are evoked by an illness, such as the fear of dying, of being mutilated, of feeling helpless, or of losing affection, or who even ignores some aspects of the disease itself, may relieve anxiety effectively in acute situations. However, chronically ill patients may become noncompliant and frustrating when they continue to ignore physical or emotional states evoked by the illness that frighten or otherwise bother them. A common response by the clinician is to attempt to confront patients with the unpleasant information regarding their disease, especially when the patients deny strong emotions. This usually frightens the patient even more, resulting in increased denial that is manifested as insistence that he will be able to accomplish some impossible goal and refusal to participate in appropriate rehabilitative efforts because the patient does not believe that he is ill.

HELPLESSNESS

Many chronically ill patients feel that they have lost control of their health and their lives. Some may adopt a passive attitude, fail to comply with appropriate treatment because they believe that nothing they do can have any significant positive impact, or refuse to exert any effort on their own behalf. Sometimes patients actively make themselves worse because they feel that, while they cannot have any influence over whether they get better, they can at least feel some control if they make themselves worse. Such behavior is often mysterious and frightening to the therapist, who may feel helpless himself when he realizes that his treatment is not having the expected effect.

Projective Identification

A patient may at times relieve himself of unpleasant emotional states by giving them to the therapist who works closely with him. Projective identification is like projection in that the patient attributes his feelings or attitudes to someone else. Through subtle forms of behavior, the patient then induces that very state in the other person. In projection, which may be seen in paranoid and organic mental states, the patient has no awareness of the feeling whatsoever. In projective identification, which is not uncommon in physically ill individuals, the patient is aware of the emotional state but experiences it as coming from someone else. For example, the patient who feels helpless may present the therapist with a list of problems that he invites advice about while rejecting each solution that is offered, making the therapist feel progressively more helpless as his interventions do not work. As the patient becomes aware of the caregiver's growing sense of frustration and helplessness, which the patient now feels are the physician's or therapist's problems, the patient becomes angry in return because he feels that he is being attacked. The therapist may therefore first become aware of the patient's emotional state by paying close attention to his own feelings, as for instance when he feels frustrated and helpless and asks himself whether the patient is attempting to gain control over feelings of helplessness by making the clinician feel even more helpless.

Splitting

A patient who has difficulty experiencing postitive and negative feelings at the same time may keep himself from becoming angry at people he likes by feeling good about some people taking care of him and bad about others. One result may be that caretakers who are "good" in the patient's eyes are treated well, while the patient is hostile toward those who arouse negative feelings, creating two groups, one that values the patient and one that resents him. Disagreements may then erupt about the patient's diagnosis, treatment, or personality, not infrequently between the physician, who may be the recipient of the patient's admiration, and nursing and allied health personnel, who may be subjected to the patient's negative feelings. By behaving differently toward different caretakers, a patient may also "split" the staff in order to focus on the disagreements between others and to avoid thinking about his illness or to feel more powerful by making others feel confused. When disagreements between health-care personnel arise, the investigation of the patient's feelings about being disabled is important, especially the assessment of the patient's feelings of helplessness and the patient's ability to express legitimate complaints toward people he depends on.

Transference

Because human beings tend to learn from their past experiences, everyone brings the effects of past relationships into interactions in the present. Most of the time, the memory of past relationships does not influence the present excessively. However, under certain circumstances someone who resembles an important individual encountered in the past may be expected to be just like that person, resulting in current behavior and feelings resembling attitudes toward the original person. This phenomenon is called *transference*, the process by which feelings about someone in the past are transferred onto someone in the present. Because transference feelings repeat past experiences, they

Table 24 – 1 Common Transference Reactions Experienced in Chronically Ill Patients

Type of Transference	Characteristics	Common Physician Reactions to Patient	Management
Eroticized	Intense romantic feelings, often mixed with covertly hostile demands for attention	Anxiety Attraction to the patient	Maintain appropriate professional distance. Discuss patient's feelings openly.
Suspicious	Hostility and attacks on interest and competence	Anger Defensiveness Wish to correct alleged mistakes	Do not take patient's attacks personally. Do not confront if the patient expresses hostility only as a means of maintaining interpersonal distance.
Entitled dependent	Attempts to assign responsibility for the patient's life to the therapist and extort special favors that are felt to be deserved because of past deprivations	Hostility Pity	Do not take responsibility for the patient's life. Encourage the patient to play a more active role in therapy.
Idealizing	Unrealistic, overestimation of the therapist's prowess	Embarrassment Acceptance of patient's praise as justified	Do not confront unless the therapist or other health-care providers are also devalued.

tend to be inflexible and inappropriate to the current situation. Transference attitudes recreate the past. For example, the chronically ill patient's dependency on the health-care provider may lead to anger, submissiveness, rebelliousness, fear, admiration, or other feelings that, because they reflect the patient's attitudes toward parental figures, are out of proportion to the clinician's behavior. Chronically ill patients are especially likely to experience transference feelings toward their caretakers because of the prolonged nature of the dependent interaction. Since transference reactions (Table 24-1) do not represent genuine feelings about the caretakers, the avoidance of a direct response is important.

Countertransference

Health-care providers' reactions to their patients may represent realistic responses to the patients' situations or to subtle or overt provocations, or they may be derived from other sources. If the clinician is tired or upset, he may be more irritable with all of his patients. However, a particular patient may evoke transference if the patient reminds the therapist of some other important person in his life. Regardless of immediate stresses on the caretaker, however, certain aspects of the management of the chronically ill patient may evoke stereotyped attitudes. For example, the intense physical interaction between therapist or nurse and patient tends to evoke strong feelings, especially attachment, while the need to encourage some behaviors and limit others often evokes parental attitudes. Commonly, caretakers identify with patients of similar age or background and assume that the patients feel what the caretakers think they would feel under similar circumstances. In addition, therapists who during training were exposed primarily to acutely ill patients who improved, died, or at least left the hospital may believe that medical care is usually terminable and then feel guilty and inadequate when faced with a condition that cannot be reversed or even ameliorated.

Clinicians who do not feel comfortable with their own dependency needs may encourage inappropriate independence in patients who need to learn how to depend on others without giving up all of their autonomy. The feelings of helplessness that are commonly evoked when no definitive treatment is available also may cause considerable distress. Finally, the capacity to ignore feelings resulting from one's best efforts having at best a palliative effect and from the eventual loss of more severely ill patients, which usually eases the task of working with the chronically ill patient, may cause difficulties if this capacity interferes with an awareness of disturbing feelings in the patient.

In addition to these general tendencies, specific unrealistic attitudes toward patients may be evoked in certain situations, resulting in "countertransference binds" in which the therapist's attitude is determined by unrealistic or inflexible attitudes.

RESCUE FANTASY

Particularly when the patient expresses the belief that only a particular person can help him, the clinician may come to believe that he can effect significant changes that nobody else has been able to achieve.

COUNTERTRANSFERENCE PITY

As opposed to empathy for the patient, pity often results from a mixture of hopelessness and covert hostility, and may result in the therapist lowering his expectations of what the patient can do for himself because he believes that the patient cannot and should not be expected to do much else.

COUNTERTRANSFERENCE HATE

Manipulative and self-destructive patients can evoke intense dislike. If the caretaker feels that it is inappropriate or bad to dislike a patient, negative feelings may be disguised by excessive efforts to please and help the patient. At the same time, hostility may be expressed covertly by forgetting appointments, seeing the patient only briefly, demanding too much or too little of the patient, or making mistakes about treatment.

DESTRUCTIVE TREATMENT EFFORTS

Patients with self-destructive tendencies may manipulate their therapists into agreeing to treatment plans that are inappropriate or harmful to both patient and clinician. This behavior may occur when strong narcotics are administered to a patient with chronic pain or the therapist agrees that a paraplegic patient will be able to walk. Although the pain remits somewhat initially, it eventually increases and the physician's reluctance to confront the patient leads to larger prescriptions as the patient becomes increasingly demanding of the medication to which he has become addicted. Similarly, the paralyzed patient is initially encouraged but soon feels disappointed and betrayed when it becomes apparent that the treatment plan was unrealistic.

Maximizing Constructive Aspects of the Therapist — Patient Relationship

Several simple guidelines should help the health-care provider to avoid destructive interactions while using emotional reactions to the patient to facilitate treatment.

1. Convey a realistically hopeful approach to the patient's emotional as well as physical health. Even when the illness cannot be cured, the patient can achieve a better adaptation to it.
2. Pay attention to all feelings about the patient, no matter how inappropriate or unacceptable they may seem. Most of the time, feelings and thoughts about a patient reflect the patient's emotional state. Intense countertransference feelings are much more likely to indicate a problem in the *patient* than in the *caretaker*. Chronically ill patients are especially likely to evoke anger, helplessness, anxiety, despair, and unrealistic optimism.
3. Consult regularly with colleagues. Regular discussion of difficult patients with other members of the health-care team aids in the recognition, before they become too severe, of reactions that the clinician is ignoring out of a natural tendency to minimize unpleasant emotions.
4. Set limits on destructive and self-destructive behavior. An agreement to treatment that may be harmful to the patient or the therapist in order to placate or humor the patient is never helpful. When patients ask for inappropriate treatments or otherwise attempt to undo therapeutic efforts, the meaning of this behavior should be pointed out to the patient and the clinician should refuse to comply.
5. Interpret the meaning of the patient's behavior. Patients communicate strong emotions through the medium of the therapist – patient relationship because patients are not aware of these feelings or are unable to express them directly. If a patient expresses feelings about his illness in words, the need to express them in action usually decreases and makes him feel that he is effective at least in his ability to make others understand him.
6. Point out inappropriate and negative aspects of the patient's behavior. When transference feelings enhance the clinician – patient relationship, caregivers need not point them out to the patient. This situation might occur when the patient expresses admiration that is not completely justified by the therapist's behavior but that helps him to continue to cooperate with therapy even when no obvious benefit is apparent. On the other hand, negative feelings should always be discussed openly. Realistic complaints should be acknowledged, while pointing out that transference is derived from another relationship. For example, when the physician reminds the patient of someone he dislikes, it may help the patient to continue to work more effectively with the physician if this transference to a previous relationship is pointed out to him.
7. Schedule regular open discussions with all members of the treatment team. Disagreements should be aired openly with the understanding that they are likely to be provoked by the patient. Everyone should agree or at least adhere to the approach that is adopted with a difficult patient.

8. Remain aware of the therapist's emotional limits. Working with chronically ill patients, especially when they are terminally ill or may be expected to follow a progressively downhill course, is extremely draining emotionally. The clinician who overestimates his emotional reserves and becomes intimately involved with too many patients whose illnesses result in their making extreme psychological demands may eventually experience frustration, anger, depression, and other signs of "burnout." If it is impossible to avoid working physically closely with a large number of severely ill or dying patients, other members of the team can be extremely helpful in sharing the emotional burden and developing more intimate relationships with patients who are encountered when the therapist is already involved with a significant number of chronically ill patients. When one has become involved with a chronically ill patient who becomes substantially worse or dies, sufficient time should be allowed to mourn the loss of the patient and to receive support from family, friends, and colleagues.

Suggested Readings

ARAONSON G: Some types of transference and countertransference. Bull Menninger Clin 38:355–359, 1974

DUBOVSKY SL: Psychotherapeutics in Primary Care. New York, Grune & Stratton, 1981

GREENSON RR: Loving, hating and indifference towards the patient. Int J Psychoanal 1:259–265, 1974

GROVES HJ: Taking care of the hateful patient. N Eng J Med 298:883–887, 1978

MALTSBERGER HT, BUIE DH: Countertransference hate in the treatment of suicidal patients. Arch Gen Psychiatry 30:625–630, 1974

Carole Ann Brammell
F. Patrick Maloney

25

Wheelchair Prescriptions

In 1977, three of every 1000 citizens of the United States used wheelchairs, representing over 500 million dollars in cost for 645,000 chairs. Many chairs are sold without prescription or professional guidance. If the need is for temporary or casual transportation, this approach may be adequate. Other wheelchairs, however, need to be prescribed with special care to meet specific patient needs.

A wheelchair is a combination posture-support system that includes a backrest, seat, armrests, and footplates; a propulsion system that includes wheels and drive mechanism; and brakes. A mobility clinic serves the needs of patients and provides education for medical and allied health personnel in the principles of wheelchair prescription.

The clinic's philosophy emphasizes independent living and quality of life for both patients and caretakers. Inadequate wheelchair prescriptions frequently occur when physicians, vendors, and families fail to consider both the precise physical needs of the patient and the social environment in which the chair will be used. Patient convenience and functional limitation may temper the resultant prescription. The expense of unnecessary wheelchair "gadgets" should be avoided. A wheelchair purchase should be made with the same care and thought as buying a car. Indeed, some motorized wheelchairs cost more than a compact car.

Roles of the Clinical Staff

Regular members of our mobility clinic team are a physician, occupational therapist, social worker, and vendor representatives. A nurse and physical therapist attend for specific cases. The responsibilities of the individual team members are as follows:

1. The *physician* has three major functions: (1) taking the patient's history and performing the physical examination; (2) evaluating the patient for support services, equipment, and vocational counseling; and (3) writing the wheelchair prescription. Consultation reports from the physical therapist, occupational therapist, and psychologist and records from previous hospitalizations are reviewed by the physician. The physician identifies medical and safety considerations and their severity, such as skin problems, focal weakness, tremors, and imparied balance.
2. The *occupational therapist* assesses a patient's functional needs, including activity of daily living skills and upper extremity function. Chairs are delivered to the occupational therapy clinic for checking the prescription's accuracy. This check includes the adjustment of footrests, head positions, hand and mouth control operation and placement for motorized chairs, and correct seat belt placement. The patient or caretaker receives instructions and practice in collapsing and lifting a manual wheelchair, in maneuvering the chair on curbs, and in transfer safety. Driving sessions for motorized wheelchairs are provided as needed.
3. The *social worker*, as coordinator of the clinic, schedules appointments, arranges transportation to the clinic, and determines insurance coverage or the availability of alternative funding sources. The social worker also is the liaison to other health-care providers, the family or caretakers, and community resources.
4. *Vendors* give valuable advice concerning the range of chair types, modifications, and accessories, and provide information about availability and cost of new and improved items. Vendors gain insight about very specific needs and the emphasis required for chair modifications and may take measurements during the clinic.

Wheelchair Features

The terminology of wheelchair features is governed by the various manufacturers and often results in confusion in wheelchair selection and purchase. Eleven basic features one must consider when ordering and fitting a chair can be applied to the manufacturers' specific coding system or systems for prescribing the proper chair. The wheelchair features given in Table 25–1 and shown in Figures 25–1 and 25–2 apply to all prescriptions.

(Text continues on p. 370)

Table 25-1   Basic Wheelchair Features for Consideration When Ordering

Features	Type	Clinical Importance
Frame style	Indoor	The chair has large wheels in the front and small casters in the back and is hard to maneuver up and down curbs and steps. An indoor frame is not recommended for patients with respiratory problems related to their illness or caused by their wheelchair propulsion efforts.
	Outdoor	An all-purpose chair with large wheels in the back and small casters in front. This chair is easy to propel on all surfaces (Fig. 25-1).
Construction	Standard	For patients weighing less than 200 lb
	Heavy-duty	For patients weighing more than 200 lb or when rugged use is expected
	Light-weight	For limited outdoor use or for light-weight persons
	Active-duty/light-weight	For patient weighing <200 lb, but allows full range of activities
Chair size	Small child Large Child Junior Adult Oversize	Each category has several sizes: some are standard but others must be customized. Measuring for proper fit is critical. See Table 25-2
Propulsion	All sizes	The patient's ability to propel wheelchair on different surfaces and whether the chair will be self-propelled (manual or electric) or by a caretaker should be considered.
	Handrims	The handrims are chrome-plated. Four clips help protect the spokes and maintain alignment. Plastic coating to increase friction is preferred for a person with poor grasp, but the coating chips. A "quad" peg or vertical projections and rotating knobs

Table 25–1 Basic Wheelchair Features for Consideration
When Ordering *(Continued)*

Features	Type	Clinical Importance
		can be added to the handrims for alternative grip needs (see Fig. 25–2).
Seating	All sizes	The seat distributes weight over the greatest possible skin area. Unless specified, the sling/hammock seat is standard. Adductor spasticity, which may be reinforced by this type of seat, may be ameliorated by a solid seat with an abductor wedge. Other types of seats available include solid seat insert, elevating seat, and folding solid seat and molded seat insert.
Armrests	All types	Armrests provide upper extremity support and are useful for posture shifts and transfers. The types of armrests available are detachable, full-length, detachable desk arm, and wrap-around arms. The desk-length arm is stepped down 5 inches in the front, which allows easy access under tables. These arms can be reversed from side to side. Detachable adjustable armrests (desk- or full-length) are the choice in most cases when continued loss of hand, arm, and shoulder function is anticipated. Wrap-around arms decrease the overall chair width by 1 ½ inches.
Legrests		A lower extremity amputee with no prosthesis is the only exception to the requirement of leg and foot support. Swing-away footrests are recommended regardless of the type of footrest and legrest to facilitate transfers, approaches to working surfaces, and easier folding for transport (see Fig. 25–2).

(continued)

Table 25–1 Basic Wheelchair Features for Consideration When Ordering (*Continued*)

Features	Type	Clinical Importance
Seat back		If the person has good head, neck, and trunk control, a standard-height back is appropriate. A reclining back is indicated for decreased respiratory function, skin problems, or general fatigue after sitting for 1 to 2 hours. A fully reclining back (from 90°—180°) is easier for the caretaker because repeated bed transfers are eliminated. A semireclining back is considered for poor sitting balance in the presence of hip and knee flexion contractures that hinder full reclining.
Steering	All chairs	Casters direct the chair. Casters 5 inches in diameter are used on a child's chair and sports' chair and work well on very hard surfaces. The standard 8-inch casters can be used on all surfaces, and come in hard rubber, pneumatic, or semipheumatic types. Hard rubber gray tires are usually preferred because they do not leave streaks on the floor.
Brakes	All chairs	Toggle brakes are easiest for the patient and are push/pull—off/on brakes. Brake extensions can be ordered when weak arms or decreased trunk balance is present. Electric wheelchairs stop and brake when the control is off or not activated (see Fig. 25–2).
Safety belts	All chairs	Safety belts are always ordered in our clinic whether they are H-strap, autometal clasp, or Velcro-fastened.

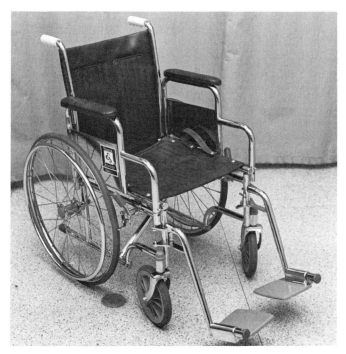

Figure 25-1 Outdoor manual wheelchair is equipped with large wheels in the rear and small casters in the front. This chair features swing-away footrests and detachable desk arms.

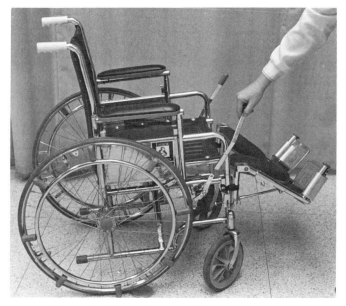

Figure 25-2 This wheelchair features detachable adjustable desk arms, swing-away elevating leg rests, vertical projections on the handrims, and brake extensions.

Wheelchair Accessories

Many accessories are available to accommodate a patient's special needs. Wheelchair accessories (Figs. 25–3 and 25–4) used most frequently with multiple sclerosis and neuromuscular patients include the following:

1. *Posture panels and inserts.* A removable or solid back and solid seat insert with foam added to a desired depth and upholstered to match the chair can be used to revamp an older stretched-out wheelchair or to provide a more solid seating surface for a person with poor trunk control.
2. *Legrest panel.* The detachable legrest panel fits between the front rigging and is especially helpful with both Duchenne muscular dystrophy and multiple sclerosis patients with knee flexor withdrawal to eliminate pressure on the feet or ankles. The panels interfere with ambulators when coming to a stand.
3. *Toe loops.* Especially useful for patients with extensor spasms (such as in multiple sclerosis), toe loops prevent forward slippage of the foot.

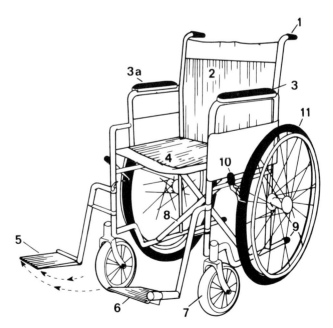

Figure 25–3 Manual wheelchair components and arm rest options. (1) Handgrips/push handles; (2) upholstered back; (3) full-length armrest; (3a) desk arm; (4) upholstered seat; (5) swing-away front-rigging; (6) footplate; (7) casters; (8) cross brace; (9) tipping lever; (10) wheel locks (brakes); and (11) wheel and handrim.

4. *Antitip bar.* Removable antitip bars prevent a wheelchair from tipping backward but can interfere with negotiating curbs.
5. *Trunk supports.* Scoliosis pads can be customized by incorporation into a molded seat or purchased as a commercially available accessory (see Figs. 17 – 9 and 25 – 2) for any manual or electric wheelchair. An extra bracket is needed on some reclining electric wheelchairs to maintain the pads at a proper height and to allow the chair to recline without hitting the power pack on the back of the chair. Scoliosis pads are used in our clinic when the curvature of the spine is less than 20 degrees. Other types of trunk supports are described in Chapters 16 and 18.
6. *Ball-bearing feeders.* This accessory is used for shoulder girdle weakness to support the forearm and to allow the hands to reach the mouth (see Fig. 17 – 6).
7. *Grade aids/hill climbers.* This device, excellent for active people, holds the wheelchair in place on grades and allows the person to reposition his hands for the next push.
8. *Wheelchair narrowing device.* A simple crank device that narrows the wheelchair up to 4 inches to negotiate narrow doors is removable and attaches to the seat and armrests when in use (Fig. 25 – 5).

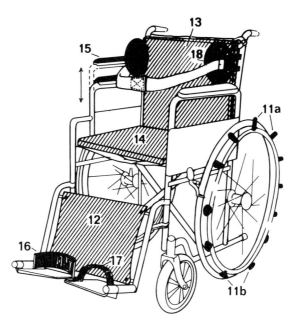

Figure 25 – 4   Manual wheelchair showing wheelchair accessories. (*11a*) Vertical projection; (*11b*) hand knobs; (*12*) detachable leg-rest panel; (*13*) solid back insert; (*14*) solid seat insert; (*15*) detachable adjustable height arm; (*16*) heel loop; (*17*) toe loop; and (*18*) scoliosis pad with belt.

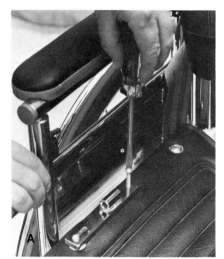
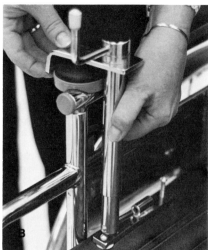
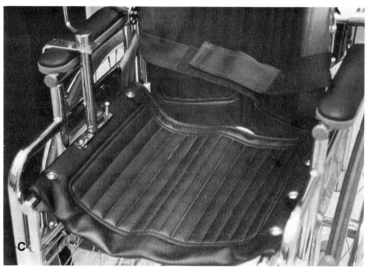

Figure 25-5 (A) Narrowing device. The narrowing device is easily installed by removing the two center bolts and nuts on the hammock seat upholstery. The adjustable oblong seat goes at the front of the seat; the bolts and nuts are then attached securely. The plate is the only permanent fixture. (B) Hook the narrowing device over the arm rest, and slip the end into the barrel on the seat plate. (C) By turning the crank on the top of the narrowing device, the chair can be narrowed up to 4 inches to get the chair through narrow doorways. The chair should be in slight motion while turning the crank to avoid stress on the cross-brace.

The chair needs to be rolled back and forth during the narrowing process.

9. *Trays.* Trays attach to the wheelchair armrest with Velcro or can be purchased in the fold-off style. Clear plastic lap trays, by allowing a child to see the rest of his body, enhance development of motor planning and perceptual skills (Fig. 25–6).

10. *Cushions.* (Fig. 25–7). A cushion, whether formed of air, water, gel, foam, or solid, decreases the danger of skin breakdown and increases comfort.

- A light-weight air cushion must be inflated enough to support the body.
- A water cushion is heavier, and more difficult to handle, and temperature changes in the water often bother patients.
- A gel cushion is also heavy, and it is cool in winter. The gel flares under pressure to accomodate the person and returns to its original shape when the pressure of the person's weight is removed.
- A foam cushion can be obtained with different densities and can be cut out for areas under pressure for relief or built up to redistribute pressures. These cushions usually need to be replaced in 6 months to 1 year.

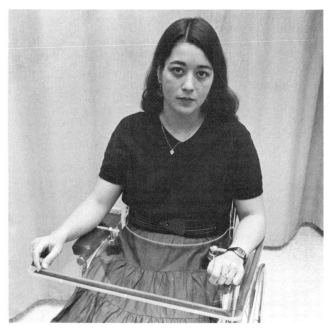

Figure 25–6 The clear lap tray is designed to enhance the person's body image.

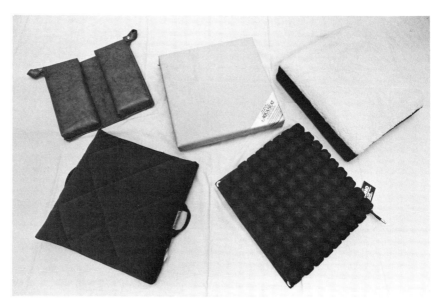

Figure 25–7 Various cushions are available for seating. (*Top, left to right*) Gibbus pad, aqua flotation pad, and foam cushion with sheepskin cover. (*Bottom, left to right*) Air cushion and low-profile Roho cushion without cover.

- A Roho cushion has fingerlike projections that are filled with air that redistributes to equalize weight on the sitting surface. This cushion has been successful in our neuromuscular clinic with patients who cannot transfer or perform hygiene activities. The constant redistribution of air caused by weight shifts makes it difficult for a person with weak arms to slide forward or use a urinal. A new low-profile Roho cushion with projections half the size of the standard Roho may ease this difficulty of sliding forward.

11. *Covers for wheelchair cushions*

- Naugahyde is washable, but is not absorbent and is often hot.
- Polyester and terry cloth are easy to launder and more absorbent, a feature beneficial for a person who has decreased sensation.
- Nylon is washable and allows sliding more easily, but it is not as absorbent as terry cloth.
- Real lambskin "breathes," distributes pressure, and is absorbent, washable, and cool both in winter and summer.
- Synthetic sheepskin must be replaced in 3 to 6 months because with continued laundering it tends to bunch, forming bare areas on the backing, leading to increased pressure and heat.

Wheelchair Measurements

The four major measurements in wheelchair prescriptions are width, depth, back height, and footrest length. Seat width and depth measurements for chairs are given in Table 25–2. A proper wheelchair should allow a person 1 inch of clearance on both sides. To check the width, opened hands with the thumbs up are placed at the patient's hips. If the hands touch the armrest panel, the chair width is too narrow. If the hands can be easily fisted, the chair is too wide and the patient will have difficulty propelling the chair simultaneously with two hands. An electric chair can be ordered slightly wider to accommodate scoliosis pads since manual propulsion is not a consideration.

The wheelchair seat depth needs to allow 2 to 4 inches of space from the back of the knee to the front of the seat upholstery (2–3 finger breadths). Circulation can be compromised if the seat is too long or if the patient habitually dangles his legs and feet by removing his footrests. The back height of the chair, if not a recliner, should be 1 inch below the scapulae.

The footrest length on a wheelchair is often overlooked because the footrest height is adjustable. Sometimes the footrest hanger that comes with a particular model of a child's chair can be too short even when adjusted to full length, particularly as a child grows. Footrest hangers on children's chairs are usually not interchangeable with adult wheelchair footrest hangers. However, some adult hangers can be used. The person ordering replacement hangers should know the type of chair the patient has and the specific brand of chair, and should work with the wheelchair vendor to match the fittings correctly.

Table 25–2 Wheelchair Basic Dimensions

| Type | Seat | |
	Width (in inches)	Depth (in inches)
Adult	18	16
Narrow adult	16	16
Slim adult	14	16
Large child	14	11½
	16	13
Small child	12	11½
	10	8

(Text continues on p. 384)

Table 25–3 Seating Features for Common Wheelchair Problems

Problem	MS	MD	Chair Type	Key Accessories	Primary Considerations	Comments
General fatigability	*	*	Manual W/C	DET desk arms SW-away Ft-rests	For traveling distances At work, school, or in crowds For partial ambulators	Fatigability usually occurs with other signs and symptoms
	**	*	Motorized scooter (see Fig. 25–8)	Basket Horn Crutch or cane holder	Disassembles easily for transportation Pts prefer appearance to conventional W/C Useful at home and at work	MS—requires sustained antigravity UE use Tremors do not necessarily contraindicate use Must have at least fair trunk balance MD—not used in Duchenne dystrophy unless controls are placed on armrest
						Mobility provided by caretaker
	***		Semirecliner (see Fig. 25–9)	DET desk arms SW-away Ft-rests DET legrest panels Chest strap Wedge cushion	MS—accomodates hip and knee flexion contractures or leg spasticity with withdrawal pattern, i.e., pts who can't fully recline	
	***	***	Full recliner (see Fig. 25–10)	DET desk arms DET ELV legrest Cushion Lumbar roll	Allows intermittent pressure relief Decreases need for transfers Frees caretaker	Used with poor head and trunk control without significant contractures Motorized recliner available with hand control or alternatives, e.g., sip n' puff
Obesity	*	*	Manual W/C	DET desk arms SW-away Ft-rests	For traveling distances	Consider oversized W/C but chair won't go through conventional door width and will require narrowing device

Pain						
Low back pain	*	***	All chairs	SW-away Ft-rests, Scoliosis pads, Lumbar roll (see Fig. 14–10)	Secures position, facilitates good posture	May be uncomfortable for thin person; may need a cushion
		*	All chairs	Solid seat and back inserts with foam padding	Comfort and body support	Total body support provides protection with sudden W/C movements
		** ****	All chairs	Solid back insert with lordosis support and contoured back padding		
Buttocks	**	**	All chairs	See under Prevention of decubitus ulcers, below	Comfort; Distributes pressure	
Foot pain	**	**	All chairs	Hammock/sling Ft-rest; Vinyl legrest panel; Cradle Ft-rest	Provides gentle, even support for the feet; Prevents foot dangling	
Chest	***	***	All chairs	H-strap; Custom harness (clavicle shoulder, etc.)	Relieves pressure on chest caused by conventional chest strap	MD—keep patient posturally balanced with custom harness and adjust according to balance and functional needs, not to patient appearance
Safety risk	*	*	All chairs	Seat Belt	Safety; Positioning	Should be used on all chairs MS and MD use on electric W/C and motorized scooters
	**	**	All chairs	Horn	Obstructed corners	
	** ****	** ****	All Chairs	Red flag or alert system	To obtain help	MD—for low speaking volume, especially if W/C batteries are dead or for falls from chair

(Continued)

377

Table 25–3 Seating Features for Common Wheelchair Problems *(Continued)*

Problem	MS	MD	Chair Type	Key Accessories	Primary Considerations	Comments
Impaired body image	**	**	All chairs	Antitip bars	Prevents electric W/C from tipping, e.g., during starts	Ensure these are detachable for negotiation of curbs by caretakers
	*	*	Manua W/C	DET Ft-rest SW-away Ft-rests Clear lap tray	For traveling distances	Clear lap tray enhances body image and self-concept
	*	*	Motorized Scooter	Horn and Basket	Enhances mobility	MD—usually not used with DMD, SMA, and ALS MS—patients prefer appearance to conventional W/C
Prevention of decubitus ulcers	*		All chairs	Foam cushion	Distributes weight to relieve pressure on buttocks	Although decubitus ulcers are not associated with MD, these pts need cushions for other reasons
Buttocks	** / ****		All chairs	Gel cushion Water cushion Air cushion Roho cushion Jay cushion (see Fig. 25–5)	Distributes weight to relieve pressure on buttocks	Consider price (ROHO most expensive) Independent transfers may be more difficult with ROHO—consider low-profile ROHO Generally depends on patients preference
Ankles	** / ***	** / ***	All chairs	Legrest panel Leg H-strap Hook on heel strap (see Figs. 25–11 and 25–12)	Supports legs Prevents feet from slipping behind footplates	MD and DMD pts like to dangle their feet behind heel loops, which causes foot pain and compromises circulation MS—seen especially with spasticity with flexor withdrawal

378

Spasticity	*	Manual W/C	DET desk arm SW-away Ft-rest	Ease in transfers	MS—useful with fixed contractures preventing full reclining
	**	Semirecliner	See General fatigability, above	Prevents person from slipping out of chair	Patient usually totally dependent
	***	Full recliner	See General fatigability, above	Allows patient to fully recline when fatigued	
	*	Motorized scooter	Basket Horn	Independent mobility	To prevent patient from entangling feet during extensor spasms, make sure there is a guard over the front-wheel drive mechanism
Poor head control	**	All chairs	Soft cervical collar	Head support and position	Clothing fits somewhat poorly; Pts may complain of choking sensation
	**		Wire frame collar (see Fig. 25–13)	Head support and position Helpful during transport Head support	Air flows freely Alleviates choking sensation Clothing fits well
	****	All chairs	DET self-centering headrest (see Fig. 25–14)	For traveling in van Fatigability	Can be used on manual standard or semi-recliner W/C
	****	Custom occiput head support (see Fig. 25–15)	Cups head, less obstruction to visual field	MD—can be attached to solid back insert	
	***	Full recliner	High-back, fully recline	Total support for trunk and head	
Trunk weakness	**	Manual or electric W/C	Scoliosis pads	Maintains position	MD—retards scoliosis
	***				
	***	Child safety travel/traveler	Trunk and head supports	Prevents falling to either side or forward	MD—child safety in transportation, ease of care, ease of feeding

(Continued)

Table 25–3 Seating Features for Common Wheelchair Problems (Continued)

Problem	MS	MD	Chair Type	Key Accessories	Primary Considerations	Comments
	*		Manual or electric W/C	Seat belt or H-strap harness Body jacket Lumbar roll	Positioning and safety Provides support and retards further curve development Safety and security in sitting position	MD—for curve >20° use body jacket; may still use scoliosis pads for balance
Impaired balance	*	*	Manual W/C Scooter	Seat belt and/or chest strap See General fatigability, above	See General fatigability, above	See General fatigability, above
	**	**				
Scoliosis		**	Manual or electric W/C	Scoliosis pads	Retards curve development Corrects sitting posture	MD—use immediately with electric W/C; even without scoliosis, child leans to the side of hand controls
		**	Manual or electric W/C	Body jacket (see Fig. 18–16)	Good trunk position	For curves >20°
		***	Manual or electric W/C	Custom-molded body/seat insert (see Figs. 16–5, 18–17, and 25–15)	Form-fitted to hold person securely in upright position	DMD—Costly; uncomfortable overcorrection and patient dissatisfaction warrant use with caution
Upper extremity Impaired dexterity	**		Manual W/C	W/C cuffs Wheelrim projections	Ease in propelling chair	MS—more problems due to tremors and sensory changes Safer with impaired sensation and fatigability
	***					

Problem	Rating	Device	Device components	Function	Comments
Proximal weakness	**	Electric W/C	DET ADJ desk arms	Raised arm height replaces need for antigravity strength	
	***		Ball-bearing feeders (see Fig. 17-6)	Supports arms; Allows free movements with limited muscle power	MD—excellent for self-feeding and ROM exercise
Distal weakness		Manual W/C	DET desk arms; SW-away FT-rests with heel loops; Crutch holder; Handrim projections	Increases Mobility; Decreases fatigue; Safety	See General fatigability, above
				See Table 25-1	
Contractures Knee—ankle—foot	**	Motorized Scooter	See General fatigability, above	See General fatigability, above	
	**	Standard manual or electric W/C	DET ELV legrest	Provides gentle constant stretch on hamstrings	MD—pts dislike; can't get W/C as close to tables, etc.; tend to not put legs on stretch because of pain
	** ***	Standard manual or electric W/C	SW-away Ft-rest with heel loops; DET legrest Panel	Keeps feet on footplate; Prevents patient from placing feet behind foot-plate and heel loops	
	***	Standard manual or electric W/C	Foot cradle or hammock/sling foot support	Keeps feet and legs from dangling; Gives support to feet but provides no stretch	MD—this is good to use with pts with fixed contractures and tender feet
	**	Electric of manual semi-recliner	SW-away Ft-rest with heel loops or DET leg rest panel; DET head support		MS—fatigue easily, but can't fully recline due to contractures; MS—DET headrest for fatigue or travel

(Continued)

Table 25–3 Seating Features for Common Wheelchair Problems (Continued)

Problem	MS	MD	Chair Type	Key Accessories	Primary Considerations	Comments
Functional Impairments						
Partial Ambulator	*	*	Manual W/C	DET desk arms SW-away Ft-rest Crutch holder	Traveling distance	
Architectural barriers	*	*	Manual W/C	W/C-narrowing device	Narrows chair up to 4 inches for narrow doors	Must roll chair back and forth while narrowing W/C to prevent stress on cross brace
	*	* **	Utility chair/ glide about	Wheel locks Removable arms	Use through narrow doors Kitchen use	Need intact trunk balance
	**	**	Stair glide seat	Seat belt	Allows person to go up and down stairs independently	User should be able to transfer independently or with minimum assistance
Ramps	**	**	Manual chair	Grade aids/hill climbers	Prevents chair from slipping on grades	
Rugged use	*	* **	Standard manual/elec-tric, or active duty chair	Puncture-resistant tires Heavy-duty frame	Chair used outside and over rough terrain Accommodates person who weighs > 200 lb	Do not order a light-weight chair for rugged active use unless chair is specified as active-duty light-weight
Auto/van	**	**	Motorized scooter	See General fatigability, above	Disassembles easily for car transport	With weakness, may need caretaker to lift parts of scooter into the car

Key: *Mild; **moderate; ***severe; ADJ, adjustable; DET, detachable; ELV, elevating; Ft, foot; SW, swing; W/C, wheelchair; ALS, amyotrophic lateral sclerosis; DMD, Duchene muscular dystrophy; MS, multiple sclerosis; MD, neuromuscular disorders; pts, patients; ROM, range of motion; SMA, spinal muscular atrophy; UE, upper extremity. All chairs should have seat belts. Most chairs should have utility bags.

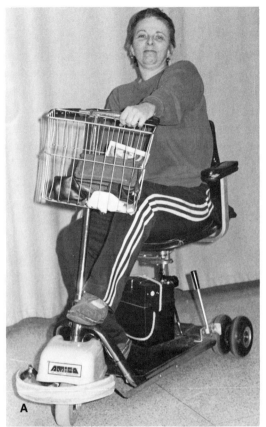

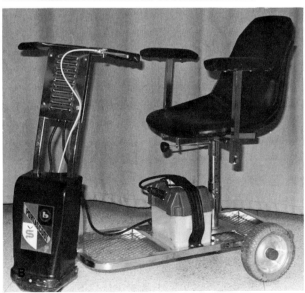

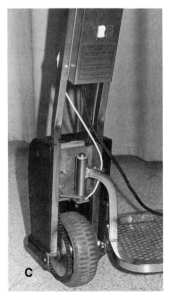

Figure 25 – 8 (A) The Amigo motorized scooter is one type of scooter frequently used by MS patients. (B) Portascoot motorized scooter, side view. (C) Portascoot motorized scooter. The front tire needs a guard, which is added for patients with extensor spasms.

Using the background information of the basic wheelchair features and accessories, Table 25–3 and Figures 25–8 through 25–15 address patient needs from a problem/solution orientation. The patient's problems are identified in the table with the degree of severity of the muscular disorder. The points of separation in degree between mild, moderate, and severe may be somewhat arbitrary, depending on the person using

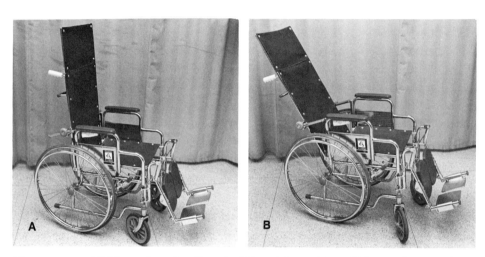

Figure 25–9 (A) Manual semirecliner in full upright position. (B) Manual semirecliner at maximum recline. The semirecliner is mostly used most with MS patients who have fixed contractures at the hips.

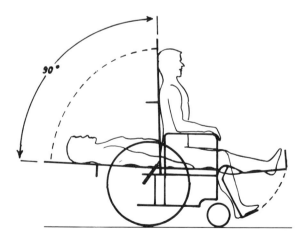

Figure 25–10 The full recliner is used with severely involved MD and MS patients. It provides intermittent pressure relief from sitting upright, decreases the need for transfers from the chair to the bed and frees the caretaker. (Adapted from The Wheelchair Catalog, p 33. USA/Welsh Graphics, January 1980)

the table, but should pose little difficulty once familiarity with the table is gained. The Jebsen Test of Hand Coordination, activities of daily living (ADL) evaluation, and specific muscle testing can be of assistance to the inexperienced (see Chaps. 8 and 17).

For multiple problems, begin with the chair type and number of accessories showing the most complete order, and then eliminate items

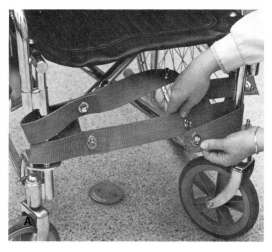
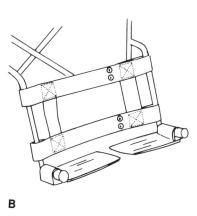

Figure 25–11 (A and B) The leg H-strap is used to prevent the patient's legs and feet from slipping behind the footplates. The H-strap can be easily removed for the person who can stand to pivot transfer. (Adapted from The Wheelchair Catalog, p 61. USA/Welsh Graphics, January 1980)

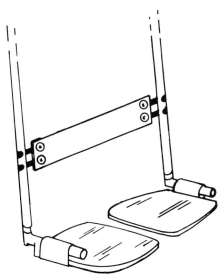

Figure 25–12 The hook on the heelstrap is an accessory to use instead of heel loops. The heelstrap is adjustable to the level of greatest patient comfort.

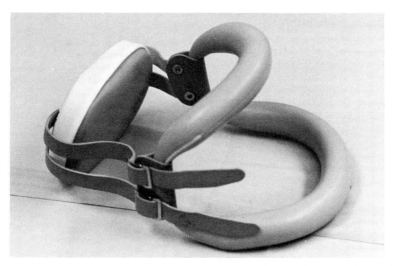

Figure 25-13 Wire frame cervical collar is used for head support for undue fatigue or for weak musculature while being transported from place to place.

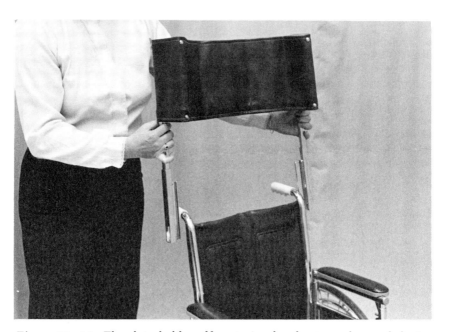

Figure 25-14 The detachable self-centering headrest can be used during transport or when a person is fatigued and needs to rest his head against a support.

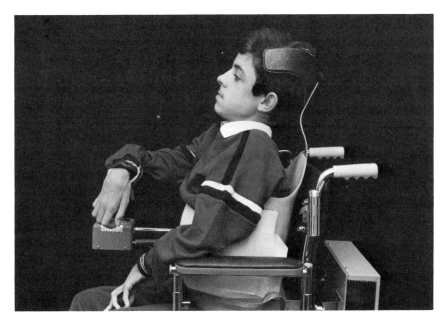

Figure 25–15   A custom head support can be attached to a molded body insert as shown or to a solid back insert. When attached to the solid seat insert, the insert can be removed and the chair can be folded easily.

as the primary use and comments are considered. Refer back to the section Wheelchair Accessories and Tables 25–1 and 25–2 for variations in equipment for final determination of an individualized prescription.

When a standard wheelchair or motorized scooter is not adequate for a patient's needs, other transport chairs are available for specific patients (according to diagnoses) and seating needs.

1. The safety travel/traveler is a seating transport system that allows a child to be positioned and supported at the head, trunk, leg, shoulder, and foot. This chair must be propelled by the caretaker but has multiple uses, since it serves as a car seat, a chair for feeding, and a place to perform fine motor activities (Fig. 25–16).
2. The Pogan or stroller is light-weight and is principally used to transport a child. One disadvantage of this chair with a neuromuscular disease patient is that it puts the child in a rounded-back position (Fig. 25–17).
3. The Mulholland wheelchair, used primarily with severely impaired cerebral palsy children, has a totally adjustable seating and support system. The chair is difficult to push because of its four small casters. If used on public transportation, this chair, as well as the safety travel

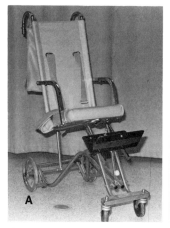 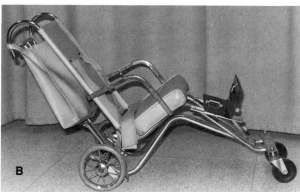

Figure 25–16 The safety travel/traveler is propelled by the caretaker and can serve as a car seat, a chair to feed the child, and a transport vehicle. The chair provides support at the head, trunk, leg, shoulder, and feet (Palmco Traveler). (A) Upright position. (B) Fully reclined position can be used for automobile car seat.

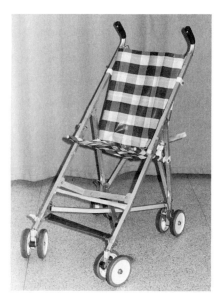 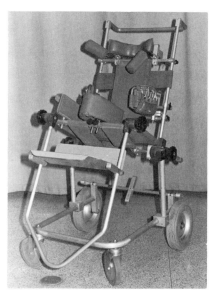

Figure 25–17 The Pogan or stroller is used for temporary seating and transport.

Figure 25–18 The Mulholland wheelchair has a totally adjustable seating and support system. The chair was designed for severely involved cerebral palsy children but has potential use with involved Werdnig-Hoffman children.

chair, requires modification of the public vehicle's fasteners (Fig. 25 – 18).

4. An adjustable posture-care positioning system by Theradyne, although not motorized and not currently available in small children's sizes, has a detachable seat, scoliosis and trunk supports, and legrests. The component parts are made of molded foam rather than vinyl-covered. The seat can be elevated to function as a wedge cushion, with the width of the abduction wedge individualized.

5. "Quickie" and "Quickie II," new light-weight chairs (20 lb lighter than the standard wheelchair, which is approximately 46 lb without front rigging), require fair to good trunk balance but are excellent for the active MS patient who uses a bus for transportation (Fig. 25 – 19).

6. The new light-weight total modular construction wheelchair works well for some patients with good arm strength and trunk balance. This 16-lb chair is totally collapsible, including each of its 3-lb detachable wheels.

7. Wheelchairs with one-arm drive are available for patients who have the use of only one arm. Alternatively, a "Poirier" chair with adjustable resistance and a push/pull technique for propulsion may be used (Fig. 25 – 20).

8. A Levo or Moto stand chair, particularly useful in spinal cord injury patients, allows a person to come to a standing position.

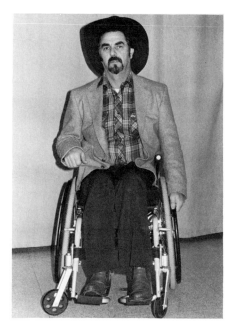

Figure 25 – 19 Pictured is the Quickie II wheelchair, which is light weight. It can be used with both MS and MD patients.

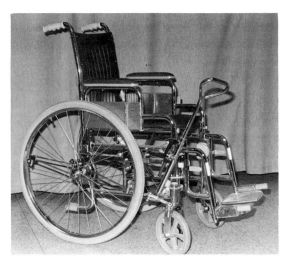

Figure 25–20   A Poirier wheelchair with adjustable resistance and push/pull technique for propulsion. The Poirer one-arm drive chair works with MS patients who are active in the indoor home situation. It is a difficult chair for the caretaker to control if the patient fatigues due to the steering set-up.

9. A new motorized Amigo scooter, the ULTA, has the control mechanism mounted on the armrest, allowing a person to drive the chair with the arm resting on the armrest. Custom scoliosis and head supports can be mounted on the chair seat. The scooter can also be modified to accomodate standard chair seats. As with all motorized scooters, the clamps and fasteners on public bus transportation do not accommodate these scooters. This chair is effectively transported by car or Ambocab.

Many manufacturers recently have added lightweight wheelchairs and motorized scooters to their inventory. Although the increased variety of options is welcome, manufacturers constantly are changing the available features, necessitating continuous updating of information. The relative importance of any of these features must be individualized for each patient. Currently, some important considerations for motorized scooters include rear or front wheel drive; adjustability of wheel bases (for stability on rough terrain); adjustability of seats; seat interchangeability with orthokinetic type; noise levels; and the types and placement options of controls.

Although many more chairs are available, the chairs described in this chapter are particularly useful with MD and MS patients. Wheelchairs need maintenance and repairs to keep them in top working order. An important consideration is the easy availability of parts, preferably in the patient's locale.

Suggested Readings

COCHRANE CM, WILSHERE ER (eds): Equipment for the Disabled. Wheelchairs. Oxford, England, Oxfordshire Health Authority, Nuffield Orthopaedic Centre, November, 1982

FAHLAND BB: Wheelchair Selection — More than Choosing a Chair with Wheels. Minneapolis, Kenny Rehabilitation Institute, 1967

HERMAN SJ, GURISH PM: Wheelchair maintenance. The Exceptional Parent 13(1):17–36, 1983

JAEGER DL, ADAMS J, BONN L, et al: Pediatric chair prescription. Clinical Management 3:28–34, 1983

KOHN J, ENDERS S, PRESTON J JR, et al: Provisions of assistive equipment for handicapped persons. Arch Phys Med Rehabil 64:378–381, 1983

PEZENIK D, ITOH M, LEE M: Wheelchair prescription. In Ruskin AP (ed): Current Therapy in Physiatry, Physical Medicine and Rehabilitation, pp 475–498. Philadelphia, WB Saunders, 1984.

26

Nan O'Neal Campbell

The Social Service Worker and the Neuromuscular Disease Patient: A Partnership in Problem-Solving

A social service worker, in cooperation with other members of the medical team, provides a neuromuscular disease patient with information and comfort to alleviate fear and confusion throughout a painful emotional process.

The experienced social worker who knows the consequences of a diagnosis of multiple sclerosis (MS) or muscular dystrophy (MD) can help the patient and his family weave through medical and social bureaucracies to find appropriate resources.

A neuromuscular disease patient may find a social worker through private health agencies, such as the Muscular Dystrophy Association (MDA) or the National Multiple Sclerosis Society (NMSS), or through a school, a hospital, or a special clinic.

Regardless of where the family finds a worker with experience in the problems of neuromuscular disease, theirs can become a partnership in problem-solving.

A successful introduction to the health-care system influences a patient's future attitude about seeking help, but, unfortunately, many patients spend months and sometimes years before finding an agency or professional knowledgeable about MD and MS. Subtle first symptoms of the illnesses complicate a patient's finding help quickly and add to frustration in the maze of community services. Friends, teachers, school nurses, or family physicians may be the first to notice mild physical signs and may refer the person to agencies and clinics, but often the family must seek help independently.

Even after a diagnosis is made, a patient and his family may know little of the consequences of the disease other than its immediate effects. A social service worker can provide and interpret information and seek to resolve misconceptions about the illness. The family's knowledge about the physical and genetic characteristics of the illness influences a host of family decisions, from buying a vehicle that can accommodate a wheelchair to having another child. Thus, accurate information is vital. A careful social worker must be sure that information given the family is correct and is also understood correctly. To ensure this, the worker must constantly ask himself "What am I saying?" "How is it being heard?" and "What have I left unsaid?"

Frequently, a worker will have repeated information so often that his answers to similar-sounding questions become automatic, but important distinctions are omitted if responses are not individualized to the patient's needs.

Medical jargon sounds mysterious and authoritative, and can be confusing or frightening to a patient. Information that is commonplace to members of the medical team is news to the patient hearing it for the first time, and the impact may be startling. When life-threatening illness is being discussed and the person hearing it is the one whose life is threatened by the illness, the impact is understandably profound.

Similarly, information may not be heard by a patient or family member who is distressed by what has been said previously. Although a physician might have spent considerable time discussing current theories about the illness and its treatment, patients in these circumstances may feel the physician was brusque and unsympathetic when explaining the diagnosis and prognosis.

The social service worker assists the physician by making medical jargon more understandable to the patient and by relating significant misunderstandings back to the physician for his clarification.

Members of a medical team who are knowledgeable about chronic, disabling disease understand communication problems and work together to ensure the patient's understanding of the illness by encouraging the patient's questions. Complicated information, such as genetic implications in some disorders, needs to be repeated several times. Written materials are useful so the patient and family can absorb information at their own pace or refer to it when they need it. Written instructions for home physical therapy increase the likelihood that exercises will be done correctly. Brochures about program benefits and maps with directions to other clinics, orthopaedic stores, and welfare agencies are helpful to families who have been given a great deal of information in a short visit or who are preoccupied with sad news of a grave prognosis.

Because of the progressive debilitation of neuromuscular disease, the complexity of problems encountered by the patient and family increases over time, necessitating frequent and prolonged consultation with a social worker. The relationship may last years and may be a partnership that exists for the duration of the patient's life.

The benefit of an extended relationship is a worker's thorough understanding of the patient's problems, but negative consequences may also occur. A patient's previous failure to heed medical instructions or pursue referrals may make a social worker reluctant to make additional plans that might not be followed.

Ideally, past failures should challenge a social worker to devise plans the patient will follow, such as simplifying instructions or making directions more specific. Referrals may need to be made to a particular person in an agency rather than to the agency in general, or the worker may need to narrow his focus and to separate one solvable problem from the morass of interrelated difficulties the patient faces.

Another difficulty in long-term patient — worker relationships arises from the progressive nature of MD and MS. The social worker may feel despair when a patient's condition worsens. However, to remain helpful, he must remember that theirs is a friendly partnership that differs from a friendship. The relationship exists for the benefit of the patient and his family, not for the benefit of the social worker.

A long-term familiarity with a patient, combined with a social worker's knowledge of the progressive stages of an illness, increases the worker's opportunities for intervention before minor problems become crises.

Periodic phone calls can monitor the loss of physical function complicating illnesses and developing social problems that need the medical team's attention. The family of a child with Duchenne muscular dystrophy, for example, may not notice the insidious development of joint stiffness that needs a therapist's attention to avoid contractures. In another case, physical care may be burdening the family beyond its capabilities and the social worker's suggestion of attendant care and home health assistance may avoid a family crisis.

The psychological depression frequently complicating myotonic dystrophy and multiple sclerosis poses special problems for the social service worker. A task as simple as keeping a clinic appointment or applying for financial aid can be overwhelming for someone whose ambition is compromised by depression.

When families have several members affected with a disorder, such as myotonic dystrophy with accompanying depression, the pervasive apathy can make problem-solving difficult. Such situations require the combined efforts of physicians, therapists, and social service workers with realistic expectations about the family's capabilities.

No health-care worker can care for a patient's every need. The coordination of services given by doctors, counselors, therapists, and agencies rests with the patient and his family. The social service worker is most helpful when he teaches the patient where to get help and how to use it.

The social service worker can teach a patient to structure services so the patient's independence is maximized. One technique is to have the patient organize a notebook in which he records names of agencies with program descriptions, eligibility qualifications, and phone numbers of contact people. Other self-help tools a worker may give a patient include catalogs picturing orthopaedic devices, magazines published for the handicapped, and newsletters from advocacy groups. Patients and families should be encouraged to keep informed about community resources and how to use them without a social worker's help. No matter how severe a person's disability may be, the patient is ultimately responsible for himself. This responsibility should be respected by the social worker and the other members of the medical team because the weakness of one's body should not mean powerlessness over one's life.

The National Multiple Sclerosis Society

The National Multiple Sclerosis Society (NMSS) has 150 local chapters, which provide information and a variety of services. Services may vary from one chapter to another because of differences in community resources and finances. Most NMSS chapters have staff members or volunteers who can provide information about medical services, resources for financial assistance, home health training, and supportive counseling.

Chapters may provide durable medical equipment if prescribed by a physician. The provision of equipment is dependent on a chapter's financial resources, but may include wheelchairs, bathroom aids, and hospital beds. Some chapters support free clinics or may suggest knowledgeable physicians. Support groups, marital counseling, and psychiatric evaluations are sponsored by some chapters to assist patients and family members in coping with emotional stress. Home care education and therapeutic recreation programs, such as yoga and swimming, are offered in some locations. NMSS has contracts with vocational rehabilitation agencies throughout the nation.

The NMSS also funds research and has established the International Federation of Multiple Sclerosis Societies to coordinate a worldwide network of organizations concerned with MS research.*

The Muscular Dystrophy Association

The Muscular Dystrophy Association (MDA) has offices in every state, as well as in the territories of Puerto Rico and Guam. The national headquarters in New York City administers the program of countrywide services. Local chapters of the MDA are authorized to pay for

*Contact National Multiple Sclerosis Society, 205 E. 42nd Street, New York, NY 10017, for information on the location of chapters and offices in a particular area, or for literature about services and research developments.

services specified in the national program, and qualifications to receive assistance are uniform for every chapter.

Any resident of the United States who has a diagnosis of one of 40 neuromuscular diseases included in the MDA's program (see list, below) may receive services. (Multiple sclerosis is not an included diagnosis.)

DISEASE INCLUDED IN THE MDA'S PROGRAM

Muscular dystrophies
   Duchenne muscular dystrophy
    (pseudohypertrophic)
   Becker muscular dystrophy
   Facioscapulohumeral muscular dystrophy
    (Landouzy-Dejerine)
   Limb-girdle muscular dystrophy
    (including juvenile dystrophy of Erb)
   Myotonic dystrophy
    (Steinert's disease)
   Congenital muscular dystrophy
   Ophthalmoplegic muscular dystrophy
   Distal muscular dystrophy
   Muscular dystrophy of late onset
Spinal muscular atrophies
   Amyotrophic lateral sclerosis (ALS)
   Infantile progressive spinal muscular atrophy
    (Werdnig-Hoffman disease)
   Juvenile progressive spinal muscular atrophy
    (Kugelberg-Welander disease)
   Benign congenital hypotonia
    (formerly called amyotonia congenita)
   Adult progressive spinal muscular atrophy
    (Aran-Duchenne type)
Inflammatory myopathies
   Polymyositis
   Dermatomyositis
   Myositis ossificans
Diseases of peripheal nerve
   Peroneal muscular atrophy
    (Charcot-Marie-Tooth disease)
   Friedreich's ataxia
   Dejerine-Sottas disease
Disease of neuromuscular junction
   Myasthenia gravis
   Eaton-Lambert (myasthenic syndrome)
Myotonias
   Myotonia congenita (Thomsen's disease)
   Paramyotonia congenita

Metabolic diseases of muscle
  Phosphorylase deficiency
    (McArdle's disease)
  Acid maltase deficiency
    (Pompe's disease)
  Phosphofructokinase deficiency
    (Tauri's disease)
  Debrancher enzyme deficiency
    (Cori's or Forbes disease)
  Carnitine deficiency
  Carnitine palmityltransferase deficiency
  Periodic paralysis
Myopathies due to endocrine abnormalities
  Hyperthyroid myopathy
  Hypothyroid myopathy
  Myopathies secondary to disorders of adrenal corticosteroids
Less common myopathies
  Central core disease
  Nemaline myopathy
  Mitochondrial disease
  Myotubular myopathy
  Idiopathic myopathy
  Malignant hyperthermia
    (hyperpyrexia)

No financial disclosure is required for services, nor does income limit eligibility. However, if a patient has insurance or if public assistance programs will pay for services, the MDA requires that those programs be billed first. This rule enables the MDA to use its funds to provide more services to more patients.

The MDA provides numerous items, such as standard wheelchairs, hospital beds, leg and back braces, hydraulic lifts, bathroom aids, and some respiratory equipment. Motorized wheelchairs are provided only for persons in school or in a work place where independent mobility is necessary (see appendix, at the end of the chapter).

Many of the over 200 MDA clinics throughout the country are located in medical colleges or are affiliated with research facilities. The MDA pays for clinic visits, diagnostic testing, and follow-up consultations, as well as for some physical, occupational, and respiratory therapy treatments.

A physician's prescription is required for the MDA to provide equipment or other medical services.*

---

*Contact Muscular Dystrophy Association, 810 Seventh Avenue, New York, NY 10019, for a complete list of clinics, addresses of local offices, or for additional information on services and illnesses covered.

Other Assistance Programs

The quality and availability of services from nongovernmental agencies vary in different communities. Agencies in urban settings far outnumber those serving patients in rural areas, but most remote communities have visiting nurses employed by either the Visiting Nurse Association (VNA, a private agency), or by county health departments (community health nurses).

VNA staff members work closely with physicians to monitor a patient's medical condition and to administer prescribed treatments. Some local VNAs have expanded their staff to include physical therapists, occupational therapists, speech pathologists, home health aides, and social service workers. VNA is a good resource for in-home assessments of health needs. A visit to the home may reveal unknown conditions that may influence the course of treatment. VNA staff members also train family members in caring for a patient at home and can recommend other services available in the community.

Other home health agencies, certified to operate in a state, provide a range of services. Some home health agencies provide in-home attendant care, educational training to increase independence in the home, and homemakers. Home health agencies may also employ registered nurses, physical therapists, and social workers.

A physician's order for home health assistance is required and must be updated periodically. A list of certified home health agencies in a state can be obtained from the state's health department.

Independent Living Centers

All states now have at least one community with an independent living center (ILC) where severely disabled people can be taught the necessary skills to live more easily in private residential settings. Most clients are young adults who want to reside apart from their families, or who have lived in institutions or nursing homes and wish to move to independent settings.

ILCs train people with any disability and have demonstrated effective alternatives to nursing-home residence for the disabled. ILCs are private agencies with a close linkage to state departments of rehabilitation through which federal funds supporting independent living programs are channeled.

In addition to individualized educational programs, ILCs provide a variety of services to handicapped people. Some have transportation services in specially equipped vans and buses. A few are also certified home health agencies and can provide attendent care in a patient's home.

Some ILCs have short-term housing facilities where clients live while learning skills, such as home economics, cooking, using public transportation, and managing a personal attendant.

Many of the social service workers employed in the centers are disabled themselves and can give first-hand advice on problems encountered by people with disabilities. ILCs are also advocates for increased integration and accessibility for people with disabilities and are good reference sources for information about community services. For information on the locations of ILCs in a state, contact the state's independent living center coordinator in the vocational rehabilitation division of the department of social services.

Summary

The social worker's vital role with patients with neuromuscular disorders is varied in setting and complexity. The complexity of these patients' needs requires flexibility, knowledge, sensitivity, interpretation, and friendliness. The social worker helps the patient to take responsibility for his own life. Assistance programs are available through organizations such as the NMSS and the MDA and a variety of health agencies. The social worker should become familiar with the benefits and limitations of each organization and be ready to initiate proper referrals.

The future promises more independence and personal control over one's health care. Computerized information and referral systems are being developed, which will increase a patient's access to resources and which may permit the immediate calculation of eligibility for program benefits.

However, machines cannot supplant someone who asks the right question at the right time. Knowledge of what questions to ask and when to ask them comes from familiarity with the illness's physical and psychological effects. The knowledge to give practical advice and sympathetic counsel and to trust intuitive feelings, combined with the ability to elicit information, makes the job of the social service worker a rewarding challenge.

Suggested Readings

BRILL NI: Working with People: The Helping Process, 2nd ed. Philadelphia, JB Lippincott, 1978

BROOKE MH: A Clinician's View of Neuromuscular Disease. Baltimore, Williams & Wilkins, 1977

NELSON M: Effective Coping with Multiple Sclerosis Denver, Multiple Sclerosis Society of Colorado, April, 1980

Appendix: The MDA Patient and Community Services*

ORTHOPAEDIC AIDS

Medical prescriptions are required from the director of the local MDA clinic or from the patient's personal physician for the following ortho-paedic aids (except for motorized wheelchairs, which require a pre-scription from an MDA clinic director). When the following aids are prescribed in relation to an individual's neuromuscular disease, the MDA provides for their purchase or rental and for reasonable repair.

- Walkers, crutches, and canes
- Selected braces: unilateral leg braces, bilateral leg braces, surgical corsets, body jackets, back braces, cervical collars, trunk support straps; no JOBST stockings
- Wheelchairs (nonmotorized) and the following accessories: ball-bearing feeders, specially padded cushions, trays, lap boards, seat belts, elevating legrests, body positioners, removable desk arms
- Wheelchairs (motorized — not to exceed the cost of a basic motorized wheelchair) only when the equipment is prescribed by an MDA clinic director and is essential to the pursuit of an educational or vocational goal as substantiated by a written statement from a school official or employer or prospective employer. Such recommendations are sub-ject to review by the Association's National Office before authoriza-tion may be given for chapter payment.
- Orthopaedic shoes when prescribed for and associated with braces
- Night splints
- Hospital beds (nonmotorized), mattresses, side rails, and overbed tables
- Hydraulic lifts and bath adapters
- Aids for daily living as follows: transfer boards, synthetic sheepskin pads, heel and elbow protectors, long-handle reachers, lamp-switch extension levers, telephone arms, book holders, hand-held or mouth-held page turners, writing aids/pencil holders, wheelchair pouches, adjustable key holders, DYCEM, closed-cell foam padding, nonskid safety stripping, doorknob levers, blanket supports, alternat-ing pressure mattresses and pumps, plastic mattress covers, shampoo and rinse trays, urinals, commodes, bedpans, external catheters and accessories, raised toilet seats, toilet-assist arms, grab bars, shower and bathtub seats, shower hoses, long-handle bath sponges, built-up and extended toothbrushes, comb and brush handles, Velcro, elastic shoelaces, button aids or loops, zipper pulls, on-and-off stocking pullers, long-handle shoehorns, universal utensil holders, built-up

* Reprinted with the permission of the Muscular Dystrophy Association.

and extended utensil handles, swivel utensils, rocker knives, cutting forks, plate guards, scoop dishes, easy-grip mugs, straw holders, manual communication boards and accessories for their use

RESPIRATORY EQUIPMENT

When prescribed for treatment of intermittent breathing difficulty due to muscle weakness, the following equipment is provided:

- Manual resuscitators
- Suction machines (aspirators)
- Nebulizers, humidifiers, compressors
- Intermittent positive-pressure breathing devices (electric)
- Accessories necessary for the use of the above equipment, such as suction catheters and positive-pressure hose assemblies (venti-collars, lip seals, mouthpieces, face masks, etc.)

Marcia B. Smith
Beth G. Wolf

27

Therapeutic Recreation

In 1977, more money was expended for leisure activities and recreation in the United States than for any other industry. Recreational hours away from work, home, or school are anticipated by most Americans. In recent years, attitudes toward the disabled and toward eliminating architectural barriers for the disabled have gradually changed in response to pressure from disabled persons for access to recreational activities. The disabled have the same right to the advantages of recreation as does any other group. While acquiring new skills and interests that may substitute for lost function, recreation provides physical and mental stimulation and helps build a sense of self-worth, promotes an opportunity for the physically disabled to interact with others, and develops social relationships and social acceptance, thus serving as an entry point to a more "normal" life. Recreation can provide a family with shared experiences whereby the disabled member changes from the focal point to only a participant. Recreation is an important ingredient for the physically disabled as they establish a functional, well-rounded life.

Recreational activities, depending on individual interests, may be passive, requiring little demand on the cardiovascular system, or active, such as outdoor activities, requiring greater muscular action. Passive indoor activities can be done despite inclement weather and whenever the inclination "moves" the person to participate. In either setting, recreation can be adapted to meet the needs of the individual (Fig. 27–1).

For ambulatory individuals with lower extremity physical dysfunction, walking is preferred over jogging because the latter is more precarious when a person cannot control ground-reaction forces at the hip, knee, or ankle. Swimming and bicycle riding, stationary or not, are also preferred gross motor activities because they provide conditioning without traumatizing joints. Selection of appropriate activities for peo-

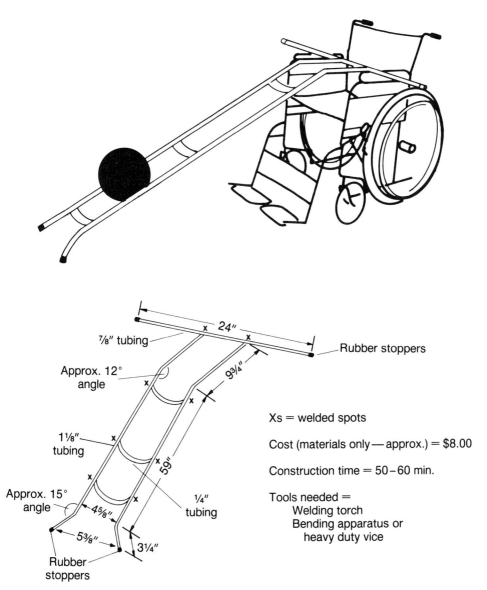

Figure 27–1   A bowling frame can rest on the arms of a wheelchair or on a bowler's lap. The ball is placed on the frame's highest point; the bowler lines up the frame to aim the ball at the pins and pushes the ball down the ramp onto the alley. Bowling frames are now commercially available but can be constructed by following the instructions. (Hale G: The Sourcebook for the Disabled. Copyright © 1979 by Imprint Books, Ltd. By permission of Bantam Books, Inc. All rights reserved.)

ple should consider the effect of the disease on performance. For example, distal weakness or tremors may make many manual skills inappropriate whereas proximal weakness or instability may interfere with physical activities requiring overhead function (tennis and volleyball). People with visual deficits may require assistance to perform an activity to compensate or to learn adapted methods. Table 27 – 1 is an overview of recreational activities with use, adaptations, and comments as applied to multiple sclerosis (MS) and muscular dystrophy (MD). Suggested definitions of levels of disability are

> For MD—functional classifications (see Chap. 16, pp. 242 – 243): mild, numbers 1 through 5; moderate, numbers 6 and 7; severe, numbers 8 and 9
> For MS—functional mobility levels (see Chap. 6, pp. 78 – 79): mild, numbers 1 and 2; moderate, numbers 3 through 7; severe, numbers 8 through 12.

Recreation and Multiple Sclerosis

For many years, physicians and other health-care personnel were opposed to physical activity for persons with MS. This philosophy has changed and physical activity is now thought to be not only appropriate but also advantageous for MS patients.

The amount of exercise and the time of day when exercise is performed, as well as body temperature during the activity, need to be considered when an MS patient participates in recreational activity. Tolerance should be developed slowly and patients need to be aware when maximum tolerated exertion is reached. For example, the patient who can walk four miles without difficulty may get blurred vision after walking five miles. The time of day of activity is equally important. Swimming in the afternoon may cause footdrop, but swimming in the morning or evening may be tolerated without difficulty. The patient must also be aware of the increased body temperature produced by an activity, monitor the physical effects, and modify the activity as needed. As long as these factors are considered, MS patients can safely engage in a wide range of recreational activities.

Gross motor recreation can serve to increase endurance, keep muscles flexible, increase tone, and strengthen muscles not affected by axon demyelination. The potential beneficial effects of aerobic exercise on the fatigue of MS patients is currently under investigation and may prove to be an interesting component of recreational activity. Psychologically, these activities serve as a boost to morale, as is apparent in this letter from an MS patient.

(Text continues on p. 411)

Table 27-1 Recreational Activities for Patients with Neuromuscular Disorders

Activity	MS*	MD*	Adaptation	Comments
Manual Skills				
Sewing	*	*	Needle threader; magnifying glass; wheelchair lap tray (see Chap. 25)	
	**	**		
Needlepoint	*	*	Magnifying glass; needle threader	Gross point or plastic canvas may be easier
	**	**		
Embroidery	*	*	Magnifying glass; needle threader; stationary hoop	
	**	**		
Knitting	*	*		
	**	**		
Crocheting	*	**		
	**			
Weaving	*	*		MD—large loom requires stability at shoulders
	**			MS—may be helpful in strengthening upper extremities
Drawing, sketching, or painting	*	*	Pencil grip; magnifying glass; bookholder for paper or canvas; easel with clamp; electric easel; wheelchair lap tray; ball-bearing feeder; built-up handles; extension handles; mouth-piece handles (see Chapts. 8 and 17)	
	**	**		
		***		
Woodburning	*	*		MS—check for limited sensation in hands
		**		
Woodworking	*	*		MD—shoulder stability needed for power tools.
		**		MS—poor sensation or dizziness may limit this activity.
Leatherworking	*	*	Built-up handle tools	Stamping requires shoulder stability
	**	**		
Ceramics	*	*	Built-up handle tools	Shoulder stability is needed to "throw clay"
	**	**		
Finger painting	*	*		
	**	**		
		***		

(Continued)

Table 27-1 Recreational Activities for Patients with Neuromuscular Disorders *(Continued)*

Activity	MS*	MD*	Adaptation	Comments
Jewelry making	*	*	Wheelchair lap tray	MS—eyesight and sensation influence this activity
		**		MD—even severely disabled can participate
		***		for short duration with adapted work area
Photography	*	*	Small tripod on wheelchair lap tray; auto-	
	**	**	matic film advancer; cable release held in	
	***		mouth	
Mosaics	*	*		
	**	**		
Model making	*	*		MS—poor eyesight and hand sensation
		**		influence this activity
		***		
Physical Activities				
Bicycling	*	*	Tce clips; three-wheel bike; if person cannot	Check balance; during winter can be done on
	**		sit astride seat, he should sit in chair and	stationary bike MD—stationary bike
			place feet on pedals	preferred
Bowling	*	*	Wheelchair ramp (Fig. 27-1); wheelchair ring	Can be done from a wheelchair; most wheel-
	**	**	to hold ball as chair is maneuvered in lanes	chair bowlers use 10-lb ball and conven-
				tional grip; shoulder stability needed if not
				using ramp
Croquet	*	*		Can be done from a wheelchair
	**	**		
Horseshoes	*	*		Can be done from a wheelchair
	**	***		
Kite flying	*	*		Can be done from a wheelchair, which would
	**	**		then require the assistance of an able-
	***			bodied person
Table tennis/ping pong	*	*	Two-handled paddle. Poor vision—ball sent	Can be done from a wheelchair; is easy to
	**	**	across surface through hole in net	learn; requires minimal strength; National
				Wheelchair Athletic Association has
				modified rules available
Shuffleboard	*	*		Can be done from a wheelchair

Activity	Rating	Equipment/Adaptations	Comments
Swimming/water activities	* ** ***	Life vests, inflatable swim suits, hydraulic pool lifts	Excellent for non-weight-bearing because water buoyancy allows increased balance and range of motion
Soccer	* ** ***		MD—Mild difficulty running or kicking. Can be done from a wheelchair, with modified rules
Football	* **		Mild MD—difficulty running
Golf	* *		
Baseball/softball	*** ***		Modified wheelchair rules
Billiards	* *	Adapted bridge to steady cue; wheeled cue to teach shooting	Can be done from wheelchair
Tennis	** ***		Can be done from wheelchair with modified rules; MD—may be unable to move quickly due to instability; may not have the proximal arm strength; National Wheelchair Tennis Association, 4000 MacArthur Blvd., Suite 420 East, Newport Beach, California 92660.
Basketball	* **		MD—difficulty running and shooting because of proximal instability; modified wheelchair rules available from National Wheelchair Basketball Association, 100 Seaton Bldg, University of Kentucky, Lexington, Kentucky
Jazzercize	* ** ***		
Yoga	* ***	Separate each posture into individual components; people assume components they can	MS—increases flexibility and relaxation
Archery	* **	Light-weight bows and other adapted equipment available from P.O. Box 268, 534 Timothy Street, Newmarket, Ontario, Canada	Can be done from a wheelchair

(Continued)

Table 27–1 Recreational Activities for Patients with Neuromuscular Disorders *(Continued)*

Activity	MS*	MD*	Adaptation	Comments
Skiing	* **		Outrigger (crutches with skiis at bottom); "ski bra" (metal latch to hold end of skiis together); walker (bar with little skiis at bottom)	MS — people who cannot walk can ski
Fishing	* **	* ** ***		Can be done from a wheelchair
Horseback riding	*	*	Adapted saddles	Check balance
Walking	* **	*		Excellent choice
Jogging	*			
Frisbee	**	**		Can be done from a wheelchair
Cultural Activities				
Writing	* **	* ** ***	Pencil grip; magnifying glass; typewriter; wheelchair lap tray; ball-bearing feeder	
Lectures	* ** ***	* ** ***		
Reading	* ** ***	* ** ***	Talking books; large-print books; bookholder; magnifying glass; electric page turner	
Music	* ** ***	* ** ***		
Social Activities				
Games	* ** ***	* ** ***	Computer	

Activity				Adaptations/equipment	Comments
Dominos	*	**			
	**	***			
Monopoly	*	**		Computer	
	**	***			
	***	***			
Checkers	***			Velcro on checkers and board; loops on checkers	
	**	*			
Chess	***			Weighted chess pieces; magnitized board and pieces; hooked mouth-piece to lift wired chess pieces	Correspondence chess league—games conducted by mail
	*	**			
	**	***			
	***	***			
Puzzles	*				
	**	***			
Card games	*			Electric card shuffler; playing card holder (see Chap. 8); braille cards	
	**	**			
	***	***			
Collecting (coins, stamps, cards, cups, etc.)	*				May require assistance, but person can choose items and enjoy looking at them; consider expense as well as interest
	**	**			
	***	***			
Gardening	*			Tools with built-up handles; short stool; extensions on tools	Consider window or other indoor gardening; can be done from a wheelchair
	**	**			
Social clubs	*				
	**	**			
	***	***			
Dancing	*				For information on wheelchair dancing and for wheelchair square dancing information, contact Supervisor of Recreation and Athletics, University of Illinois, 136 Rehabilitation Education Center, Oak Street at Stadium Drive, Champaign, Illinois 61820
	**	**			
Parties/visiting	*				
	**	**			
	***	***			

(Continued)

Table 27–1 Recreational Activities for Patients with Neuromuscular Disorders (Continued)

Activity	MS*	MD*	Adaptation	Comments
Dramatics	* **	* ** ***		
Camping	* **	* ** ***		List of accessible camping areas is available from National Park Guide for the Handicapped, National Park Service, Department of the Interior; "Camping in a Wheelchair" Accent on Living, Summer, 1974
Scouting	NA	* ** ***		Manual for leaders is available from Boyscouts of America, North Brunswick, New Jersey, 08902
Traveling	* ** ***	* ** ***		Access National Parks—A Guide for Handicapped Visitors, 1978, National Park Service, Washington, D.C., Government Printing Office; Wheelchair travel—Annaud Enterprizes, Milford New Hampshire, 150-page guide for disabled travelers; free information service available from the extensive library of facts, Moss Rehabilitation Hospital, 12th Street and Tabor Road, Philadelphia, PA 19141
Hayrides	* **	* ** ***		MD—done during summer camp

* * = mild; ** = moderate; *** = severe.

". . . The equipment is all done [made] especially for my handicap which is MS. I now ski with sort of a walker [bar with little skis attached at the bottom], and . . . with a bra [a metal latch at the end of the skis] attached to my skis to keep the tips together . . . then these neat ski instructors ski with us. Since I have no equilibrium, they place their right ski between my skis and hold me by the hips. They check my speed and make sure I don't ski out of control. I swear I ski better now — even better then pre-MS days . . . They also help me sit when my legs do give out and then pull me back up and off we go . . . thank . . . you . . . for giving me the opportunity to realize that . . . after 24 years of MS [I] could ski again. I did have the spirit to do it, but I needed . . . help [to] achieve it."

Recreation and Neuromuscular Disease

Activities for children or adults that involve recreational sports will generally be performed over a longer period of years than formal calisthenic exercise programs because the former brings enjoyment to the individual. Specific activities can be chosen that will meet the need for strengthening without appearing to be an exercise program *per se.* For instance, throwing and catching a frisbee not only enhances upper extremity range of motion and strength but is enjoyable as well.

Perhaps the most notable recreation for the patient with neuromuscular disease is the Muscular Dystrophy Association's camp sessions. From a pilot project begun in 1955, the camping program now has over 92 camps that serve over 3,000 campers. The one-week camps are for children ranging in age from 6 to 21 years. The camp, away from parental charge, is a time of relaxation for both child and parent and creates bonds of communication between people from disparate backgrounds as well as between the disabled and their able-bodied attendants. Adult weekend "camps," sponsored for both the disabled and their spouses, are held at resort facilities in urban or country sites. Both indoor and outdoor activities are done in all camps, and because expertise exists in many localities, the activities can be resumed at home.

The camps not only meet the goals of recreation, but also allow increased socialization with friendly competition. One camp held a pinewood derby where children designed, carved, and painted racing cars from pinewood blocks and entered them in competition. On another day, ambulatory and wheelchair contestants showed enhanced comaraderie when assigned to the same relay team.

Recent legislation, PL 94–142, the Education for All Handicapped Children Act (1975), and Section 504 of the Rehabilitation Act (1975), mandated that handicapped children should be mainstreamed into the least restrictive environment, which in the school system includes physical education (see Chap. 20). For the child with muscular dystrophy, adaptive physical education programs emphasize fun, success, enthusiasm, and positive reinforcement. In many states this program may be called *positive physical education*, which has able-bodied students working one-to-one with the handicapped in the physical education setting. Games played during adaptive physical education should allow rule changes, such as decreased time periods for lessened stamina or an adjustment in the size of the playing area (see Table 27–1). The class may adopt games in which everybody participates and nobody loses such as those found in *The New Games Book*. Other programs may be held in addition to regular physical education classes for those students requiring more specific help.

In summary, recreational activities can be enjoyed alone, in small groups, or in teams. Recreation may be impromptu or require greater planning; may be competitive, passive, or active; and provides increased self-expression and aesthetic enjoyment. Recreation means different things to different people, but for all who choose to participate, it provides an enjoyable way to enrich life.

Suggested Readings

BRUCK L: Access: The Guide to a Better Life for Disabled Americans. New York, Random House, 1978

FLUEGELMAN A (ed): The New Games Book. New York, Doubleday Dolphin, 1976

KRAUS R: Therapeutic Recreation Service: Principles and Practice. Philadelphia, WB Saunders, 1973

Recreation for Disabled People: I. Physiotherapy 64(10):289–301, 1978

Recreation for Disabled People: II. Physiotherapy 64(11):324–329, 1978

This Is Patient Service: Recreation. New York, Muscular Dystrophy Association, Spring, 1977

This Is Patient Service: Recreation New York, Muscular Dystrophy Association, Fall, 1981.

28

Mark E. Litvin

Vocational Rehabilitation and Social Security Disability Programs

LIST OF ABBREVIATIONS USED IN CHAPTER 28

ALJ = Administrative Law Judge
DDS = Disability Determination Services
DI = Disability Insurance
HHS = Health & Human Services
NEPH = National Employ the Handicapped (week)
OHA = Office of Hearings & Appeals
POMS = Program Operations Manual System
RFC = Residual functional capacity
SGA = Substantial gainful activity
SSA = Social Security Administration
SSDI = Social Security Disability Insurance
SSI = Social Security Income

The Public Vocational Rehabilitation Program

Attitudes in the United States have gradually evolved into the acceptance of the vocational rehabilitation concept. Since 1808, various types of assistance to veterans of war have been under federal jurisdiction. However, these programs represented hard-fought victories over the doctrine that the government had no business providing services to individuals. The support did not come from a feeling of compassion and responsibility, but from a fear of a draft resistance for the next year.

Worker's compensation as a social responsibility of the state first began in Wisconsin in 1909, and gradually spread to other states. In

413

1917, the federal government authorized grant-in-aid support to the states for a vocational education program. This move established a precedent, which is currently under attack, for federal support of human services programs. The closely related civilian vocational rehabilitation program of the federal government began in 1920, and consisted of grants-in-aid to the states to encourage the provision of services through their state board for vocational education. Over the next 60 years the program has expanded considerably.

ELIGIBILITY

State vocational rehabilitation agencies have been established to serve eligible physically and mentally handicapped persons. Although basic criteria are specified by federal statute, responsibility for determining the eligibility of individuals for these services rests solely with the state agency. The criteria of eligibility for vocational rehabilitation are as follows:

1. The presence of a physical or mental disability that constitutes or results in a substantial handicap to employment; and
2. A reasonable expectation that vocational rehabilitation services may benefit the individual in terms of employability.

The current Program Regulation Guide (guideline chapters) includes the following clarifying paragraph:

In view of the priority to serve the severely handicapped established by the Rehabilitation Act of 1973, particular care will be necessary in predicting rehabilitation potential for individuals with impairments for which current medical science may not be able to provide precise prognoses as to future functional capacities and limitations. Such impairments include, but are not limited to, multiple sclerosis, rheumatoid arthritis, some forms of mental illness, and certain types of cancer; e.g., Hodgkin's disease. In reaching a judgment on whether applicants disabled by conditions of this kind can reasonably be expected to benefit in terms of employability from vocational rehabilitation services, it is necessary that appropriate consideration be given to the probability of the applicant's undergoing periods of remission, exacerbation, and relative stability in the course of the disease. Medical advisory committees and specialized consultants to state vocational rehabilitation agencies can assist counselors in making sound decisions in cases where the "state of the art" does not permit precise prognoses by development guidelines based on the best available individual and group experience with such impairments. The medically oriented Research and Training Centers may, in certain instances, be a useful resource in this program area.

SERVICES

The following services are made available for the purpose of assisting handicapped persons to prepare for employment:

1. Evaluation of rehabilitation potential, including diagnostic and related services incidental to the determination of eligibility for the nature and scope of services to be provided
2. Counseling and guidance, including personal adjustment counseling, to maintain a counseling relationship throughout a handicapped individual's program of services, and referral necessary to help handicapped individuals secure needed services from other agencies when such services are not available under the Act
3. Physical and mental restoration services
4. Vocational and other training services, such as vocational, prevocational, and personal and vocational adjustment, including work experience, books, tools, and other training materials
5. Maintenance not exceeding the estimated cost of subsistence during rehabilitation
6. Transportation in connection with the rendering of any vocational rehabilitation service
7. Services to members of a handicapped individual's family when such services are necessary to the adjustment of rehabilitation of the handicapped individual
8. Telecommunications and sensory and other technological aids and devices
9. Recruitment and treatment services to provide new employment opportunities in the fields of rehabilitation, health, welfare, public safety, law enforcement, and other appropriate public service employment
10. Placement in suitable employment
11. Postemployment and follow-along services necessary to assist handicapped individuals to maintain their employment
12. Occupational licenses, tools, equipment, initial stocks (including livestock) and supplies
13. Other goods and services that can reasonably be expected to benefit a handicapped individual in terms of employability

VOCATIONAL EVALUATION

The vocational evaluation portion listed under Services, above, "evaluation of rehabilitation potential," is important and generally not fully understood.

Vocational evaluation is a service or program that is provided systematically and on an organized basis for the purpose of determining individual vocational objectives. Vocational evaluation typically includes a study of assets, limitations, and behaviors in the context of work environments in which the individual might function and specific recommendations that may be used in the development of the individual's program plan. Vocational evaluation is a comprehensive process that utilizes work, real or simulated, as the focal point for assessment and vocational counseling to assist individuals in vocational development. Good vocational evaluation should incorporate medical, psychological, social, vocational, educational, cultural, and economic data to assist in the attainment of the goals of the evaluative process.

The purpose of vocational evaluation is to provide an assessment of individuals who are vocationally handicapped or who may be vocationally handicapped at the time they enter the employment market. (This statement is not to imply that the work evaluation approach is not applicable for nonhandicapped people.) These individuals may have a physical or mental disability (emotional problem or retardation) or the vocational handicap may have resulted from cultural or social deprivation. They may be clients of a rehabilitation facility, patients in a hospital, public offenders (in or out of an institution), or students in a public school. While work evaluation clients are a diverse and heterogeneous group, their common characteristic is that they all appear to need evaluative services and vocational direction for a number of reasons (i.e., inability to obtain or hold jobs, lack of vocational goals, lack of motivation, etc.).

In order to estimate the vocational potential (strengths and limitations) of individuals, the work evaluator uses real or simulated work tasks, supplemented by medical, social, educational, vocational, and psychological data from other sources. These sources may include the referring agent, other professionals working with the client, family, lay people who are acquainted with the client, and the client himself.

Vocational potential is a global concept and incorporates many factors and characteristics. To determine vocational potential, the work evaluator needs to assess specific and general skills and abilities, aptitudes and interests, personality and temperament, values and attitudes, motivation and needs, physical capacity and work tolerance, educability and trainability, social skills and work habits, work adjustment and employability, placeability, and rehabilitation/habilitation potential. In other words, the work evaluator needs to understand the client as he exists and functions in a multidimensional life space. If the goal of vocational rehabilitation is to assist the client to achieve his highest level of vocational potential, then the goal of work evaluation is to accurately determine that potential. In order to accomplish this goal, the work evaluator not only needs a high degree of professional skill, but also the appropriate tools, equipment, materials, and work space.

A COLORADO EXPERIENCE

The State of Colorado, Division of Rehabilitation, has taken a progressive role in an attempt to provide vocational rehabilitation services to individuals with neuromuscular disorders. The vocational rehabilitation case service reporting system does not record specific diagnostic data beyond the general categories of muscular dystrophy and multiple sclerosis. However, each of these diagnostic categories is differentiated according to three levels of severity. During 1982, the agency served 56 persons diagnosed as having muscular dystrophy and 233 diagnosed as having multiple sclerosis. Of these cases, 52 were successfully rehabilitated (i.e., employed). Some examples of the types of employment and the weekly wages earned were

Accountant — $150.00
Sales — $200.00
Cosmetologist — $200.00
Pharmacy — $134.00
Mechanic — $160.00
Drafting — $244.00
Janitor — $240.00
File clerk — $196.00
Telephone operator — $300.00
Laborer — $408.00

Because of the nature of neuromuscular disabilities and their sometimes progressive, degenerative, and unstable characteristics, they pose particular problems for vocational rehabilitation. The disability can disrupt training, make placement difficult or impossible, require placement unrelated to training provided, and generally frustrate the vocational rehabilitation process. Vocational rehabilitation counselors often prefer to work with clients who have a more traumatic disability, such as a spinal cord injury, because of the relative stability of the disability. However, research and practice have shown that many persons with neuromuscular diseases can benefit from vocational rehabilitation services and this option should be explored. The state vocational rehabilitation agency including its local offices, is listed in the telephone directory, usually under "State Government."

It is illegal for any state vocational rehabilitation agency to discriminate based on a person's disability. Therefore, any person who believes that he is qualified but is being denied services because of a neuromuscular disability should appeal that decision. All state vocational rehabilitation agencies are required by federal law to have an appeal process for all major decisions, including acceptance for service, during the vocational rehabilitation process.

Social Security Disability Programs

Title XVI of the Social Security Act, known as the Supplemental Security Income (SSI) program, and Title II, known as Social Security Disability Insurance (SSDI) program, are two major programs that provide basic income support to many persons who are disabled by neuromuscular disease. The purpose of the SSI program is to provide direct cash payments to low-income elderly people and disabled children or adults whose income and resources are below specified levels. Case assistance in the form of monthly checks from the Social Security Administration (SSA) is provided to eligible people. In addition, most states supplement the SSI payment for certain recipients. The purpose of the SSDI program is to provide direct cash payments to (1) eligible disabled people with a record of Social Security-covered employment and their dependents throughout the period of disability; (2) retired workers and their eligible dependents; and (3) surviving dependents of deceased workers. The SSI program is an income-assistance program for disabled people with low incomes. The SSDI program is an insurance program for people and dependents covered by Social Security. It is possible to be simultaneously eligible for both programs (see Table 28–1).

The decision as to whether a person's disability meets the eligibility criteria of either program is made by a state agency, usually known as the Disability Determination Services (DDS). The DDS is often a unit of the state vocational rehabilitation agency. The total operating costs of the DDS are paid by the SSA. The administration of these programs has created a controversy in the past two years.

The SSDI program, which provides cash benefits to disabled workers age 50 years and older, was established by Congress in 1956. Dependent's benefits were added in 1958, and the age-50 requirement was eliminated in 1960.

An individual must meet certain insured-status requirements to qualify for benefits. These requirements have been modified over the years, but still require that workers, with the exception of blind workers, who are disabled after age 31 must have worked in employment or self-employment covered by Social Security for 5 out of 10 years prior to their disability. For workers under the age of 25, the minimum requirement is one and one-half years of work out of the three years prior to disability; for workers age 25 through 31, progressively more years of coverage are required. A worker is required to wait five full calendar months after the onset of disability before benefits are payable.

The Social Security Amendments of 1972 federalized the state public assistance programs for the needy aged, blind, and disabled into the Title XVI SSI program. This program pays federal benefits, under uniform rules, financed from general revenues. Payments under the SSI program, which started in January 1974, may be supplemented by the individual states. Under SSI, disabled or blind persons on the state programs before July 1973 were automatically "grandfathered in" under the state's own definitions of disability. New applicants and applicants who were placed on the welfare rolls after June 1973 must meet the same definition of disability as applicants under the Disability Insurance (DI) program. However, they are not subject to any waiting period.

DEFINITION OF DISABILITY

The statutory definition of disability originally required that the worker be unable "to engage in any substantial gainful activity [SGA] by reason of any medically determinable physical or mental impairment which can be expected to result in death or be of long-continued and indefinite duration." In 1965 the statutory language was changed to stipulate a duration requirement of at least 12 months in place of the previous "long-continued and indefinite duration" requirement. Amendments in 1967 further specified that an individual's physical or mental impairments must be ". . . of such severity that he is not only unable to do his previous work but can not, considering his age, education and work experience, engage in any kind of substantial gainful work which exists in the national economy, regardless of whether such work exists in the immediate area in which he lives, or whether a specific job vacancy exists for him, or whether he would be hired if he applied for work."

THE DISABILITY DECISION—A SEQUENTIAL EVALUATION PROCESS

The standards for evaluating disability claims are not further defined in the statute itself, but are set forth in SSA Regulations and written guidelines. The Regulations are intended to ensure uniformity and fairness in the disability-determination process. The standards provide a sequence of steps and criteria for determining whether or not an applicant meets the definition of disability in the law.

The first step is to determine whether the claimant is currently engaged in SGA. The law required the Secretary of Health and Human Services (HHS) to prescribe, by Regulation, the criteria for determining when services or earnings from services demonstrate an individual's ability to engage in SGA. The Regulations establish dollar amounts of earnings. Earnings above these amounts ordinarily show that an individual is engaged in SGA and therefore is not disabled for purposes of the Social Security definition. This amount is currently $300 a month.

The next step in the sequence is to determine whether the claimant has a severe impairment. The Regulations define "severe impairment"

Table 28-1 The Social Security Act, as Amended (Selected Titles)

Title	Date Enacted Effective	Program Name	Who Is/ Was Served	Purpose	Current Status	Type of Program
I	1935	Old Age Assistance (OAA)	Needy Aged	Income and medical assistance	Repealed. Still in effect in Puerto Rico, Guam, and Virgin Islands	Assistance
II	1935 1939 1957	Old Age, Survivors, and Disability Insurance (OASDI)	Retired wives, husbands, children, widows, widowers, and parents	Income	In effect	Insurance
III	1940	Unemploy- ment Compensa- tion	Unemployed	Income	In effect	Insurance
IV-A	1935	Aid to Families with Dependent Children (AFDC)	Needy dependent children and their families	Income	In effect	Assistance
	1961	Aid to Families with Dependent Children of Unem- ployed Fa- thers (AFDC-UF)				
IV-B*	1968	Child Welfare Services (CWS)	Children needing protection, foster care, etc.	Service	In effect	Formula grant-in-aid to states for services
IV-C	1972	Work Incentive Program (WIN)	Employable AFDC family members	Training and Child care	In effect	Assistance
IV-D	1975	Child Support and Establish- ment of Paternity	Needy dependent children and their families	Enforcing support ob- ligations of parents of AFDC families	In effect	Assistance
V*	1969	Maternal and Child Health, and Crippled Childrens Services (MCH) (CCS)	Mothers, infants and crippled children	Medical care	In effect	Formula grant-in-aid to states for services

Title	Date Enacted Effective	Program Name	Who Is/ Was Served	Purpose	Current Status	Type of Program
X	1958	Aid to the Blind (AB)	Needy blind	Income	Repealed but still in effect in Puerto Rico, Guam, and Virgin Islands	Assistance
XIV	1950	Aid to the Permanently and Totally Disabled (APTD)	Needy disabled	Income	Repealed but still in effect in Puerto Rico, Guam, and Virgin Islands	Assistance
Old XVI	1962	Aid to Aged, Blind and Disabled (ABD)	Needy aged, blind, and disabled	Income	Amended by PL92–603; applies only to Puerto Rico, Guam, and Virgin Islands	Assistance
New XVI	1972 1974	Supplemental Security Income, for the Aged, Blind and Disabled (SSI)	Needy aged, blind, and disabled	Income	In effect except for Puerto Rico, Guam, and Virgin Islands	Assistance
XVII	1963	Planning to Combat Mental Retardation	The mentally retarded and their families	Grants to states to develop comprehensive plans for services for mentally retarded	In effect but not funded. Precursor of the Developmental Disabilities Act	Grants for planning
XVIII	1966	Medicare	Aged and disabled OASDI beneficiaries	Cost of medical care	In effect	Health Insurance
XIX	1966	Medicaid	SSI and AFDC recipients; other needy, optional	Costs of medical care, including intermediate care facilities	In effect	Medical assistance
XX	1975	Social Services	Individuals and families below 80% of median income	Services	In effect	Formula grants for social services

* Note: there are no mandatory means tests in IV-B or V.

as one that "significantly limits physical or mental ability to do basic work activities." If the claimant does not have an impairment that is considered severe, the claim is denied on medical consideration alone.

If the claimant does have a severe impairment that meets the duration requirement, the next step is to determine whether the impairment meets or equals the degree of severity in the Medical Listing of Impairments. This rule, commonly referred to as the "Medical Listings," is published in Regulations. The Medical Listings describe specific diagnostic signs, symptoms, and clinical laboratory findings for various common impairments that are considered severe enough to ordinarily prevent a person from any gainful activity on an ongoing basis. If the signs, symptoms, and findings for the claimant's impairment meet those listed in the Regulations, the claimant is allowed benefits on the basis of meeting the criteria of the Medical Listings. If not, but if the claimant suffers from several impairments, the claimant may be found to be disabled on the basis that these two or more impairments equal in severity one impairment found in the Medical Listings.

If the claimant is not found to be disabled on the basis of the medical criteria in the Medical Listings, a determination is made of the claimant's residual functional capacity (RFC). RFC is the claimant's physical and mental ability to perform various types of work-related functions. Assessment of RFC requires consideration of both exertional impairments (those limiting strength) and nonexertional impairments (e.g., mental, sensory, or skin impairments). Once the claimant's RFC has been established, a judgment is made as to whether the claimant is able to perform his relevant past work. If it is found that the past work can be performed, the claim is denied.

If the claimant is found unable to do his previous work, the next step in the process is to evaluate the factors of age, education, training, and work experience in conjunction with whatever RFC the claimant has. This assessment, in turn, is used in deciding whether the claimant can perform any other jobs that exist in significant numbers in the national economy. The medical–vocational rules that guide this last step in the evaluation are set forth in Regulations.

There are three tables in the medical–vocational rules, one for each of three levels of RFC—ability to do medium work, light work, or only sedentary work. Impairments that do not preclude performance of heavy work are generally considered to be nondisabling. Administrative notice has been taken of the fact that a number of jobs exist in the national economy that can be performed by persons with each level of RFC. In addition, the tables relate the requirements of such jobs to the vocational factors of age, education, and prior work experience. The Regulations specify that the medical–vocational rules will direct decisions of cases in which a claimant's RFC is significantly affected only by exertional impairments and the claimant's RFC, age, education, and work experience match those attributes in the table. The guidelines do not direct decisions on disability for claimants with solely nonexertional impairments and do not specifically direct conclusions on disability for claimants with combinations of exertional and nonexertional impairments. In these cases, the medical–vocational rules are to be used as a guide, or framework, for determining disability.

THE DISABILITY DECISION SYSTEM — STRUCTURE AND PROCESS

The disability determination process, which is essentially the same for both DI and SSI disability and blindness claims, can involve decisions at five distinct levels. The structure and procedures of each decision level (prior to PL 96–265) are discussed briefly below.

Initial Determination by SSA District Offices and State Agencies

Applications for DI and SSI disability benefits are filed by claimants in one of the SSA's district offices. The district offices accept applications, obtain the names of the physicians, hospitals, or clinics that have treated the claimants, and make all the nonmedical eligibility determinations based on such factors as insured status, work activity, and, for SSI claims, income and resources. If the claim is denied because the applicant does not meet those nonmedical eligibility requirements, a formal notice is sent.

A claimant's application, any medical records he may have provided, lists of sources of medical evidence, and other background information obtained during the district office interview, are forwarded to the DDS in the claimant's home state.

The DDS requests detailed medical reports from physicians who have treated the claimant. This procedure uses clinical and laboratory findings in the files of treating physicians and has been successful in expediting the gathering of complete medical information and in limiting the need for purchased examinations. However, if sufficient medical information can not be obtained in this manner, the DDS may purchase a consultative examination — that is, ask the claimant to be seen by a private physician selected by the DDS. The DDS may also seek more information from the claimant pertaining to the claimant's education and work experience.

After the required evidence has been obtained, a two-person DDS team consisting of a physician and a lay disability examiner makes a decision on the claim. From the medical evidence, the DDS physician determines the extent to which physical or mental limitations exist and whether the impairment meets or equals the Medical Listings, and, when required, assesses residual functional capacity. The DDS lay examiner determines whether, with some limitations, the claimant can or cannot perform SGA in jobs that exist in the national economy, based on the claimant's age, education, and work experience. DDS determinations are then issued as federal decisions and the claimant is notified of the decision. If the claim is denied, the formal notice indicates the reasons and advises the applicant of his or her appeal rights.

Reconsideration by State Agencies

Claimants whose applications are denied have a right to have their claims reconsidered, but they must file for reconsideration within 60 days of receiving notice of the denial. The reconsideration decision is also made by the DDS. Additional evidence may be submitted by the claimant or requested by the DDS. The reconsideration decision process is similar to the initial disability decision process except that, after the district office updates the claimant's file, a different DDS team reviews the claim. If denied again, the claimant is given notice and advised of further appeal rights.

Hearing Before an Administrative Law Judge

If the DDS reconsideration team upholds the initial denial, the claimant may request a formal hearing before an Administrative Law Judge (ALJ) in the SSA Office of Hearings and Appeals (OHA). The claimant must file a request for the hearing within 60 days of receiving notice of the reconsideration determination. These requests are forwarded to one of SSA's hearing offices located across the nation and are assigned to individual ALJs. Hearings are held as soon after the request as possible.

The ALJ is an experienced attorney who has received training in adjudicating disability claims. The ALJ is responsible for perfecting the evidentiary record, holds face-to-face nonadversary hearings, and issues decisions. At the hearings, the claimant appears for the first time before a decision-maker. Testimony is taken under oath and recorded verbatim. The ALJ may request the appearance of medical and vocational experts at the hearing and can require claimants to undergo consultative medical examinations. Claimants may submit additional evidence, produce witnesses, and be represented by legal counselor or lay persons. The hearing is nonadversarial, whether or not the claimant is represented. There is no charge for a hearing.

Appeals Council Review

Following an ALJ's decision to deny a claim, the claimant may, within 60 days of notification, request the Appeals Council to review the decision. The Appeals Council is a 15-member body located in the OHA. The Appeals Council may deny or grant a request for review of an ALJ's action. If the Council agrees to review, it may uphold or change the ALJ's action or it may remand the case to an ALJ for further consideration. It may also review any ALJ action on its own motion within 60 days of the date of the ALJ's action.

Federal District Court

The Appeals Council Review represents the Secretary's final decision and is the claimant's last administrative remedy. If the Council affirms the denial of benefits or refuses to review the claim, further appeal may only be made through the federal district courts.

Appeals

A major source of inequity and adverse publicity in the program is the disparity in the manner in which claims are adjudicated nationwide at the state agency levels and at the hearings levels. The extent of this problem is illustrated in Table 28 – 1. In short, the states are held by law, regulations, SSA policies issues in the Program Operations Manual System (POMS) and related documents, and by stringent federal review to a severe application of the law. Increasingly, decisions rendered by OHA are being subjected to review in an effort to require more uniform application of the law. Many legislative approaches to this problem have been offered, but it is essential to keep in mind that if state agency decisions are to move in the direction of the more liberal OHA posture, substantial funding increases for benefits will be necessary.

Suggested Readings

BROOK JR: Recent studies on multiple sclerosis: Inferences on rehabilitation and employability. Mayo Clin Proc 44:758–765, 1969

FULTON TW: Multiple sclerosis: A social-psychological perspective. Phys Ther 57:170–173, 1977

NELSON L, THOMPSON D: Psychological issues in adjustment to multiple sclerosis: A review of selected literature. Psychosom Med (submitted for publication)

PRUITT W: Vocational (Work) Evaluation. Walter Pruitt and Associates, 1977

ROZIN, R, SCHIFF Y, KAHANA E, et al: Vocational status of multiple sclerosis patients in Israel. Arch Phys Med Rehabil 56:300–304, 1975

TOWNE A: Multiple sclerosis: Rehab insights and outlook. Rehabilitation Record 11:1–6, 1970

WRIGHT G: Total Rehabilitation. Boston, Little, Brown & Co, 1980

The Budgetary Process

Most programs and services available to disabled persons can neither function nor be provided without money. It is particularly important for advocates and professionals interested in the rehabilitation process of disabled people to be aware of funding mechanisms in order to be in a position to secure research treatment and service funding. In a country where most basic service-delivery programs are heavily subsidized with federal funds, it is important for people to understand the basics of these systems. This statement is based on a belief and an assumption: the belief is that the right kind of information is a powerful asset; the assumption is that if we give people information about how to apply and adapt existing resources, the result will be improved services of all types for disabled people. This chapter will outline how federal programs are funded and how the money is made available through various channels. The discussion will deal solely with the expenditure side of the budget process and does not attempt to treat the other portions of the federal budget process, the raising of revenue. Readers will be directed through the maze of the federal budget and funding system. (This process is displayed sequentially in Fig. 29-1.)

The federal budget process defines and reflects our priorities as a country. Whether these priorities will include services to persons with disabilities depends on the complex interaction of private citizens and organizations, state and local governments, executive branch policy-makers, and members of Congress. Advocates for disabled persons must understand how to have an impact on the budget process to ensure that appropriate services and benefits will be included in the federal budget. The first step requires understanding the fundamentals of the complex process.

(Text continues on p. 430)

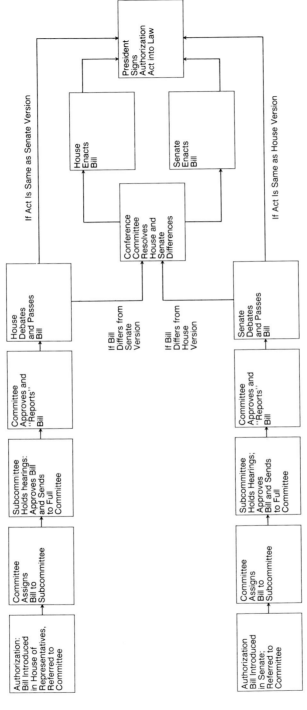

Figure 29–1 Federal government authorization process for one program. The same process simultaneously repeated for other federal programs. The figure represents the ideal and does not attempt to show what happens if a bill runs into problems along the way, for example, if it is vetoed by the President.

(continued)

Figure 29-1 (continued)

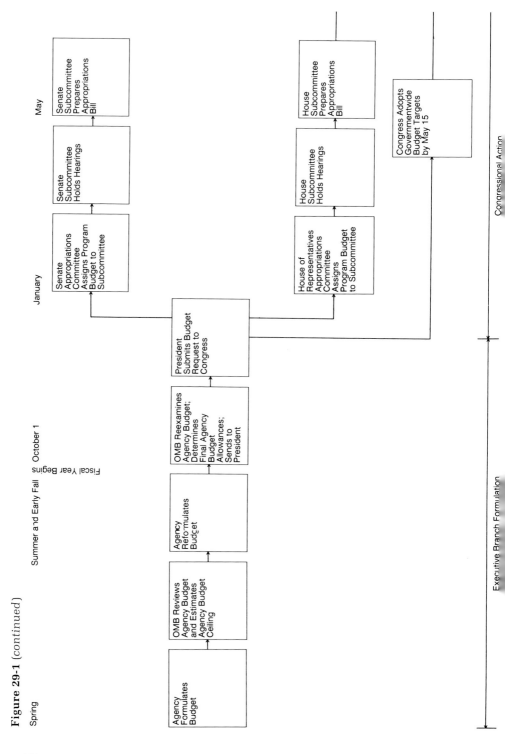

Spring   Summer and Early Fall   October 1   January   May

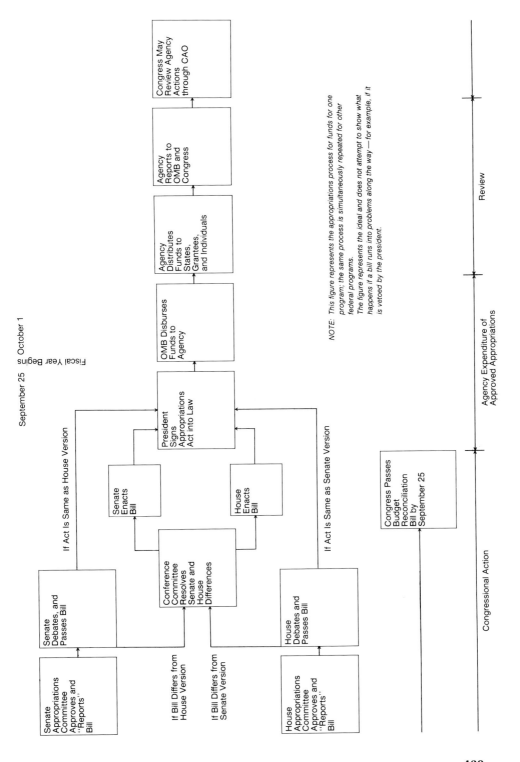

September 25   October 1

Fiscal Year Begins

Senate Appropriations Committee Approves and "Reports" Bill

Senate Debates, and Passes Bill

If Act Is Same as House Version

Senate Enacts Bill

If Bill Differs from House Version

Conference Committee Resolves Senate and House Differences

President Signs Appropriations Act into Law

If Bill Differs from Senate Version

House Enacts Bill

House Debates and Passes Bill

If Act Is Same as Senate Version

House Appropriations Committee Approves and "Reports" Bill

OMB Disburses Funds to Agency

Agency Distributes Funds to States, Grantees, and Individuals

Agency Reports to OMB and Congress

Congress May Review Agency Actions through CAO

Congress Passes Budget Reconciliation Bill by September 25

NOTE: This figure represents the appropriations process for funds for one program; the same process is simultaneously repeated for other federal programs.
The figure represents the ideal and does not attempt to show what happens if a bill runs into problems along the way — for example, if it is vetoed by the president.

Congressional Action

Agency Expenditure of Approved Appropriations

Review

The federal funding cycle has four main phases: (1) Executive Branch formulation; (2) congressional action; (3) agency expenditure of the approved appropriations; and (4) review to ascertain that the funds are used correctly and for approved objectives. Most people think this process begins in January, when the President's budget message and proposed budget for the following fiscal year are officially delivered to Congress. The public announcement of the next fiscal year's budget proposals, however, is only one step in a continuing process that begins much earlier and out of public view.

The Federal Budget Process

EXECUTIVE BRANCH FORMULATION

Every spring the Executive Branch agencies work on the budget, which will be presented to Congress the following January. Each agency determines a tentative budget figure for programs that the central administration wishes to fund. It then submits the projected figures to the Office of Management and Budget, which has the responsibility for Executive Branch budget functions.

The President and his advisers review the agencies' budget figures while also considering the administration's goals and the state of the economy. Tentative determinations on the amount of money each agency may spend are made and given to agencies as guidelines for the final preparation of their budgets.

In the summer and early fall, the agencies, using these guidelines, formulate their budgets for the coming year and submit them to the Office of Management and Budget a second time. After final review and approval by the President, the budget is sent to Congress.

CONGRESSIONAL ACTION

The law provides that Congress must receive the President's budget request in January within 15 days after the start of each new congressional session. The funding process in Congress usually involves two elements: authorizations and appropriations.

Authorizations and Appropriations

Authorization laws, such as the Rehabilitation Act of 1973, are those laws that establish a federal program or services (see Fig. 29–1), while appropriations legislation actually provides the money with which to operate programs (see Fig. 29–1). With a few exceptions, programs are authorized (or voted into law, which is signed by the President) and then funded (*i.e.*, the program existence is approved before funds are granted). A few programs automatically include the appropriation of funds and release of those monies from the Treasury at the time the law is enacted. Others have funds appropriated separately, but the appropriations are for long periods of time and are called "permanent appropriations." The *standard* process requires a yearly appropriation for each federal program, which is voted on separately following the authorization process.

Authorization laws usually set a dollar ceiling figure for a program. No additional money can subsequently be appropriated by Congress without a change in the program's authorization. However, most program budgets are usually pared beneath the authorization level during the budget development and appropriations process. Advocates for a particular program should follow the appropriations process as it applies to that program to ensure that it has adequate funds with which to operate. Some programs exist only on paper because no funds are appropriated to make them functional.

The Appropriations Process

Sections of Congress begin their involvement in the appropriations process as early as October, well before the President submits his budget. For instance, the Senate Subcommittee on Health, Education, and Welfare starts at that time to determine the issues and emphasis of its hearings, which will be held in the following spring. Suggestions made by all Senators are seriously considered in this determination, so it is important for interested Senators to become involved at this early stage.

Official congressional appropriations activities begin once the President's budget has been received by Congress. The budget is scrutinized by two kinds of committees: the Budget Committees in the Senate and the House of Representatives, and the Appropriations Committees in the two bodies.

The Budget Committee takes an active role in congressional decisions that affect the budget. The two Budget Committees consider budget totals and goals of individual program appropriations in mid-March prior to consideration by Congress. Each committee makes recommendations to its respective legislative chamber, the Senate or the House of Representatives. By May 15th the Senate and the House must agree on and adopt the first budget resolution containing government-wide budget targets for revenues and expenditures.

Each of the Appropriations Committees divides the various programs among its 13 subcommittees for deliberations. The subcommittees' recommendations are usually upheld by the full committee. The subcommittees hold hearings in which persons from Executive Branch agencies appear in order to justify their budget requests for the coming year. Citizens and representatives of special interest groups may also testify about programs of interest to them. Witnesses must establish the validity of their requests for money not only with the congressional subcommittee members, but also with the professional staff members of the subcommittee who are generally familiar with the actual workings of the programs being reviewed.

Subcommittees of the Appropriations Committees, using the targeted spending goals adopted earlier by the Congress, approve and send the bills to the full Appropriations Committee. The full committee may make changes in the bill, and the full committee subsequently comments on and sends the bills to the House of Representatives and Senate, where they are debated, possibly amended, and passed. At this point, the measure technically ceases to be called a bill and is instead called "an act," signifying that it is the act of one body of the Congress. Popularly, it continues to be referred to as a bill.

If the Senate and House versions of the act are different, a Conference Committee, consisting of representatives from the Appropriations Committees of both chambers, meets to resolve differences. The Conference Committee's compromise recommendations must then be passed by both the Senate and the House so that a newly created appropriations act will contain identical provisions. Once a measure has been passed by both bodies, it is ready to be transmitted to the President for approval or veto.

The deliberative process for appropriations takes place from July 1 to October 1. This gives Congress 9 months to act on budgets submitted by the President. The act also mandates that a second resolution by the two Budget Committees on the budget's totals of monies to be raised and spent be recommended to Congress by September 15; a budget reconciliation bill binding Congress to those revenues and spending levels must be adopted by both bodies no later than September 25 of each year.

Additional requests for money for emergencies or new programs can be submitted to Congress any time during the year in a supplemental appropriation request. Requests for supplemental money are handled in the same manner as the major budget request.

The President can make two other types of requests to Congress with respect to appropriated funds: rescissions and deferrals. These requests generally are made if the President and Congress are at political odds. A rescission cancels an appropriation, which allows the Executive Branch to withhold money from the program for which it was intended. To deny a request for rescission, both chambers simply take no action on the measure for 45 working days. A deferral is a request to delay, usually for a fiscal year, the flow of appropriated money to a program. To stop such a deferral request, one chamber of Congress must pass a specific resolution denying the request.

Agency Expenditure of Approved Appropriations

The third portion of the budget cycle, the apportionment of the money to agencies of government, begins after the appropriations acts have been signed into law by the President. The President directs the Office of Management and Budget to disburse the appropriated funds to agencies of the Executive Branch for the purposes which Congress outlined. Money is usually released to the agencies on a quarterly basis. Some federal agencies use this money to provide services and do not distribute funds, while others disburse money to the private sector and to state, local, and foreign governments in the form of grants, contracts, benefits to individuals (such as Social Security), direct loans, guaranteed insured loans, direct insurance programs, direct payments programs, donations of property and goods, and general revenue sharing. The "grants" referred to here are usually either formula grants or block grants and differ from the type of grants referred to in the next section.

Formula grants apportion funds in accordance with a formula established by law or regulation. The considerations that determine the amount of money a state or locality may receive are based on such factors as that area's population characteristics, per capita income, substandard housing, or rate of unemployment. Occasionally, the amount of money available for a particular recipient is also influenced by a hold-harmless provision in the law. This means the amount of the recipients previous awards is taken into account in determining how much money that recipient will receive for a period in the future. Therefore, a sudden and harmful decrease in grant funds will not occur.

Generally, formula grant funds are not automatically sent to eligible recipients. The formulas indicate the total to which recipients are entitled if the criteria or law is met. These requirements may include a state plan for the program, maintenance of effort comparable to a previous time period, planning and coordination activities, provisions that the recipients share a portion of the total cost of the program or project, or conformance with various civil rights activities.

Block grants are awards of money for various purposes and focus on functional areas such as health, transportation, education, or community development. These grants allow recipients, usually states, latitude in deciding how to spend the money within general guidelines established by congressional and Executive Branch regulations. Block grants have been particularly popular with the Reagan Administration, and initially Congress approved the creation of new block grant allocations. However, because the block grant mechanism is usually accompanied by elimination of federal regulation and enforcement for specific programs that puts programs for specific populations in potential competition and jeopardy, there has been a strong political resistance from the disabled community to the block grant concept.

Grants and Contracts

Grants and contracts are two major channels through which federal funds flow to state and local governments, institutions, agencies, organizations, and individuals. An understanding of grants is particularly important for advocates and professionals working for disabled people. Grant funds are usually made available to help start or support activities outside of the basic service-delivery system. Research is a good example. Most research is funded by the grant or contract outside of the funding channels for basic services. Unless you are aware of the basics of funding, the places to look for funding, and the application process, you may miss many good opportunities for program service or research development. A number of programs distribute money by one or both of these mechanisms. The fundamental differences between grants and contracts are contrasted in Table 29-1.

A PRIMER ON GRANTS

The following discussion outlines the standard procedures commonly used for awarding federal grants. Each agency may vary or modify this process. The two methods for application are by one's own initiative, which is called an *unsolicited proposal*, or in response to a grant announcement.

Step 1

Identify a program that awards project grants in response to unsolicited proposals. Find out what agency administers the program, and locate its nearest office. Contact the office to find out if and when the agency funds projects in the area of interest. If the agency is not interested in the idea for a proposal, and if no other federal programs deal with that area of interest, federal funding may not be available. If the agency does award grants in the area of interest, then the application process for unsolicited proposals is the same basic procedure that applies to solicited proposals.

Step 2

Solicitations for proposals are published in the *Commerce Business Daily* (for awards over $5,000) or in the *Federal Register*. Most agencies publish grant announcements in the *Federal Register*. These notices usually inform a prospective applicant of specific requirements, the closing date for receipt of all applications, where to find more detailed information, occasionally the total amount of money available, and the average award for each grant.

Agencies may also maintain announcement mailing lists of prospec-

Table 29-1 Fundamental Difference Between Grants and Contracts

Grants	Contracts
1. Grant awards are based on the priorities established by an agency for activities it wishes to support. The government allows the grantee substantial latitude in carrying out the activities supported under the grant.	1. Contracted activities are very specifically defined tasks that must be accomplished within a definite time frame and comply with criteria the government specifies.
2. Grant proposals may be one of a kind.	2. Contract proposals are very competitive, (i.e., many proposals may be submitted that address one specific type of activity or project).
3. Grant projects are generally negotiated with program office staff prior to submitting the formal application.	3. With contracts, there can be no contact with program officials once a RFP is published. All communication must be directed to the contracts officer.
4. The grant application and award process usually vary.	4. Proposals for contracts are generally due 30 days after the announcement of a RFP in the *Commerce Business Daily*.
5. Grant proposals must document the need for the services the grantee intends to provide.	5. Contract proposals do not justify the need for an activity since it has already been determined by the agency. With contracts, emphasis is placed on the documentation of methodology and procedures, and on budget estimates.
6. Grant applications often include letters of support.	6. Contract proposals do not include letters of support.
7. Grants are awarded at specific times during the course of the year, such as quarterly, biannually, or annually.	7. Contracts are awarded on a continuing basis at any time during the years.

tive applicants, and one can request that one's name be placed on the pertinent lists of agencies to contact.

In some instances, institutions and public and private organizations are eligible for grant awards, although there may be restrictions for profit-making organizations. Most programs that affect disabled persons do not award grants to individuals and profit-making organizations.

Step 3

If a person thinks he or she would qualify as an applicant based on the grant announcement, an application kit, which contains forms and instructions for the completion of the proposal, should be obtained. Ask for regulations and guidelines that detail how the program operates.

Step 4

It is helpful to write or call the federal official who administers the program before drawing up a proposal outline. Inform the official about the proposal, including its goals and why it's necessary and why it needs federal money, to determine if such a project elicits interest and matches the agency's priorities for grant awards. Any questions about regulations and the application process should be asked at this time, and it should be determined if the agency will review a proposal outline.

Step 5

Draft a proposal outline and forward it to the agency contact. The proposal outline should include information in the following areas:

- Objectives and need for this assistance
- Target population
- Hypotheses and results or benefits
- Methodology

Step 6

Request the support of others in the community who are supportive of having the request for a grant approved. Community resources might include locally elected officials, local and state agencies, and others who will be directly affected by the grant activity. Forward copies of the outline to all persons whose support is sought. If possible, suggest that they contact the federal agency to express their support. Include written statements of support as attachments to the proposal. Letters of support should be used judiciously and should document how the agency, organization, or group will support the activity with matching contributions, volunteers, staff time, and involvement in the grant activities. If and when it is deemed appropriate, one might ask his or her Congressperson or Senator for help.

Step 7

Prepare a formal proposal based on the outline. Ask federal officials to clarify any part of the process that isn't understood, and ask for suggestions to improve the proposal.

The applicant's credibility is an important factor in the application outcome. Federal officials will scrutinize any applicant's record to determine if the services or goods promised in the application can be delivered; therefore, it is important that the proposal reflect the capabilities to perform proposed tasks.

OTHER ISSUES TO CONSIDER

Attempt to determine from the federal agency contacts what the internal review process is, how funds flow inside the agency, and the extent to which money is currently available for the project. Inquire if there is a required review process that involves local, state, or private entities comments on the merits of the proposal, and ask for the date of award notification.

Be prepared to negotiate specific items such as budget figures. Only the individual submitting the proposal can decide if and how to compromise the original proposal, because that person probably knows the needs of the disabled persons to be served better than the government agency does.

There are advantages to draw up a proposal, even if it is not approved. Competition for federal dollars is keen, and rejection of a proposal does not necessarily mean that it was a poor idea or a poor proposal. It simply may have met with too much competition for limited funds. You can rewrite and submit it at a later date if changes may improve the prospects of your proposal. A rejected proposal can form the basis for new proposals in response to solicitation notices.

The time frame between the allocation and deadline of proposals also has an impact on approval or rejection of proposals. Grant announcements are frequently issued with less than a month's time allowed for the final date on which bids or applications are accepted, particularly near the end of the fiscal year when agencies must obligate money they have left in their budget or the dollars will be lost to them. Inexperienced organizations may not be able to produce, in a short time, a skillfully formulated proposal that can compete with professionally written ones. Accordingly, one should think about the types of services desired, research them, and prepare a draft proposal outline so it can be quickly tailored to a specific solicitation. Check this approach with an agency official to see if it is likely that such a solicitation notice will be issued.

Do not jeopardize a grant by committing an error or oversight. Ask the awarding officials for all the rules and regulations and then make certain that they are observed. An example of such a rule is that all grant proposals must contain assurances for affirmative action that ensure equal opportunity and nondiscrimination.

Further assurances must be given that no project will violate Title VI of the Civil Rights Act of 1964, which prohibits discrimination on the basis of race, color, or national origin, or Section 504 of Title V of the

Rehabilitation Act of 1973, which prohibits discrimination against otherwise qualified disabled individuals.

If the proposal is rejected, request a written explanation. In most instances, the Freedom of Information Act assures you the right to see the terms of the grant that won the award. If, after comparing the proposals with the agency's explanation, it is believed the proposal was treated unfairly, a formal complaint can be lodged to the agency's higher-level authority.

A PRIMER ON CONTRACTS

This discussion outlines the standard procedures used for awarding a contract by the federal government through its central or regional offices where such offices exist. However, each agency may modify this process to some degree.

Step 1

During the previous fiscal year, each program within a federal agency establishes priorities as the basis for the next year's projects for grants or contracts. Specific activities are described in a plan, the Research and Evaluation Strategy. Based on this plan, the agency designs specific projects and drafts a 20- to 25-page work statement for each.

Step 2

After internal review of the work statement, it is developed into a Request for Proposal (RFP) by the agency's contracts office.

Step 3

The contracts office then publishes a notice of the Request for Proposal in the *Commerce Business Daily*. This is usually a short statement that gives the title of the contract to be awarded, the contact person, when and for how long the Request for Proposal will be available, and the deadline for submission of proposals. No cost figures are announced. This statement is the only public notification of a Request for Proposal.

Step 4

An interested applicant would write to the contracts offices for a copy of the Request for Proposal. The Request for Proposal, which incorporates the work statement, is a detailed, technical document. Instructions for responding to the Request for Proposal, the criteria by which all proposals will be evaluated, and deadlines for proposals are given.

Step 5

An applicant then sends a technical proposal that responds to the project outline described in the work statement to the contracts office. The proposal specifies how the work requested will be accomplished. A separate budget proposal is submitted simultaneously. It must reflect cost estimates, including a detailed budget, for accomplishing the task.

Step 6

The program office that developed the work statement convenes a Technical Review Panel consisting of three to five people to review and evaluate all the technical proposals submitted in response to the Request for Proposal. Two of the panel members should be from outside the program office. Proposals are generally evaluated according to the following criteria:

- Understanding the problem: the bidder shows how much knowledge he or she is bringing to the project and the depth of technical expertise.
- Technical approach: this requires a detailed plan on how a bidder proposes to accomplish the task.
- Management capabilities: the kinds of staff, amount of staff time to be devoted to each task, and the staff qualifications must be indicated.
- Organization qualifications: this includes an account of successful work on similar or related projects.

The results are forwarded to the contracts office. The Technical Review Panel then reviews the budget proposals. Based on these reviews, the proposals are ranked and decisions are made for acceptance or rejection of proposals.

Step 7

The chairperson of the Technical Review Panel and the project officer assigned to a project may contact the acceptable bidders to clarify issues or cost estimates not adequately addressed in the Request for Proposal. The bidder must frequently submit written responses within 24 hours. This process is referred to as *negotiation*.

Step 8

The Technical Review Panel meets again and reviews responses or amendments (known as *resubmissions*) to the original proposal, and rescores the proposals.

Step 9

Acceptable bidders are again contacted to clarify any further questions and are requested to submit best and final offer.

Step 10

The Technical Review Panel reconvenes and develops a final ranking of the acceptable proposals. Because the contracts office has the authority to make the final decision, the applicant is notified of the decision by that office.

OTHER ISSUES TO CONSIDER

All statements pertaining to grants apply to contracts as well.

Index

Page numbers in *italics* indicate illustrations; those followed by *t* indicate tables.

441